D0958516

Also by Gary Null

Clearer, Cleaner, Safer, Greener
Gary Null's Complete Guide to Healing Your Body Naturally
The Complete Handbook of Health and Nutrition
Body Pollution
The New Vegetarian
The New Vegetarian Cookbook
Vegetarian Eating for Good Health
Good Food Good Mood
The Joy of Juicing Cookbook
The Foot & Leg Care Handbook
The Egg Project
The Vegetarian Handbook

No More Allergies

No More Allergies

Identifying and Eliminating Allergies and Sensitivity Reactions to Everything in Your Environment

▲

▲

▲

Gary Null

With an Introduction by Dr. Martin Feldman, Environmental Medicine and Allergy Specialist

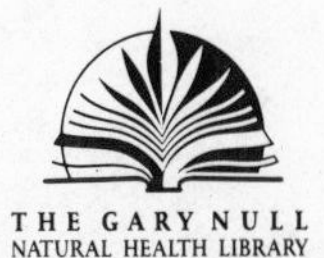

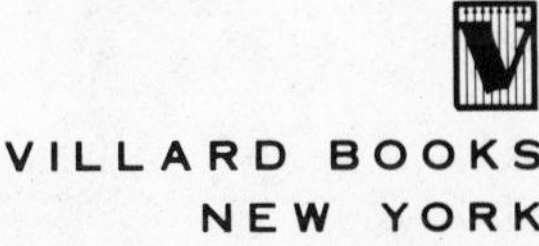

VILLARD BOOKS
NEW YORK

 Published in the United States by Villard Books, a division of Random House, Inc., New York, and simultaneously in Canada by Random House of Canada Limited, Toronto.

Library of Congress Cataloging-in-Publication Data

Null, Gary.

No more allergies : identifying and eliminating allergies and sensitivity reactions to everything in your environment / by Gary Null.—1st ed.

p. cm.

Includes bibliographical references.

ISBN 0-679-74310-3

1. Allergy. 2. Environmentally induced diseases. 3. Allergy—Homeopathic treatment. I. Title.

RC584.N86 1992

616.97—dc20 92-50149

Manufactured in the United States of America on acid-free paper

9 8 7 6 5

Preface

Environmental medicine—dealing with the effects of our surroundings on our health—is one of the most exciting and important fields in health care today. As an approach to allergy diagnosis, prevention, and treatment, environmental medicine takes into account not only the effects of inhaled substances—such as pollens, chemicals, molds, and animal danders—but also foods, as well as home and work surroundings where we may be exposed to various allergy-causing substances. Recent advances in our knowledge about the environment increase our ability to achieve the best possible health.

The concept of understanding how our bodies interact with our surroundings is not new. It is, however, all too often overlooked. As our daily contacts with foreign substances, allergens, and irritants increase, and as our communities and workplaces continue to expose us to synthetic and dangerous substances, we need to critically examine the effects on our health. It seems to me that the traditional "symptom treatment" approach to illness is backward. We are taking various prescription medications to improve our symptoms without learning about the cause of illness or learning about our bodies.

Everyone, especially physicians, should first and foremost learn about ourselves, our environment, and the relationship between the two. We need to understand how we are chemically, physically, and emotionally individual and then modify our behavior and tailor treatment accordingly. We must assess and maximize our nutritional status as well as our physical and emotional well-being. All of this plays an important role in achieving optimal health. Alternate methods of testing for substance sensitivity and an expanded definition of its causes can only add to the information-gathering process of the holistic approach to health care.

Education has always been Gary Null's passion, and this book enables the layperson to fully understand the effects of allergies, pollution, chemicals, and toxins on our health. The chapters on immune functions, nutrients, and herbs are replete with useful and important information on maintaining proper health. This is not a casual compilation of biased material so often found in traditional or conservative texts and reports. This is a thorough, scientific examination of past and current literature and clinical experience, something rarely offered by educators or physicians.

This book is not only a primer, but a guide and resource. With the knowledge contained herein, we can keep ourselves healthier and meet the challenges that our environment presents.

Another job well done.

Christopher L. Calapai, D.O.

Acknowledgments

I would like to thank YongSoo Ha for his very special presence in assisting with many of the receipts and I appreciate the hundreds of hours of dictation and editing given by Eileen Davis and Lois Zinn.

Contents

Introduction

There is a revolution of medicine afoot in which some of us are returning to "old-fashioned" remedies such as herbs, simple minerals, homeopathic remedies, and foods. Allergy sufferers of the world would do well to learn about these therapies. Although modern-day pharmaceuticals are becoming more and more sophisticated, they tend to have side or rebound effects, which will be discussed later. The practitioners of complementary medicine—i.e., those who view treatments as filling out or completing the body's own systems—coming from many separate fields of specialization share the common philosophy that observing patient responses is more important than relying only upon laboratory computer printouts. In the field of allergy, this is a great philosophical advance, although, in a sense, it is a throwback to a less-technological and less-specialized practice of medicine.

Actually, most complementary physicians tend to be generalists who see patients with problems of any organ system. As such, they can save a lot of burdensome traveling from one medical office to another; for instance, for a problem of frequent urination a gynecologist, a urologist, and a psychiatrist could all be involved even though the disorder may be nothing more than an allergic or immune-system process. The same might be true of a patient suffering from joint pains who would be traditionally treated by an orthopedist, a rheumatologist, and an internist.

Complementary physicians are a natural choice for those suffering from known allergic disorders as well. If you are in the midst of weekly or less-frequent allergy infections, these practioners offer a new type of therapy you can administer to yourself at home. They can test for irritants such as perfumes, automobile exhaust, and newsprint. You might be asked to reduce your intake of such foods as wheat, corn, egg, milk products, citrus, and others. If you have yeast overgrowth and might be sensitive or intolerant to your body's yeast, known as candida, natural, nondrug symptom relievers are available.

The field of allergy diagnosis and therapy has a new breed of practitioners who tend to take a more empirical and less dogmatic view of how to diagnose and treat problems related to allergic processes. This book summarizes the current knowledge of these physicians who might be described as environmental medicine detectives.

DIAGNOSED AND UNDIAGNOSED ALLERGY DISORDERS

Allergy in the population is so prevalent that you very likely have some allergic processes at some level. How do you fit into the following spectrum of allergy-related problems?

Obvious allergy that is clearly diagnosed, such as hay fever;

Immediate reactions to specific allergens, such as when exposure to a cat leads to reddened skin or a dusty room provokes running nose and tearing eyes;

Well-known classical symptoms of allergy where the agents have not been identified yet the allergic process is obvious—nasal congestion, sinus congestion, postnasal drip;

Mysterious agents, which may provoke less-obvious allergic reactions than the above, and which might be solved by an environmental medicine detective. Mysterious agents can range from chemicals at the workplace, such as from a photocopying machine, to molds growing in the home.

Functional problems or irritations of almost any target organ such that symptoms are annoying and uncomfortable, but not classical disease states. Sufferers of functional problems are usually not diagnosed as allergic and discomfort usually continues for a long time. Symptoms include tinnitus (ringing in the ears), frequent urination, muscle aches and pains, and heart palpitations.

Obesity and fatigue states, which have an underlying relationship to immune-system dysfunction of the allergy type;

Disease states, which may have an underlying or immune-system dysfunction as a factor that is often unrecognized. Rheumatoid arthritis, osteoarthritis, asthma, migraine headaches, irritable bowel syndrome, and many skin inflammations are all symptoms of an allergy disorder.

Food-related reactions, such as hives resulting from eating shrimp. These reactions may occur immediately. However, many more food sensitivities provoke symptoms hours or even a day or two later.

A COMPLEMENTARY PHYSICIAN'S VANTAGE POINT

I would describe myself as a physician practicing a complementary style of medicine. A complementary practitioner employs all available medical technology and methodology to ascertain the diagnosis. In addition to all of this diagnostic technology, he or she uses natural nondrug therapies to complement any traditional therapies.

The complementary approach tends to rely upon using what works. If an herbal preparation effectively reduces allergic activity, this natural mode would be employed even though the reason why it works may be unknown. The practice of complementary medicine relies upon patients self-monitoring their reactions. Patients know their own health better than anyone else. They report changes in symptoms in the context of environmental exposures, food exposures, or exposure to stressful situations. A traditional physician trained as a neurologist, I come from the background of a specialty in which the observation of body function is the essence of the neurological examination. The observations that patients relate to me have served as a textbook of allergy information. Neurology involves detective work to determine what part of the nervous system is not working and why. The detective job in allergy disorders involves finding out what part of the entire body may be reacting to allergic processes and which antigens or substances are provoking the symptoms. Outside of the lab, the patients are the source of information in the real world.

IT'S NOT "IN YOUR HEAD"

The traditional physician tends to rely upon the general physical examination and often a standardized battery of laboratory tests including the SMA-24, which profiles such items as cholesterol, liver functions, calcium, sodium, potassium, and glucose. The white blood and red blood counts are also routinely tested, and urinalysis is performed. When this data comes back from the laboratory within the normal range and when the physical examination reveals no obvious findings, the tendency is for the physician to diagnose "no organic findings." When there are "no organic findings" traditional physicians tend to consider the patient a hypochondriac, a neurotic, or worse. I have found in my practice, day in and day out, that such patients with disorders of function but no proven disease have a high probability of immune-system or glucose-control-system malfunction.

The first order of business in this regard is to raise the physician's level of consciousness to at least consider the possibility of the dysfunction's being a result of allergic processes. Also, we may have to go directly to the consumers—such as the readers of this book. This book deals with the controversies between the traditional allergists and the more contemporary allergists, but we need to involve the entire medical community, especially primary-care practitioners, family practitioners, and internists. Although the total percentage of health-care expenditures dealing with classical allergy illnesses in adults and children, such as allergic rhinitis, allergic sinusitis, allergic skin disease, hay fever, and the like, is surprisingly high, I conclude from my patient population that there are even more sufferers who have never been considered allergic. Admittedly, my sampling is somewhat skewed since most patients who seek out a complementary physician such as myself have not been helped or diagnosed by traditional practitioners. On the other hand, with my new patients, who don't consider me an allergist, I do see a large variety of problems much as any primary-care physician would.

The allergic process may target any area of the body and cause any number of symptoms. Some unusual examples with which I have had firsthand experience are tinnitus or ringing in the ear; frequent urination; pains that do not follow nerve-distribution patterns; chest pains without heart disease; muscle spasms; palpitations or erratic or rapid heartbeat not from heart disease.

COMMON MISDIAGNOSED ALLERGY-RELATED MALADIES

Are you suffering from any of the following, which may be allergy related?

Fatigue

Fatigue states rob millions of people of energy to enjoy life, function at home or work, or have many hours of high-level performance per day. In the extreme case of low energy, this situation may be mistaken for "depression," and a multitude of psychological explanations may be offered by therapists of differing disciplines. Another example, far to the extreme end of the spectrum, is "chronic fatigue syndrome." Actually, its more proper designation is CFIDS, which stands for chronic fatigue immune dysfunction syndrome. In this energy-deficient condition, there are one or more viral infections that stress and weaken the immune system leading to an immunity breakdown. This immunity imbalance leads to a drain on the body's energy mechanism. My private practice has presented many patients whose conditions are examples of interactions between the immune system imbalanced by allergy and the state of diminished energy.

The most common pattern of low energy is difficulty in getting out of bed in the morning. Even though the sleep time may be seven, eight, or more hours, upon awakening the person is still tired and not refreshed.

The second most common pattern I see is the two, three, or four P.M. letdown. The least-severe energy deficit is the pattern of having a tired feeling at seven or eight P.M. While there are many factors that drain total body energies, I usually diagnose immune and allergic conditions.

Obesity

While some obese patients have sluggish thyroid activity with concomitant lowered basal metabolic rate (the rate at which energy is used up by a person at complete rest), the majority just eat too much and/or have relatively low activity levels and thus burn low calories. Why do they eat so much? Some overeaters have a tendency toward reduced glucose levels in their circulating blood, which impels them to eat in an attempt to raise their low sugar level. Although this sounds very mechanistic, hypoglycemia (the condition of having decreased blood sugar) may interact with food allergy. (See discussion of hypoglycemia, page xxxiv.)

A more common mechanism is that of "food addiction." If the body has an immunity to a food such as wheat or corn, there may be an obvious reaction when this food is eaten or there may be an internal or unrecognized biochemical reaction. The nature of this process is such that when the wheat or corn is not eaten for many hours, the body goes into withdrawal. Evidently, food intolerance complexes act in some ways similar to an addictive drug. Thus, at some level the appetite mechanism impels the person to seek out and eat more of the "addictive" foodstuff.

Headaches

Migraine and other headaches may result from foods eaten even as much as twenty-four hours prior to onset. Whereas most practitioners and even very prestigious medical school headache clinics treat via drugs to suppress pain, medical detective will usually uncover hidden food or environmental allergens. Incidentally, there is often an additional problem of structural imbalance of the neck and skull bones and/or related muscles.

Digestive Symptoms

Digestive symptoms of all types, including diarrhea and constipation, burping, belching, flatulence, abdominal discomfort, nausea, and indigestion may occur at one time or another in most people, who ordinarily would not seek a physician's advice. Yet these symptoms may reflect an irritation of the digestive apparatus and over time may lead to more severe symptoms of digestive problems. Even if the person is distressed enough to seek out an internist or gastroenterologist, the current medical model does not seem to include sensitivity to foods as being high on the list of conditions to diagnose or treat.

Brain-Related Reactions

Brain-related reactions such as diminished concentration, a brain "fog" with a general impairment of clear thinking, a "fuzzy" or "spacey" sensation, and episodic memory problems are a class of conditions of which the alert medical detective will want to take note. As a classically trained neurologist, I have always found these subclinical or ill-defined impairments of function that do not have very precise diagnostic labels of great interest. As a complementary physician who looks beyond the classical disease entities, I have tested many such patients and have found that the brain is reacting to allergens. There is a growing body of medical literature regarding these cerebral allergy phenomena. The allergens may be hard to uncover, so a detective-type investigation may be called for.

Skin Problems

Many skin problems such as rashes, a reddish discoloration, patches of roughness, and even the presence of fungi or molds may have an underlying relationship to an intolerance or allergy whereby the skin is the target organ.

WHY IS THE ROLE OF FOOD ALLERGY NOT WIDELY RECOGNIZED?

Approximately 10 percent of food sensitivity is classical-allergy mediated with an immediate response as soon as the food is ingested. Thus, after you eat a shrimp or strawberry there is an instant reaction such as hives or a headache. It is easy to diagnose the food allergy both because the symptoms occur so close in time to the exposure to the food and because these immediate reactions tend to happen each time the food is eaten. This type 1, or fixed, allergy response is mediated via IgE antibodies (see glossary) everpresent in the circulating bloodstream. Unfortunately, mankind suffers from another type of food sensitivity, which has been described as type 2—masked or cyclic allergy. The majority of food reactions are type 2 and are not immediate nor of the same character at each exposure; they are not IgE mediated. Most of the available laboratory equipment measures only IgE levels of specific antigens so that the reports from the "official" laboratory instruments have data limited to this subgroup.

Newer avenues of measurement include IgG food antibody levels or white blood cell reactions to antigens. The difficulty in monitoring some of the reactions relates to the need to observe these cells under a microscope by a skilled and dedicated technician. Instrumentation that measures these cellular reactions by the "eyes" of the instrument are more reliable; however, they are very expensive and not in wide use. (If and when instrumentation becomes generally available that would quantitate those food-sensitive metabolites in the blood, there would be a revolution in classical allergy medicine.)

Beyond the problem of tracking down and measuring the components of food allergy, we have the puzzle of variability of food reactivity: The same person may react with different responses to the identical food at different times. On one day, milk may result in diarrhea; on another day, headache; and on another day, mental confusion. Also, different concentrations or quantities of the food may serve as triggers at different times. In addition, the elapsed time between ingestion and reaction may vary from an hour or two to even a day later.

The pattern from patient to patient may be quite different as well. For example, one patient may exhibit only wheezing from the ingestion of any one of ten allergenic foods. Similarly, another patient reacts with only runny nose from eating twenty different allergenic foods. Other patients may have combinations of symptoms referable to two or more target organs, such as increased urination and runny nose. Another pattern may be provocation of different symptoms with different foods, such as egg causing itching; wheat, headache; beef, wheezing.

Quiz: Are You Food Sensitive?*

Check any symptom(s) you have experienced under each target area.

Skin

__ hives __ blotches __ angry red blemishes
__ itching __ burning __ flushing __ tingling
__ sweating, without exertion

Ear, Nose, and Throat

__ nasal congestion __ sneezing __ nasal itching
__ runny nose __ postnasal drip __ clearing throat
__ sore, dry, or tickling throat __ itching palate
__ hoarseness __ fullness, ringing, or popping of ears
__ earache __ intermittent dizziness

*Adapted from *Food Allergy* by Joseph B. Miller, M.D., Mobile, Alabama.

Eyes

__ watery eyes __ blurring of vision __ glare hurts eyes __ eyelids twitching, itching, drooping, or swollen __ redness and swelling of inner angle of lower lid

Respiratory

__ mucus formation in bronchial tubes __ cough __ shortness of breath __ wheeze

Cardiovascular

__ heart pounding __ increased pulse rate __ skipped beats __ flushing __ paleness __ warm flashes __ tingling __ redness or blueness of hands __ faintness

Gastrointestinal

__ dryness of mouth __ canker sores __ stinging tongue __ burping __ retasting __ heartburn __ indigestion __ nausea __ vomiting __ difficulty in swallowing __ rumbling in abdomen __ abdominal pain __ cramps __ diarrhea __ itching or burning of rectum

Genitourinary

__ frequent, urgent, or painful urination __ inability to control bladder __ vaginal itching or discharge

Muscular

__ generalized muscular weakness __ muscle and joint pain __ stiffness __ soreness __ backache __ neck muscle spasm

Nervous System

__ headache, migraine __ sleepiness __ drowsiness __ grogginess __ slowness __ sluggishness

__ dullness __ crying __ tension __ anxiety __ overstimulation __ overactivity __ restlessness __ jitters __ head feels full or enlarged __ sensation of floating __ giddiness __ inability to concentrate __ feeling of alienation from others __ amnesia for words, numbers, or names __ stammering speech

Quiz: Do You Eat These Foods Frequently?*

Most Common Hidden Food Allergens

Beef	Peanut
Chicken	Potato
Chocolate	Pork
Coffee	Soybean
Corn	Wheat
Egg	Yeast, Baker's
Orange	Yeast, Brewer's

Moderately Common Hidden Food Allergens

Apple	Malt
Beet Sugar	Mustard
Cane Sugar	Oats
Cinnamon	Onion
Coconut	Peas
Garlic	Rice
Lemon	Tea
Lettuce	Tomato

*Adapted from *Food Allergy* by Joseph B. Miller, M.D., (1972, Mobile, Alabama, C. C. Thomas)

HAVE YOU A MILD OR RECENTLY ACQUIRED ALLERGY PROCESS?

Allergic sensitivities may appear at any age. My experience from patient histories has been that allergic processes tend to progress once they begin. Since we have nutritional avenues for rebalancing an immune system that has become overactive with any of the allergic processes—including the mild type—it is worth the time and effort to take this approach in putting the body back into balance. The process of immune-system analysis requires profiling the immune-related nutrients, which include vitamin A, zinc, vitamin C, bioflavonoids, vitamin E, gamma linoleic acid, essential fatty acids, and selenium. Many of these are the building blocks of immune-system function. Nourishing the body with these basic nutrients via foods and food supplements is a simple process in the hands of a health practitioner who is knowledgeable. Step one is the testing of the body's stores of these vitamins. Step two is the replacement via food and food supplements of the nutrients found to be in short supply.

An experienced practitioner must select the dose of each nutrient as well as the exact formulation to be ingested. For example, recent studies have revealed that zinc combined with picolinic acid to form a zinc-picolinate complex is a well-absorbed and very effective form of this mineral. Since we are discussing persons with the first stages of allergy symptoms, we must test vitamin or mineral supplements as we might have to test for food sensitivity or food intolerance. It has been my experience that patients may be sensitive to, or may react to, any nutrient formula, even a simple mineral or vitamin preparation.

It is a question of probabilities, so that with experience

the practitioner will develop a statistical profile of which nutritional products tend to be less and which tend to be more sensitizing.

IS YOUR IMMUNE POWER DECLINING?

When your immune system starts to weaken, there is an increased probability that you will develop allergic processes related to environmental and/or food allergens. Even if this does not happen, wouldn't you prefer to have an efficiently functioning immunity? The rebalancing of the underactive immune system requires the same building blocks as that of the overactive system. The early signs to watch for are frequent colds, lingering colds, recurring "fever blisters," which are actually virus lesions, eye sties, bladder infections and vaginal yeast. A more complex immune problem is that of recurrent general herpes outbreaks, which signal a lowered resistive capacity.

Each time the immune system weakens below a certain level, the usually dormant herpes virus emerges from hiding. The process of yeast infection is similar since the body harbors the *Candida albicans* type of yeast and it grows excessively in numbers when the digestive environment allows it to and/or when the immune system weakens enough to permit overgrowth. In other words, the pathogen is only part of the equation; very often, it is the resistance of the host that is more important. The same philosophy holds for all mixed viral infections, since the human body is exposed to a myriad of viruses throughout life.

HYPOGLYCEMIA AND ALLERGY

My testing of patients has often uncovered a hidden tendency toward erratic glucose levels in the circulating blood. Problems arise when the erratic glucose-control machinery in your body allows the glucose to fall rapidly or to reach a low level of concentration such as 50 mg/dl. A subpopulation of persons with allergic processes have blood-sugar control problems and the two malfunctions interact. In other words, exposure to sensitive allergens such as ragweed pollen, cat hair, chemicals, or even foods may provoke changes in blood sugar. The traditional medical community is grudgingly accepting the concept of hypoglycemia since glucose-tolerance tests generate blood-sugar data with numbers demonstrating the rise and, more important, the fall. This interaction between allergic reactivity and lowered blood sugar is a doubly complex ailment since it involves two functional systems, whereby either one alone could be overlooked or not even considered.

ARE YOU HYPOGLYCEMIC?

The key word to describe hypoglycemia—the abnormal decrease in blood sugar that creates symptoms—is *episodic.* That is, the symptoms occur erractically and have a pattern of striking and then receding. These symptoms may appear without any obvious provocation. Some examples are intermittent headaches; panic-type attacks; sweating; racing or pounding heart or erratic heartbeat; anxiety unrelated to circumstances; attacks of irritability or crying; and impaired concentration.

A family history of diabetes skews your odds of developing a hypoglycemic tendency to a higher-than-average probability.

My experience has been that patients with diagnosed hypoglycemic tendencies who have not been treated over the span of many years will tend toward the dysregulation of glucose metabolism of *hyper*glycemia, or uncontrolled sugar levels, which we term diabetes. There is a spectrum of disorders relating to the metabolism of starch and sugar of which hypoglycemic tendencies are a milder form that may precede actual overt diabetes. Sugar craving is a very common correlate of hypoglycemia.

Patients who notice reactions when they eat sugar are likely to have hypoglycemic tendencies. In addition to the usual white sugar, which is easy to see, there are many foods with hidden forms of sugar that could cause trouble for such patients. As a matter of fact, there is growing use of corn-derived sugar, where we now have a "double whammy"—difficulty metabolizing the sugar molecules plus the common development of allergy to corn. Here are some examples of the hidden sugars in food: 1 tablespoon of catsup has approximately 1 teaspoon of sugar; an 8-ounce soft drink may have as much as 5 teaspoons of sugar; an ice cream cone, 3½ teaspoons of sugar; a 2-ounce chocolate bar, 8 teaspoons of sugar.

WHAT IS NEW ABOUT ENVIRONMENTAL MEDICINE?

The contemporary allergy medicine practiced by environmental physicians is a departure in a new direction for three reasons:

1. The patient's medical history will be more extensive, taking into account exposures to dust, molds, trees, grasses, animals, chemicals, and pollutants of all kinds—at home and in the workplace.
2. This new branch considers body processes that react on target organs as valid medical symptoms even though they may not be mediated by IgE antibodies.
3. Environmental Medicine Academy members tend to be more empirical in their approach such that there is no dogmatic methodology, but rather a willingness to see what works and to use the same with or without a certainty of *why* it works. Part of this empirical acceptance is the use of the serial end point dilution technique.

IS NEW BETTER?

Not always, but in the context of allergic patients' suffering, the new methods are more effective. The experience in day-to-day therapy that I have had the great fortune to be a part of is quite satisfying. I do not have a control comparison using the classical method, but many of my colleagues do and report increased effectiveness. Many of these pioneers are quoted extensively throughout this book. You the consumer may need to accelerate the change in allergy development within the medical community by inquiring about the environmental medicine approach. Some of the practical advantages of the serial end point dilution testing and resultant neutralization therapy are: (1) Since the patient is taught to self-administer the neutralizing formula and is given the appropriate vials to take home, the weekly, biweekly, or monthly trips to the doctor's office are eliminated; (2) Since there are fewer medical office visits, there are fewer medical fees to pay, which reduces the cost of therapy significantly; (3) The correction of the patient's sensitivity to the specific antigens treated is more rapid since the dilutions of antigens administered are custom made for that patient. As a matter of fact, the dilution of each and every antigen is determined individually. For instance, the neutralizing dose for ragweed may be at one level and that for molds and yeast may be at very different levels for the same person.

WHO PROVIDES THE NEW THERAPY AND WHERE DO WE FIND THEM?

A list of environmentally oriented health-care practitioners and organizations is included in Part Three of this book (see page 312). It is of interest that many of the practitioners are board certified in one or even two medical specialties. Many started out as traditional specialists in the field of allergy; many are ear, nose, and throat specialists; some are pediatricians; and many others arrived via their interest in complementary medicine and natural therapies.

TAKING CONTROL VIA "NATURAL LIVING" IDEAS

This book is, in part, an extension of one of the best of the increasingly popular radio programs devoted to nutrition and related health topics: namely, Gary Null's "Natural Living." The material in this book reflects the quality and in-depth knowledge imparted by Null's carefully selected guest interviewees.

Each person suffering from mild or moderately severe allergic processes would benefit from some of the underlying philosophies of the "Natural Living" radio programs and related books. The "Natural Living" approach emphasizes enhancing health as opposed to simply fighting disease. It also takes a new view of disease so that rather than having a cancer, you are "cancering." The current medical model in America is that of isolating and defining pathological and atomical or laboratory entities given specific names. Part of the compartmentalization of the American specialists' system even goes so far as to define allergy as only those processes that can be proven to be mediated by the IgE antibodies. However, it is actually the whole body—including the mind—that is part of every disease process. This is particularly relevant to the field of allergy-related problems in that the mind is a major factor in such ailments as fatigue states, asthma, headaches, "nervous stomach," and irritable bowel syndrome. The "Natural Living" approach represents the growing interest in psychoneuroimmunology, the study of the relationship between psychological aspects and immune-system function or dysfunction.

Here are some of the "Natural Living" philosophy's basic tenets:

Strive Toward Mental Balance Millions of allergy sufferers attest to the fact that stressors, whether real or perceived, may aggravate or even precipitate allergic-type reactions. The concept of "allergic burden" usually refers to the individual antigen exposures or cumulative environmental insults per day. When this burden overwhelms the immune system, a headache or wheezing or diarrhea results. However, psychic stressors should be considered as part of this process. As such, patients need to incorporate stress-reducing techniques into their daily life-style.

Enhance Food Selection Consider vegetarianism. The good part about this choice is that the exclusion of beef and chicken removes sources of impurities from your diet but also gets rid of possible intolerance, sensitivity, or allergy to these foods. On the other side of the coin, there is a growing incidence of sensitivity to soybeans, wheat, and corn when eaten frequently. Good food choices include live foods with fresh enzymes (i.e., fruits and vegetables), which enhance the entire body's health.

Modern technology is improving upon juice-producing appliances that are now available at modest cost and should be present in every kitchen. Information is becoming available regarding the pulp part of the juicing process, which can be used in cooking.

Exercise Intelligently Promote overall body fitness by exercising and, in turn, benefit the immune system. There is much research to support the view that aerobic exercise, which increases the heart rate into the target range, should be performed for at least twenty minutes, three times a week. Brisk walking, swimming, running, race walking, bicycling, and rebounding are some of the more popular activities. A different aspect of body fitness involves weight lifting or Nautilus-type individual muscle development or strengthening. Although exercise has great benefit, potential problems for the patient with allergy include increased exposure to allergenic substances in the air such as pollen, trees, weeds, or mold substances and possibly vehicle exhaust and other pollutants. Actually, one of the benefits of reducing allergic sensitivity is being able to engage in more vigorous outdoor exercise.

Detoxify the Body This is a major emphasis of the "Natural Living" way to optimize health. In my experience as a physician, having seen allergy sufferers before and after a food cleansing (or detoxification) program, the majority have had reduction in allergic sensitivity. In many instances where I tested the immune system status before and after a one-week juice-and-food cleansing program, the immune system was in better balance and the patient had fewer and less-severe symptoms. Whereas juice-or-food cleansing programs are generalized body cleansers, more specific programs are available that target the removal of toxins such as heavy metals, including lead, copper, or mercury. In my practice, I have been puzzled by how many patients have these heavy metals in their bodies. Very often, lead or copper enters their household water from pipes. The current laboratory technology is such that small quantities of toxins can be detected in tap water for a moderate lab fee. There is no question that toxins impair immune system function and thus enhance the problems of immune sensitivity or allergy.

NUTRITIONAL SYNERGY FOR ALLERGY CONTROL

The ideal approach to allergy would be via the combination of life-style changes, psychological work, detoxification, and ingesting immune-related nutrients at dosages to correct antigen sensitivity. However, the reader may have to assume some personal responsibility. It is rare to find a health practitioner who is equally skilled in the allergy testing and treatment areas and the somewhat different areas of nutrition, life-style, mental health, and detoxification. All these paths must be traveled for optimum health. Read on to see how you can increase your role in the process and start on the path to well-being.

Martin Feldman, M.D.

Part One

Allergies: Causes, Symptoms, and Treatments

▲

▲

▲

1

ALLERGIES AND THE OVERAGGRESSIVE IMMUNE SYSTEM

In today's complex environment, some 40 million Americans—and that number is growing—suffer from allergies to one degree or another. Allergies can manifest in various ways, appearing not only as skin problems and hay fever but also as bladder conditions, brain problems, respiratory ailments, digestive problems, and other conditions. Since the body's systems work as a unit, allergic reactions can occur anywhere throughout those systems.

Allergies are brought on by multiple factors. It is commonly presumed that most allergies come from pollens, grasses, and animals. But what many people, including doctors, fail to consider as possible culprits are common foods you eat and chemicals you breathe. The presence of allergies is not always obvious. You may not even realize you have an allergy when, in fact, you are allergic to many everyday things around you.

Allergies occur when your immune system is overaggressive. If you do not have an allergy to dust, for example, you can enter a dusty room and have no reaction. Your immune system will gobble up the dust and remove it from your system. But if you have a dust sensitivity, you will have an allergic reaction when you enter that same room because your immune system makes a big fuss without good reason. This may bring on symptoms in any area of the body, including the nose, ears, eyes, lungs, and even the brain.

By contrast, an underaggressive immune system can create other types of problems. Reduced immune function can make you susceptible to various conditions such as colds that linger, multiple infections, and recurrent bronchitis. Both the weak immune system and the overactive one require rebalancing.

Dr. Warren Levin, a doctor of environmental medicine in New York City, describes the difference between an overactive and underactive immune system and explains autoimmune disease. When the body's antibody defense system turns against healthy body tissues, the result is an autoimmune reaction:

> The immune system is responsible for fighting infections—that is, an outside invasion—and for fighting cancer—that is, an inside invasion. It is also responsible for the production of what we now know to be autoimmune disease. Autoimmunity means we are behaving as though we are allergic to ourselves, our own organs. For example, President and Mrs. Bush are both suffering from a condition in which they have become allergic to their own thyroid glands. The doctors say it is just a one-in-a-million coincidence, but as a clinical ecologist and environmental medicine specialist my belief is that it is much more likely due to some common exposure, especially since their dog even has an autoimmune disturbance. The immune system functions in many different ways. If it is overactive you get one kind of response and if it is underactive you get an-

other. An overactive response to an external substance is an allergy.[1]

To overcome the problems created by a hypervigilant or an underactive immunity, you must do more than treat symptoms. You must look at how the immune system becomes dysfunctional and learn how to build it up again. The immune system comprises an intricate, interdependent network of cells, organs, glands, and biochemical processes. For example, the thymus gland directs white blood cells, appropriately termed T cells, which direct the white blood cells derived from bone marrow, called B cells. The B cells, in turn, produce biochemical antibodies as part of the defensive mechanism. Other cells such as eosinophiles, basophiles, and mast cells produce various chemical substances as part of immune protection. Any interruption or breakdown in these and other immune system links may lead to malfunction.

THE GERM DISEASE MYTH

Multiple factors can cause your immunity to weaken, no one factor alone causes disease. Thus, the germ disease theory Pasteur set forth is not holding up today. Pasteur's seemingly revolutionary concept states that many diseases are solely the result of invading pathogenic bacteria poisoning the host. This theory is helpful in explaining illnesses such as staphylococcus pneumonia or *E. coli* bladder infection. However, we now understand that bacteria are omnipresent in our environment and even inhabiting our bodies at all times. Thus it is not so much Pasteur's invaders that result in illness, but rather the host's weakness that allows the residing bacteria to multiply. It is not humanly possible, after all, to live in a world that has no viruses, bacteria, fungi, and molds. Every time someone coughs, sneezes, or even talks loudly in your direction particles can be projected up to sixty feet. Some of these germs can get into your eyes or mouth. Your body then creates an antibody reaction to the germs. In all likelihood, that reaction kills the invaders and you do not become infected. Because of this you can end up with countless different antibodies.

At some point down the road, you may develop a problem such as chronic fatigue or some other debilitating condition. The culprit is not a new virus, however, but the continual stress that challenges the immune system and does not allow it to rest and recover. For example, chronic fatigue syndrome does not appear until years after you have been living recklessly and pushing the throttle to the fullest. Many years of this type of abuse is enough to wear down the best of immune systems. While a viral-related illness may surface at any time, the virus has usually been dormant in the body for many years. Only after sufficient wear and tear to the immune system do viruses start to manifest as different disease states.

As a result, it is difficult to restore long-term health by treating the symptoms of a disorder only, as allopathic medicine does. The immune system remains as weak as ever. Even if the symptoms are temporarily eliminated, they frequently return in the same or another form.

WHY THE IMMUNE SYSTEM BREAKS DOWN

Multiple Assaults to the Body

Over time, multiple assaults to the body weaken the immune system through their cumulative effects. For example, various factors that may have weakened the immunity of the baby boomer generation include the following: the above-ground atomic explosions of the 1960s, the massive vaccine programs of the same era, the large consumption of meat that was and still is contaminated with viruses, long-term effects of pesticide toxicity, exposure to lead and mercury, and the widespread use of recreational drugs like marijuana and cocaine. To this list we can add an unhealthy exposure to electromagnetic fields and other sources of low-level radiation at home and at work, as well as exposure to various chemicals on a day-to-day basis. Indeed, thousands of little things that you are not even aware of add up over the years. And then one day you no longer feel fine. Your body has finally passed its threshold barrier and has difficulty repairing itself.

Environmental physician Dr. John Trowbridge of Humble, Texas, explains how this process can produce a "sudden" illness in a seemingly healthy individual:

> One thing doesn't just happen to make your body say, "Wow, that was horrible." Instead, the small daily insults to your body accumulate over time until finally something catastrophic happens. An infection doesn't heal; an unexpected heart attack occurs; joints suddenly hurt and won't stop hurting.[2]

As your immune system weakens and your tolerance level lowers, you may become allergic to things that previously didn't bother you. This can create a mushroom effect. First, you are allergic to one thing, and then to two, ten, or even twenty substances. Before, you could tolerate molds, yeast, and fungi. Now you can't. As you become allergic or sensitive to more individual allergens, there is often a progressively greater stress upon your immune-allergy mechanism. When the allergic burden produces a stress on the system, "the straw that breaks the camel's back" leads to other sensitivities. Dr. William Rea, a cardiologist and leading environmental medicine expert from Dallas, Texas, offers this example of how a toxic overload from one substance can cause other sensitivities:

> I recently saw a physician colleague of mine who had been working in a laboratory where she was exposed to a substance called xylene. This chemical is used in slide fixatives and in different solvents. It is also present in automobile exhaust and in glue. She started having aches and pains from this, as well as poor memory and flulike symptoms. Then she was exposed to carbon monoxide at very high levels and got quite ill. When I saw her she could hardly walk across the room and could barely talk at all. We found that she became sensitive to all foods, which was a secondary phenomenon to the chemical overload. She was a classic example of someone who became exposed to different chemicals while doing her routine job, and as a result became nonfunctional.[3]

Dr. Marjorie Siebert, a nutritionally oriented physician in New York, says there are two types of immune-system breakdown: immune dysregulation and immune dysfunction. With immune dysregulation, the system actively creates autoimmune conditions, such as colitis, Crohn's disease, rheumatoid arthritis, lupus, thyroid disease, multiple sclerosis, and reactions to common chemicals, pollens, and molds. With the second type of breakdown, immune dysfunction, the immune system is weak and underactive and therefore unable to operate normally or effectively. Often this occurs from a deficiency of certain specific nutrients such as vitamin B_6, zinc, or even protein. Immune dysfunction can result in such conditions as chronic candida overgrowth or chronic viral activity. Viruses that may develop include cytomegalovirus, Epstein-Barr, human herpes VI, and, if carried a bit further, full-blown immune insufficiency syndrome and cancer. Immune dysregulation and immune dysfunction can happen either simultaneously or at different times. The same agents can be responsible for both types of disorders.

Nutritional Deficiencies

In addition to the chemical onslaught we face, our lack of nutrition also causes our immune systems to break down. Part of the problem is that we do not get enough nutrients in the foods we eat, even when we attempt to eat well. The other factor is that we suffer from "pollutant injury." We are exposed to an array of pollutants in the environment such as automobile exhaust, acid rain, hydrocarbons from spray cans, glue fumes, and the outgassing of chemicals from carpets. All of these toxins can injure or weaken our immune mechanism.

Lack of Trace Minerals

Whereas there is a widespread understanding of the role of essential minerals in the body such as calcium, sodium, and phosphorus, the scientific community is just learning about elements present in minute amounts. Today, we are experiencing global deficiencies of the trace minerals, such as selenium, molybdenum, and manganese that the body needs to detoxify chemicals. One explanation for this deficiency can be found in *Empty Harvest*, by John Anderson. In this book, the author shows that our lack of minerals stems, in large part, from the soil erosion created by bad farming practices such as choosing to grow foods on synthetically fertilized soil.

Some of the more common minerals in which you may be deficient are as follows:

Magnesium Magnesium helps to detoxify the chemicals in your body. Without it, the immune system may malfunction. And yet, about 66 percent of people do not even get the Recommended Daily Allowance (RDA) of this mineral. A committee of scientists meets periodically to form a consensus regarding minimum quantities of minerals and vitamins required by the human body of different sexes and ages; these levels are very conservative and err toward inadequate levels. If your immune system needs repair or help in fighting off all the new chemicals being introduced into your body, two to three times more than the basic RDA may be required.

Molybdenum People are generally deficient in molybdenum as well. This mineral is important in the functioning of aldehyde oxidase, an enzyme that metabolizes and rids the body of formaldehyde. It also helps to eliminate sulfites from the body.

Manganese Many people lack sufficient amounts of manganese. This deficiency has been associated with almost all illnesses, including heart disease, cancer, and rheumatoid ailments. The type of disease to which someone with a manganese deficiency becomes predisposed will depend upon his or her genetic weaknesses. Manganese also competes with mercury, which means that mercury toxicity will have a more damaging effect if you are deficient in manganese.

Poor Absorption of Trace Minerals

Even if you receive enough minerals, you may have a difficult time absorbing them. One factor that may affect absorption is the ingestion of antibiotics at high doses and over prolonged periods of time such that the bacterial environment of the colon becomes unbalanced, which lessens its effectiveness in absorbing. Poor absorption can also occur during times of psychosocial stress, when stomach acid and enzymes are not being properly produced. The minerals may be coming in, but they are not properly absorbed because the body is in a hyperactive state that does not allow for the assimilation of food.

Poor Dietary Habits

Our poor approach to eating in the United States has weakened our immune systems and undermined our health. Sugar, in particular, is weakening our nation because it is being consumed in extreme amounts. Teenagers, for example, may drink an 8-ounce bottle of soda a day, which could contain about 7 teaspoons of sugar. Over time, all this sugar can make them more susceptible to infection and to the development of allergies.

Excess sugar in the diet can harm us for a number of reasons. As the body metabolizes ingested sugar, the pancreas produces insulin to remove excess sugar from the circulating blood. The oversecretion of insulin then causes a large drop in blood sugar, or hypoglycemia, and sets the stage for heart disease. For this process, the pancreas requires zinc and manganese. Chromium is utilized to escort the circulating glucose—blood sugar—into cells. The B-complex vitamins are also part of this sugar-processing system. These nutrients are thus "used up" as the body struggles with the sugar overload.

Too much sugar can cause blood pressure elevation as well. It decreases our blood circulation by depositing plaque in our blood vessels. Sugar can also decrease function of red blood cells and monocytes (cells that engulf by entering foreign material and consume debris) by entering into them. And it can damage nerve function too.

Even when we attempt to eat well, it's a difficult task because today's foods are not as nutrient dense as those of the past due to poor growing conditions. A store-bought tomato does not feel, look, or taste like one that is homegrown. That could be a sign that it was harvested immature, as well as lacks minerals and other nutrients. Some studies indicate that consumers now avoid fresh fruits and vegetables because of pesticide contamination. One study conducted at the University of California found that 7 percent of the population had decreased its consumption of fruits and vegetables for this reason.

If you put these two factors together—our poor dietary habits and the lack of nutritious foods—it is easy to see why we run a greater risk of developing health problems as we get older.

Dr. William Rea believes that since our daily diets lack essential nutrients, we need to take supplements such as vitamins A, C, and E, various B vitamins, minerals such as calcium, magnesium, zinc, manganese, and selenium, and some of the amino acids. (Supplementary nutrients are discussed in detail on page 293.)

Environmental Stressors

Other environmental factors that can contribute to our overall stress load include geophysical disturbances of the earth and heavy exposures to electromagnetic contamination. The earth has a magnetic field that pulses or vibrates at an eight-cycles-per-second frequency. The evolution of the human organism has adapted us to this natural frequency whereas the sixty-cycle-per-second frequency of our electrical power systems is foreign to the human organism and disturbs our natural biological rhythms. Since we cannot see or feel this part of the energy spectrum, we are, for the most part, unaware of this influence. (Electromagnetic radiation is discussed further on pages 81 and 117.)

Psychoallergenic Reactions

When you have a psychoallergenic reaction, your state of mind directly affects your susceptibility to allergies and other sensitivities. For example, you are more likely to become ill when you are depressed than when you are happy. You may even want to become ill to free yourself from various responsibilities. Conversely, if you become environmentally ill you are likely to become depressed as well, because the quality of your life diminishes. This condition can make recovery more difficult.

Your state of mind is more powerful than your physical state. Even if you were to get all the nutrients you need and to live in a clean environment, any negative beliefs you harbor would very well lead to sickness. Indeed, every thought you have, constructive or destructive, sets the stage within milliseconds for a positive or negative affirmation of life within your cells. (One book that expands on how "negative beliefs" lead to sickness is *The Aquarian Conspiracy* by Marilyn Ferguson.) Most people carry around a great deal of negativity, yet they have few ways of dealing with problems constructively. These psychological factors deserve more investigation in the health-care field.

THE ROLE OF ENVIRONMENTAL MEDICINE

Environmental medicine is the study of the relationship between the environment and the individual. It is an old concept, since people all through the ages have realized that certain environmental aspects caused them to have problems. It was discovered several thousand years ago, for example, that some people would become ill from foods they ate more than once a day. Other people found that if they drank wine out of pewter cups they would become ill, but if they drank it out of goatskin bags they would have no problem. This finding was described by Hippocrates, the great Greek physician, in the fourth century B.C.

More recently, in the past seventy-five years, environmental medicine has focused on the effects of environmental factors like bacteria and viruses upon the individual. It has become quite clear that these elements can play a role in many of the problems we experience today. And other substances have crept into our modern-day surroundings that increase our total body load and weaken our immune system. These include exposures to chemicals, electromagnetic radiation, weather phenomena, radon, and radar.

Environmental medicine works on the principle of biochemical individuality—the idea that people are unique in the ways in which they react to environmental toxins or other burdens, such as stress. One person might get a headache, another might get a heart irregularity, and still another might get asthma, colon problems, or a skin disorder. Sensitive reactions can take many forms, some of which are described in chapter three.

Fifty percent of doctors practicing environmental medicine today are board certified in one specialty. This means they are not just ordinary doctors but specialists in pediatrics; ear, nose, and throat; internal medicine; allergy medicine; and other medical areas. And approximately 19 to 20 percent of them are board certified in two specialties. Most are physicians who became disillusioned when their patients did not respond to conventional drug therapy.

One physician, Dr. William Philpott, explains the course of his evolution from conventional psychiatry to the practice of environmental medicine:

> Like most doctors, I was trained to believe that mental problems had no relationship to physical ones. We thought they were due to different messages given to the child by both parents, which left the child in a double bind and resulted in a neurosis or psychosis. Often the treatments consisted of bringing fathers and mothers in for group therapy and spending hundreds of hours trying to convince them that their double messages were causing a schizophrenic child. Nobody thought of the possibility of a wheat reaction or a viral infection.
>
> By 1965 . . . I had given approximately sixty thousand electric shock treatments. Then tranquilizers and antidepressants came into the picture and I used them by the bushel, but they had all kinds of side effects. I was getting very frustrated and disappointed with the poor results, especially in the psychotic patients.
>
> I began to think of the neurologists who reported that their patients with brain tumors sometimes had hallucina-

tions and that schizophrenia was like any other organic illness. Since they were not psychiatrists and their bias was organically based, I had previously dismissed their focus but now I began to wonder if they were right.

I started to take a look at people's chemistries and became party to the first double-blind study done in this area, which impressed me. Then I began looking at the energy system and inquiring about the role of certain nutrients like magnesium, calcium, and certain vitamins mentioned in the literature I was reading.

That led me to a professor of biochemistry at the University of Georgetown Medical School whom I worked with as a consultant, and he outlined the kinds of testing I should do. He taught me how a stress load could disorder the nutritional state, and I found that without a doubt, most patients had nutritional deficiencies while under stress. I then learned how to isolate reactive foods, to remove them from the diet and rotate them back in, and to restore nutrients that were lacking.

I had excellent results with these methods. My patients stayed well twice as often as those treated with traditional tranquilizers, antidepressants, and so forth.[4]

Other physicians, like Dr. Albert Robbins, first began practicing environmental medicine when they themselves became victims of an environmental illness. Dr. Robbins tells his story:

For about ten years I practiced medicine in a very conventional way. Then I became sensitive when I moved into a new office building with new carpeting, and I developed multiple symptoms. When I found out why, I turned my practice around and started to recognize this illness in other people. Since that time I have developed a large following of individuals who have developed these unusual types of allergic diseases.[5]

Unfortunately, most of today's physicians are not being trained to test or treat patients with this approach. Therefore, many patients with environmentally induced problems are considered to be hypochondriacs by their physicians, who tell them their problems are "all in their head." Oftentimes, these doctors refer such patients to a psychiatrist because medical schools still teach doctors to believe in the law of parsimony, which states that every single illness has a single cause. While this may be true of some isolated problems, it rarely applies to the types of chronic problems resulting today from multiple stress factors. Environmental medicine is not widely practiced today for economic and political reasons as well. For more on this, see chapter seven.

WHO IS THE CLASSIC PATIENT WITH ENVIRONMENTAL ILLNESS?

According to Dr. Albert Robbins, anyone is capable of becoming environmentally ill in this day and age. But the classic patients with this disorder share some common environmental factors. Often, these people either work in a sealed and confined energy-efficient building that lacks windows and, thus, good ventilation, or they have just moved into a new home. Generally, this exposure causes them to develop an insidious type of illness with typical symptoms of fatigue and respiratory-tract or nervous-system problems.

In addition, people often become sick because of the type of work they do. Examples of those in high-risk professions include people who work with chemicals (like printers), people who work with computer chips, and people who work around gasoline or formaldehyde. Beauty salon operators and artists commonly suffer from environmental illness.

Finally, the list of classic patients includes people who have been on courses of multiple antibiotics—drugs, and especially antibiotics, are chemicals that can sensitize the body—and people whose bodies have been weakened from viral illnesses and may have never really recovered.

2

Allergies vs. Chemical Poisoning

▲
▲
▲

Dr. A. Lockyer, who practices internal medicine with a special interest in the role of environmental medicine, toxins, and allergens, believes the term *allergy* is used somewhat loosely these days. The health problems that result from toxic chemical exposures, he says, are actually more of a chemical response than a true allergy. People working in modern unventilated buildings, for example, may become ill from the cumulative effects of concentrated chemicals inhaled that, over time, destroy bodily tissue. This is different from an allergic reaction. "People may get ill from the various chemicals in the carpets," says Dr. Lockyer, "but since the body cannot make antibodies to man-made synthetics, because the body does not recognize these things, it cannot create allergic antibodies to them."[1] The difference between an allergic reaction and a toxic reaction is a matter of dose, since a very minute quantity of pollen or dust may trigger a severe nasal or lung reaction, whereas the level of certain chemicals would have to be many times more concentrated to produce a straight-out poisoning of the body.

However, Dr. John Boyles of Dayton, Ohio, former president of the American Academy of Environmental Medicine, considers sensitivities to chemicals a valid part of allergy medicine. He describes three types of allergies one may develop—to inhalants, to foods, and to chemicals.

TYPES OF ALLERGIES

Inhalant Allergies

According to Dr. Boyles, this category of allergy is recognized by all schools of thought. Inhalant allergies are reactions to things you breathe in that either were or are alive. They include sensitivities to pollens, dusts, molds, spores, and animal danders. Drugs can be effective in controlling this type of allergy. It is also the easiest type of allergy to diagnose with traditional skin testing or with the new Radio Allergo Sorbency Test (RAST), a blood test that measures the specific quantity of IgE antibodies to specific antigens. The ratio of antibody to inhalants correlates well with the allergenicity or sensitivity.

Most traditional allergists will define an allergy only when determined by an acute inflammatory skin reaction to a substance injected intradermally or by elevated specific IgE antibody levels in the patient's blood. The traditional treatment approach incorporates prescription medications and allergy shots to remove symptoms. Its effectiveness is limited, however, because it does not focus on eliminating the *cause* of the problem.

A screening test for inhalant allergies will include the thirteen most common substances in the air in your geographical environment. If you don't react to any of these things, inhalants are probably not responsible for your allergies and you should be tested for an allergy to foods.

Food Allergies

Food allergies are much more difficult to diagnose than inhalant allergies because they are not as well understood from a physiological or a chemical standpoint. A food allergy is still within the realm of proper diagnosis and treatment, however, because there may be many foods to which you could be reacting.

Even so, food allergies create a lot of controversy within the field of allergy medicine, in part because the standard IgE diagnostic tests used are not accurate indicators of food-type allergies. While IgE antibody levels do mediate very many allergic sensitivities, there are lots of other sensitivities—in fact, the bulk of our allergic responses to foods—that are mediated by other means more difficult to detect.

Food allergies have not gained widespread acceptance for another reason as well. Many people simply do not understand the concept since the connection between the foods they eat and the allergies they develop is not usually that obvious. If you eat shrimp and get a skin rash several times in a row, you will know to stop eating shrimp. The person with an allergy to shrimp has very high levels of circulating IgE antibodies to protein constituents of shrimp. When these antibodies sense and attack the ingested shrimp, a cascade of immune-related biochemical substances such as histamine is released.

If you slowly develop an allergy to a food you eat every day, however, then your reactions to that food become masked by each succeeding dose until you no longer realize that the food has an adverse effect on you. Foods that tend to become allergenic over time are those most commonly eaten in the American diet, such as wheat, corn, egg, and dairy products.

In addition, delayed reactions can occur days after eating, and it can take time for an immune response to occur. Even after the stool leaves the body, reactions can continue.

How Food Allergies Work

Dr. Doris Rapp, a board-certified doctor of allergy and pediatrics in Buffalo, New York, explains the mechanisms of a food allergy as follows: When the protective coating in your gut is wiped away and you do not have sufficient digestive enzymes and nutrients to keep out allergens, you may be absorbing large particles of undigested food rather than small digested particles. These large particles are apt to go directly into your system, thereby causing allergies.

Once the antigen or substance that creates an illness enters your body, it combines with something called an antibody, according to Dr. Rapp. The antibody and antigen join together like a lock and key causing your body to give off certain chemical mediators such as histamine, leukotrienes, bradykinin, and other mediators of the allergic response. The circulating antibody-antigen complex can affect any target area such as brain, muscle, or blood vessels.

Causes of Food Allergies

Food allergies have been associated with repetitious eating. In the American diet, the six most common foods to which people develop allergies are yeast, milk, corn, wheat, soy, and egg. These are the foods we eat all the time, of course.

You may even have them without realizing it because they are hidden in other food products, particularly processed foods. If you buy a commercial food that contains sugar, for example, the sugar most likely comes from corn, not cane. And soy may be found in any kind of food with protein extenders.

Our eating patterns are more repetitious than those of our predecessors, according to Dr. Boyles: "Our ancestors didn't eat the same things every day because they couldn't," he says. "There was no refrigeration and no way of storing anything. Different animals passed through their regions at different times, according to their migratory patterns, and different plants bloomed at different times."[2] The trouble began ten thousand years ago with the invention of agriculture. We learned how to grow and store grain and how to domesticate animals, which changed protein to unhealthful, saturated fat. That is when allergies to foods and other chronic disease patterns began to manifest.

Our ancestors also did not drink milk, which Dr. Boyles says is not a natural food for man. He points out that no other mammal drinks milk as an adult except for human beings, and that we don't even drink our own milk. Instead, we drink cow's milk, which was designed for baby cows. Dr. Boyles says the consumption of milk was pushed by the American Dairy Council in the 1930s as part of the basic four food groups concept.

Repetitious eating can create food addictions. In fact, the food you crave most often causes the most trouble. The mechanisms of food addiction parallel those of drug addiction. You begin to crave foods to which you are allergic because these foods cause your body to produce narcotic substances called endorphins. As a result, you feel the same type of "high" produced by a drug. Some time after the foods have been digested, however, you experience withdrawal because your endorphins drop to a lower level. At this point, you feel discomfort and begin to crave the same foods that will make you feel "better" again. If you can't live without your egg, your corn, or your cheese, that food may very well be the cause of your allergy.

In addition, you may crave processed foods because they lack essential nutrients. With natural substances, such as bananas or dates, a craving is quickly satiated when you become full.

Remember, too, that you may be allergic to chemical additives rather than to the foods themselves. Dr. Marjorie Siebert says that it is difficult to get organically grown food today in the United States. "There are fungicides on grains, antibiotics in milk, and waxes on fruits and vegetables," she says. "Some of the waxes are derived from petrochemicals and fungicides. So you're not playing with just wheat or just milk or just apples."[3] Asthmatics may have a severe sensitivity to sulfites, for example, which are the preservatives used in salad bars. Some people have even died from eating them. Recently it was found that people with such a sensitivity may be deficient in a certain enzyme. By taking vitamin B_{12} and molybdenum, their reaction to sulfites can improve. Dr. William Rea adds: "People can react to additives, preservatives, colorings, maybe to the food itself, or to the natural toxins in foods. And finally, you may have water pollutants which a person can react to."[4]

Dr. Siebert notes that several internal factors may be linked to food allergies as well. One is a low level of immunoglobulin-A, the antibody present in tears, saliva, respiratory mucus, and genital secretions. Its purpose is to prevent foreign substances from gaining entry into the body. Hence, when immunoglobulin-A is low, more foreign substances can enter your body and incompletely digested bits of food can enter your circulation.

Another internal factor to consider is adrenal insufficiency. Adrenal glands make cortisol, which helps to combat and reduce a hypervigilant immune response that might be accompanied by skin irritation, lung-muscle contraction, wheezing, or mucus flow in the nose. Constant stress can deplete your supply of this hormone, so if you are under the gun all the time you will diminish your supply of naturally occurring cortisol. Cortisol also can be depleted by excess sugar ingestion and by heavy metal toxicity.

Dr. Siebert also associates food allergy with an underactive thyroid state (hypothyroidism), which is occurring in epidemic proportions today. The high incidence of this disorder is probaly due in part to an autoimmune reaction stimulated by vaccines and other agents such as formaldehyde and radiation exposure.

Testing and Treating Food Allergies

According to Dr. I-Tsu Chao, a doctor of allergy and environmental medicine in Brooklyn, New York, modern allergy medicine developed in the last forty years has failed to detect food allergies because the problems often occur when a food has been digested and absorbed but not completely metabolized. At that point, it becomes an antigen, or a foreign body, which your system rejects. The resulting problem can occur anywhere in the body, such as in the chest as asthma, in the skin as hives, or in the joints as arthritis.

Dr. Chao believes the only way to find the cause of an allergy is to treat patients individually. He does so by having them keep a food diary in which they write down what they eat every day, when they eat it, and what symptoms occur. Along with the patient, he then studies the relationship between the food and the ailment and can usually identify the cause of the problem. He gives one successful example of this approach:

> A patient who came to me about fifteen years ago was prepared to have a stomach operation, a subtotal gastrotomy, where most of her stomach was to be removed. I found that her pain was due to an allergy to dairy products and asked her to stop drinking milk and to stop eating dairy. She did so and her abdominal pain disappeared completely. She canceled the operation and fifteen years later still has a perfect stomach.[5]

By correcting the diet in this way, says Dr. Chao, we can enhance the immune system. "The immune system is wonderful, but eating the wrong foods, where the foods can't break down properly, forces the immune system to treat foods like foreign bodies," he says. "This takes away all the immune power and then the viruses can cause trouble. But when we take care of ourselves so that our immune systems don't have to do too much work, we can do very well."[6]

Dr. John Boyles says the two best methods of testing for food allergy include challenging yourself with certain foods and using provocative-neutralization testing, both of which are discussed in chapter six. Also, the IgG test may be an accurate way to diagnose food allergies. Most allergists, however, ignore this procedure. What they do not realize is that the IgG does not have to indicate an acute or immediate reaction to a particular food to identify a problem.

Chemical Allergies

This last category of allergies is especially difficult to diagnose since today's complex environment contains thousands of chemicals. According to Dr. William Rea, there are about sixty-thousand organic chemicals in the air, food, and water. These include substances such as pesticides, herbicides, food additives, car exhaust, formaldehydes, phenols, and plastics. To this we can add the inorganic chemicals and heavy metals, including lead, cadmium, and aluminum, among others.

Blood tests on many chemically sensitive individuals often reveal high levels of toxic substances in their blood. These substances may include trichlorethylene, which is found in dry-cleaning fluid, or other modern-day solvents, such as toluene, xylene, or styrene. Chemically sensitive people also develop many secondary problems, such as allergies to various foods and an intolerance of alcohol. In addition, they are likely to become sensitive to weather changes since weather may affect the airborne levels of pollen or may promote the growth of molds via higher moisture levels.

How Chemical Sensitivities Work

Multiple systems of your body can be affected by an overload of chemicals. The chemicals you ingest or inhale get stored in your fat until this storage capacity is full. Then they travel throughout the body via the circulatory system. According to Dr. Francis Waickman of Akron, Ohio, who studied 12,100 charts of patients tested for food allergies, fifty-six different symptoms were identified, including everything from headaches and problems with thought processes to joint pains in the little toe. The numerous possible variations these symptoms can produce make the illness difficult to diagnose. But we do know that this type of allergy is most commonly expressed through the central nervous system. Dr. Albert Robbins, who practices internal and occupational medicine and directs the Robbins Environmental Medicine Center in Boca Raton, Florida, points out that 50 percent of hospital beds are occupied by mentally ill patients. He believes there is a connection between the high number of mentally disordered people and chemical allergies.

The second most common place for a chemical allergy to manifest is in the gastrointestinal tract, where it can cause irritable bowel syndrome, constipation, and the like. Mainstream doctors generally do not consider these types of symptoms to be associated with allergic problems.

Individuals with chemical sensitivities have difficulty tolerating low-level chemical exposures. Exposures to common chemicals, found in perfumes, pesticides, and food preservatives, affect them severely. To make matters worse, these people do not respond well to the medications doctors normally prescribe. In fact, some of these medications only complicate the illness. Dr. Albert Robbins offers this example of how chemical allergies affect the body systems:

> Recently a patient came to me after having seen many other physicians. She had developed an illness that affected almost every organ system of her body, including the nervous system, and she was taking multiple medications. She was having difficulty thinking and concentrating and also was having respiratory tract problems with asthmatic-type symptoms. In addition, she had developed some joint and muscle aches and was walking with a cane.
>
> After evaluating her history, I determined that she had become sick after a pesticide exposure, and as a result of this exposure, one symptom led to another. She became

sensitized to a number of common everyday products that prior to the sensitization process she was not allergic to. She also became sensitized to perfumes that she normally wore, to scented moisturizing creams, to fabric softeners which she used in her clothing and to hair sprays and other low levels of chemicals. Even the chemicals in the drugs she was taking were actually making her condition worse.[7]

The area of chemical allergies stirs hot debate, since some special-interest groups would not like people to know that the allergies exist. Some traditionally trained allergists argue that the disorder that people call a chemical allergy is really a psychological reaction. But nothing could be further from the truth—multiple chemical sensitivity is a horrible disease that causes tremendous suffering.

ALLERGIC LOAD PHENOMENON

Dr. Boyles defines the "allergic load" phenomenon as a synergistic reaction between different elements to which you are exposed, all of which can take a toll on your immune system.

Consider the person who gets up one morning when the pollen count is high, uses chemical hair spray, eats cornflakes, and then gets sick. The next day, there is no pollen in the air and she does not use the chemical spray. She eats the corn flakes as usual, but nothing happens. The patient is confused about whether or not she is allergic. The truth is that it takes a combination of substances to set off her allergic reaction. Some people with hay fever, for example, cannot eat certain foods in hay-fever season that they can eat during the rest of the year.

3

How Allergies Can Manifest

Allergies and other sensitivities can attack any organ system or multiple systems at once. Some people will develop asthma, some will develop gastrointestinal problems, and others will develop joint pains or nervous-system illnesses. It often depends on which part of the body is most susceptible. The weak area may be related to a genetic inheritance or it may result from weakening via environmental or other external factors during life.

The doctors of environmental medicine who originally studied allergies about seventy years ago did quite a bit of research into the effects of allergens (substances that induce an allergic reaction). They classified the various ways in which people could react to an antigen (a substance that stimulates an immune response). They found that allergens typically had a stimulating effect followed by a degenerative one. These initial two categories—stimulating and degenerative—were then broken down into levels.

The first stimulating reaction, called +1, would leave you relatively symptom free. You would be active, alert, alive, and responsive, and generally would exhibit normal behavior. At the +2 stage, you would become hyperactive, irritable, hungry, thirsty, tense, jittery, revved up, talkative, argumentative, and overly sensitive. A +3 reaction would make you hypomanic, toxic, anxious, egocentric, aggressive, loquacious, clumsy, anxious, fearful, and apprehensive. And if you were to have an extreme +4 stimulating reaction, you would become fully manic, distraught, excited, agitated, and even possibly convulsive.

At the degenerative end of the scale, a −1 reaction would give you allergic manifestations that might include a runny nose, hives, gas, diarrhea, frequent urination, or various eye and ear syndromes. At the −2 stage, you would have systemic allergic reactions exhibited as tiredness, mild depression, swelling, pain syndromes, and cardiovascular effects. With a −3 reaction, you would get depression, disturbed mental processes, confusion, moodiness, sadness, and withdrawal. Finally, at the −4 stage, you would have severe depression, with or without altered consciousness, and possible paranoia and even suicidal tendencies.

As allergies take form, some of the specific ways in which they manifest are detailed below.

ALLERGIC ARTHRITIS

Allergic arthritis occurs when foods and chemicals set off joint pains. Dr. Trowbridge believes this condition is quite common and that almost all arthritis patients treated early on from a nutritional standpoint will get better. He says that these patients often have nutritional deficiencies and need such things as extra magnesium and essential fatty acids.

Dr. Albert Robbins adds that allergic arthritis can be

triggered by moldy rooms, by chemicals like formaldehyde, and by many foods. One such food is pork, which has a predilection for affecting joints. Whether it is in the form of ham, bacon, or any food cooked in lard (and this is hidden in many restaurant foods), pork can trigger a joint response in individuals who are allergic to it. In many cases, however, the trigger will cause a delayed reaction. You could eat a food containing pork on Monday but not experience a reaction in the joints until Thursday or Friday.

The usual treatments for arthritis and other inflammatory conditions are cortisone and other extremely toxic medications that do not cure the problem. The best they can do is to alleviate symptoms temporarily. And ultimately, they make you worse. Dr. James Miller tells of one such experience with an arthritic patient:

> One patient who had arthritis was given the customary treatments, which caused him to develop an ulcer and ultimately to need an emergency operation to have his stomach taken out because it was bleeding.
>
> I saw him when he was about ready to retire because of his pain. He was unable to use his hands and unable to work. I proposed to put him into our hospital environment to see if we could find the cause of his arthritis. That program involved putting him in a room where he could be kept free of all chemical exposures. We put him on a fast for about five days until all his symptoms resolved and we gave him only chemically free spring water to drink. On this program his symptoms did diminish considerably.
>
> Then we broke the fast and started to feed him a single food per meal, all of which were free from chemical additives and contaminants. Nothing had been sprayed or exposed to plastic. We found that several foods provoked severe pain, swelling, and redness in the joints, particularly

in the fingers. Two of the main culprits were wheat and pork.

By eliminating those foods from the diet, the patient was able to go back to work after his release from the hospital and finish his career before retiring. He is now living in Florida and no longer suffering from arthritis.[1]

A small percentage of people with arthritis need to avoid the "nightshade vegetables": potatoes, tomatoes, and eggplants. You can tell if these foods affect you by staying away from them for thirty days and then eating all of them in one day. If you do not feel any worse after challenging yourself in this way, then you need not worry. If your joint pain worsens, on the other hand, your body is telling you to stay away from the nightshade family.

According to Dr. Doris Rapp, allergic arthritis can also be attributed to foods such as milk and other dairy products, red meat, and tobacco.

ASTHMA

Dr. Magid Ali, associate professor of pathology at Columbia College of Physicians and Surgeons, and director of laboratories, pathology, and immunology at Holy Name Hospital in Teaneck, New Jersey, says that while conventional wisdom maintains that asthma is an inflammatory disease, it is actually an allergic predisposition. While every allergic individual is not asthmatic, every asthmatic person is clearly allergic. If your bronchial tree forms the weakest link in your biological makeup, you will respond by getting asthma whenever the molecular burden reaches a certain point. "When the body is under stress, all of the organs get together and elect a spokesorgan that will yell out for help," says Dr. Ali. "In the case of asthma, the bronchial tubes have been elected to communicate biological stress."[2]

He adds that many people become asthmatic for the first time following a major trauma such as a family tragedy, a bad viral infection, or the first time they are prescribed a drug for some other condition. Thereafter, asthma is induced and people become frightened. Not being able to breathe is the most stressful situation of all. Fear, in itself, can cause spasms to get worse. Eventually the bronchial tube can become plugged up with mucus, which creates a life-threatening situation. In recent years, the death rate from asthma has increased.

Dr. Ali says the external stressors responsible for asthma basically include foods to which you are allergic and substances you inhale from the air, such as molds, pollens, and chemicals. The pollens are somewhat less burdensome, he says, because they stay airborne for relatively short periods of time. By contrast, you eat most foods all year long and molds are in the air all the time. In addition, he believes the chemicals we continuously breathe in—pesticides, insecticides, and other poisons—pose an even more important problem.

Fortunately, asthma can be completely reversed in most instances with preventive measures such as nutrient therapy, stress management, and environmental counseling. Dr. Ali came to this conclusion when he conducted a study of asthmatic patients in which seven out of ten subjects were taken off all drugs entirely following this type of therapy. All of the patients had previously been quite sick and were receiving extended pharmaceutical treatments for asthma: state-of-the-art medicines given by specialists. About one-third had been to the intensive care unit for a long-lasting asthma attack (status asthmaticus). They had been hospitalized and put on various drugs to help them breathe. A follow-up to his study revealed that twenty-eight of the forty-eight patients who were weaned off all drugs were able to breathe freely without any medication one year later.

Dr. Albert Robbins gives this example of how chemical exposures produced asthma in one of his young patients and how removing the offending substances reversed his condition:

> I had a little child in here recently with asthma who had been to a number of physicians in the area. They were ready to put him into the hospital but I talked to his mother and said that we should try and find what was contributing to his problem before putting him into the hospital. I asked her about the use of fragrances in the home and she said she used a lot of them. Her husband used aftershaves and colognes and she sprayed fragrance products throughout the home. Just by eliminating those fragrance products, we were able to get the little boy off most of his asthma medications and we eliminated the need for cortisone medications and the need for further hospitalization.[3]

Dr. Ali cautions, however, that asthma patients must be careful not to stop their drugs cold turkey because the effects could be dangerous. Instead, they must work with a skilled physician who can help them to identify their environmental triggers, like molds and chemicals, and the foods to which they are allergic. Ordinarily, allergy-producing foods must be eliminated for a time before they can be safely rotated back into the diet. Patients also must learn which nutrients to add to their diets, how to breathe properly, and how to use imagery exercises. Some of these practices can help to release spasms so that breathing can return to normal without drugs. Since it is impossible to avoid all stressful triggers all of the time, certain breathing exercises can be especially helpful when a patient gets that initial tightness in the chest. Asthma sufferers can usually prevent the spasms from happening in the first place, says Dr. Ali, because they tend to panic when they can't breathe, thereby releasing a lot of adrenaline and other catecholamines (compounds that function as hormones and/or neurotransmitters) into the body. The outpouring of all these chemicals raises the metabolic thermostat so that patients will react to every trigger that comes their way. Through self-regulation exercises they can effectively lower their thermostat. But patients must build themselves up internally and externally before they can reach the goal of no drugs.

The External Regulation of Asthma

Dr. Ali's therapy initially consists of giving patients intravenous antioxidants, substances that decrease oxidation or free-radical (see glossary) damage of tissues, such as vitamins A, C, E, and beta carotene, to provide the cells with more nutrients. The antioxidant complex of nutrients scavenge and neutralize harmful free radicals that occur in the body. The main components of his intravenous cocktail are vitamin C (10 to 15 grams), magnesium (1,000 mg or more), and vitamin B_{12} (up to 500 mcg). His oral supplement program includes manganese, zinc, cobalt, vitamin B complex, vitamin A, bioflavonoids, pantothenic acid, omega-3's, omega-6's, and GLA (gamma linoeic acid), all of which help to stabilize cell membranes.

The amount of nutrients must be adjusted to each patient's individual needs. For most serious cases of asthma, however, three to six months of injection therapy prove very useful. For less-serious problems, injections of the cocktail once a week for a month are all that's needed. Once the patient has obtained the control needed to breathe normally without drugs, he moves from injections to drops placed directly under the tongue (sublingual route of administration), which continue to help.

Dr. Ali says that a nutritional approach to the treatment of asthma has been recognized for a long time. *The Journal of the American Medical Association* has even published a paper about the use of intravenous magnesium therapy in hospital settings as a last-resort approach after Adrenalin has failed. Adrenalin, or epinephrine, is a widely used, standard, powerful pharmaceutical that functions via alteration or reduction of the spasms of the large air channels of the lungs. It is a potent stimulant of adrenergic (activated by adrenaline) alpha- and beta-receptors, which results in relaxation of bronchiolar smooth muscle. Unfortunately, alternative approaches have not been picked up, by and large, in the medical mainstream. Traditional doctors seem to be accustomed to the use of, and philosophically in favor of, pharmaceuticals instead of more natural therapies such as minerals, herbs, vitamins, and homeopathics.

Dr. John Boyles offers this example of how traditional solutions fail many allergy patients:

> A very intelligent mother brought her little boy to me. She was frustrated with her inability to control his hyperactivity, his asthma, his drooling, his lack of coordination, his mood swings and his constant runny nose.
>
> She had taken her son to her pediatrician, who diag-

> nosed him as having asthma and gave a pediatric theophylline preparation, a drug commonly used. Pediatric drugs are always highly colored and contain lots of sugar.
>
> When he got an asthma attack she gave him this medication, which only made him worse. She called the pediatrician, who told her to give him more. The child was getting huge amounts of this medication and getting much worse.
>
> Finally, she gave up on the pediatrician and found our office. Sure enough, the child was allergic to corn syrup and red dye, which that medication contained in large amounts. The medicine was actually making the child sick. But this is the common approach to chronic symptoms in American medicine today.
>
> The child became very well adjusted after we found all the foods and chemicals he was allergic to. This is just one example of literally hundreds of children who are, in essence, poisoned by our diet and by the medications they take.[4]

Not all patients, however, can eliminate their asthma medications, particularly in cases where too much lung function has been lost. These people usually have been taking cortisone for many years or have suffered advanced structural damage to their lungs from years and years of smoking, emphysema, or tuberculosis.

For the most part, though, Dr. Ali believes that people can be helped without the use of drugs and that medicine is shifting in that direction. Two factors account for this shift, he says: People have become more and more intolerant of drugs because of their destructive nature, and the cost of medicine has continued to soar.

BRAIN ALLERGIES

The central nervous system, and particularly the brain, provides a major target for an allergic response. Indeed, a brain allergy is the ultimate mind/body disharmony disease. It can lead to any number of reactions, including depression, hyperactivity in children, fatigue, headaches, and an inability to think clearly. Even serious psychotic problems can result.

Brain allergies can occur because many molecules you breathe in have the potential to pass from the blood into the brain. Although past teachings regarding brain function proposed that the brain featured a barrier that prevented many chemicals and pathogenic organisms in the circulating blood from entering the central nervous system, current data suggests that many molecules you breathe have the potential to pass this barrier, known as the blood-brain barrier. Once inside your brain, these foreign substances can interfere with enzymes and produce all sorts of biochemical changes. Chemicals, and especially solvents, are mainly neurotoxins that can anesthetize your brain so that it cannot function properly. Cognitive function may be affected to the point that you cannot dial the phone, put your thoughts into proper sequence, or even remember names.

Most conventionally trained doctors don't understand the connection between brain allergies and physical/emotional symptoms. One reason may be that these connections are difficult to discern. When you have a brain allergy, you appear to have a mental disorder when in reality you are having a physical allergic reaction. Quite commonly, these doctors will diagnose you as being psychologically depressed when they can't find a disease to match your complaints. They will say it is all in your head, recommend you see a psychiatrist or psychologist, and let you go with a prescription for antidepressants. Dr. Trowbridge explains why this approach can never solve the real problem: "Instead of coaxing a chemical reaction inside the brain to return to normal, an antidepressant drug simply squashes a different chemical reaction to make you appear normal without repairing the underlying problem."[5] Dr. William Rea adds, "It is needless suffering. In my mind, you don't put people on tranquilizers and say it's all in their heads until you have done a good environmental medicine workup to prove cause and effect."[6]

Environmental physicians who understand the concept of brain allergy recognize that the brain, like any other organ of the body, may be susceptible to adverse reactions. This doctor will look for such factors as responses to certain foods and chemicals, imbalances in minerals, heavy metals in the body, and the by-products of yeast overgrowth, which, according to Japanese studies, have been shown to attach to nerve transmitters inside the brain and to block normal nerve transmission.

Dr. Michael B. Schachter, an environmentally trained physician and board-certified psychiatrist in Suffern, New York, notes that people who suffer from these disorders can lessen or completely alleviate the problem by avoiding the substances to which they are allergic. "I had one so-called schizophrenic patient who, when stopping wheat and dairy, also stopped hallucinating," he says. "In another case, a patient of mine who was severely depressed had an unusual allergy to cinnamon where the elimination of the cinnamon completely cleared the depression."[7] Dr. Schachter believes the clearing of these allergies can be best accomplished by combining proper nutrients in proper quantity and by eliminating the offending substances.

Dr. Albert Robbins treats patients with brain allergies in a similar fashion. He also recommends that they avoid products that are chemicalized. They fare much better on organically grown food, for example. In addition, they need to buffer their immune systems, their gastrointestinal tracts, and their nervous systems by utilizing certain nutrients that help to stabilize the body. Dr. Robbins recommends a wide variety of B vitamins, vitamins C and A, and certain trace minerals like zinc, manganese, and selenium, which are vital to the functioning of the body's detoxification pathways. He also recommends a range of nutrients, including borage oil or evening primrose oil (which contain gamma linoleic acid, essential to restoring immune function), as well as niacin, which he says can have a dramatically positive effect. And he pays particular attention to the home and office environments and recommends regular physical exercise to help eliminate toxins.

As Dr. Lockyer points out, the link between environmental factors and brain allergies may be difficult to prove medically but easy to discern with some common sense. He tells the story of a twenty-year-old who developed central-nervous-system abnormalities from his job of painting the underside of boats. The patient used a fungicide to prevent fungi from growing on the boats, which clearly destroyed his immune system and evoked neurological symptoms. He developed paresthesia (a sense of tingling or prickling on the skin), a loss of sensation in his legs, muscle atrophy in his extremities, and decreased thinking ability. Dr. Lockyer says, "I know this was caused by his job because I had known the patient for at least ten years prior to this job. Therefore, I knew his mental state well."[8]

Clearly, brain allergies are a real problem for many people. Some of the forms they may take are as follows:

Autism

According to Dr. Doris Rapp, some autistic children stop being autistic when they no longer consume milk and dairy products. The actual number of children who have autism from food allergies may only be one in one thousand. But, if your child is that one, as she points out, that's 100 percent.

Chronic Fatigue Syndrome

Chronic fatigue syndrome is a wastebasket diagnosis used to describe individuals who cannot get out of bed, cannot think clearly or concentrate, have difficulty with their memory, and experience confusion. These patients have such little energy that they cannot drive a car and may even fall asleep during their medical evaluation.

Dr. Alfred Zamm of Kingston, New York, says that a combination of genetic and environmental factors determines whether or not a person gets this disorder. "With chronic fatigue we need to talk about *A* times *B* because *A* or *B* alone won't work. *A* may be mercury fillings and *B* the genetic inability of that person to function in a reasonable capacity. The inability may never show up unless that bit of reserve is taken away from that poor soul by poisoning him."[9] He says the same holds true for the Epstein-Barr virus and similar environmental disorders.

The traditional treatment for chronic fatigue is antibiotics, but these drugs may actually worsen the condition. Dr. James Miller comments:

> When you give a patient antibiotics for a while, you kill off all the normal microorganisms in the GI [gastrointestinal] tract but you don't kill off the yeast. So for two weeks the yeast gets a chance to grow without any competition. The patient gets large exposures to yeast and might become sensitive to it. If that occurs, the person will be sensitive to something twenty-four hours a day. That can wear down the immune system, impair the defense system, and create situations where he or she is more likely to become sensitive to other substances.[10]

A more effective approach might be to place the patient on allergy vaccines and special nutrients. One such nutrient, niacin, may be especially helpful for chronic fatigue syndrome and for other brain allergy conditions because it has a natural antihistamine effect on the brain.

Rob McCaleb, director of the Herb Research Foundation in Boulder, Colorado, says that along with herbal therapy (see pages 301–311 on herbs), other supplements can help you to recover from chronic fatigue. Some of these include coenzyme Q_{10}, vitamin C, and antioxidant vitamins such as E and beta carotene, a precursor of A, which the body converts only as much as is needed. Since free radicals appear in the body as a result of, among other things, exposures to background radiation, electrical fields, excess sunlight at high degrees, and slightly rancid oils and fats, the body is constantly struggling to neutralize these attackers. The vitamins A, C, and E are classified as antioxidants since they actively neutralize free radicals. They do so by helping to prevent damage to cell membranes and keeping cells from wearing out too fast.

Dementia

The causes of dementia, which can take several forms, generally are not known. Experts believe, however, that since cognitive dysfunction frequently occurs in people who have a history of allergies, the cumulative effects of these symptoms as a person ages can result in diminished brain function. It is possible, therefore, that many people with allergies, who comprise one-third of the population, will suffer from adversely affected brain functioning later in life.

Epilepsy

To date, there is no hard proof relating epilepsy to food and chemical sensitivity or to unusual reactions to dusts, molds, and pollens, says Dr. Doris Rapp. And yet, every once in a while someone stops eating eggs, coffee, or their favorite foods and their seizures cease.

Dr. Rapp tells one story of a young boy who was having convulsions repeatedly from eating eggs. He was also sensitive to molds and lived in a city where a cheese factory polluted the air with molds. This caused him to have convulsions all the time.

Schizophrenia

At present, two theories attempt to explain the development of schizophrenia. One hypothesis claims that a viral infection causes the disease early in life, while the other theory states that a vitamin B_6 deficiency early in life prevents the brain from developing properly. It is interesting to note that when epidemiologists study the frequency and distribution of diseases in human populations, they find that schizophrenia occurs in a pattern similar to multiple sclerosis. While a discussion linking the causes of the two diseases is wildly speculative, it's worth going into to provoke some philosophical inquiries.

To begin with, there are many viruses that inhabit the human body. Some of the more common viruses we harbor are the Epstein-Barr, which is a herpes-type virus, and the cytomegalovirus, which is a member of a group of large herpes-type viruses, both of which can cause infectious mononucleosis. Additionally, human herpes virus VI was recently isolated and found to react in much the same way.

These viruses infect the B lymphocytes of the immune system, which produce our antibodies. The cells, once infected, begin to behave abnormally by making antibodies at inappropriate times. They also can attack the neurons of the brain and the spinal cord. (Multiple sclerosis is a condition marked by patches of hardened tissue on the brain or spinal cord!)

Most people have one or more of these viruses at some point in their lives. They contract them by breathing in airborne particles or by being exposed to an actively infected carrier. Once infected, they never fully get over them. They only partially recover to the point that the virus is dormant. During times of stress, viruses often reactivate because the immune system usually weakens and functions less efficiently and the body's protective mechanism against the internal virus falters.

A virus can even be transmitted to a child through the mother. The stress of pregnancy may cause a virus in the mother to flare up and then transmit to her fetus. However, she does not even need to get an acute illness to transmit the virus. And sometimes the child can pick up the virus in another way during its formative years.

Whatever the origin, the virus first appears some time in early life. Although it is just a theory, the virus might be related to a schizophrenic-type process common in the adolescent. The schizophrenia usually shows up at this stage of life for several reasons. First, adolescence is a stressful time for teenagers—society puts a great deal of pressure on them and expects them to start behaving like adults. At the same time, adolescence is the time teenagers usually begin to eat poorly. Their diets often consist of things like colas, beef, and breads made of wheat, which add even more stress to their immune systems. The caffeine in colas and other soft drinks, for example, is a chemical that directly weakens immune function. Beef contains saturated fats with attendant chemicals so that the body may be weakened by this food. Bread containing wheat and yeast eaten frequently and in large quantities tends to result in sensitivity or allergy so that the body attacks this food instead of receiving nourishment. This type of diet can also make teenagers more susceptible to food addictions. It is possible that learning disabilities arise from the same cause.

Other environmental stressors may activate these viruses. If you live near high-tension wires or breathe in toxins, for example, you will weaken your system, thereby making it more possible for these reactions to occur. Any one such stressor may be just enough to tip the scales and make a difference between having symptoms and not having symptoms.

Also, patients with mental disorders like schizophrenia demonstrate a higher percentage of other degenerative disease conditions—including arthritis, lupus, and diabetes—than does the general population.

Dr. Philpott has found that since stress depletes the body of nutrition, his psychiatric patients can improve once nutrients are restored. He has achieved excellent results by removing the foods to which a patient reacts from his or her diet, rotating them back into the diet once the patient's metabolism has settled down, and supplementing the diet with specific nutrients, such as vitamin C, magnesium, folic acid, B_6, and certain amino acids. Dr. Philpott says the patients were truly well and did not battle with hallucinations, depressions, and other symptoms. In fact, he found that 75 percent of the patients who were diagnosed as psychotic remained well and that only 25 percent—those who would not follow his treatment plan—had to be rehospitalized.

Dr. Robbins also believes that an environmental approach can be extremely helpful with schizophrenic patients. He has reported success in helping people to stop taking Thorazine and Valium. With his treatment, patients eliminate all scented items, eat a clean diet, engage in regular exercise, and take certain nutritional supplements. He says that individuals who have been on these drugs for long periods of time require large doses of niacin and may benefit from extra magnesium and B_6 as well. A blood analysis is also done to identify any deficiencies in vitamins, minerals, and amino acids. Two other substances that may be helpful are glutamine and dl-phenylalanine, provided the patient is not allergic to them, and that they are given by an experienced environmental medical specialist.

Tourette's Syndrome

Sufferers of Tourette's syndrome manifest a large number of tics, including twitches of the eyes and of different muscle groups. They also exhibit unusual behavior patterns and may even slap themselves.

Generally, Tourette's syndrome is not considered to be

related to allergies. But Dr. Robbins found through skin and blood testing that two of his patients, who were previously diagnosed with this condition by a neurologist, were highly allergic and very chemically sensitive. He changed their environments, taught them to avoid certain products, altered their diets, and put them on allergy vaccines. As a result, the patients responded dramatically and were able to gain control of their lives. They no longer have these neurological symptoms and now function quite well.

Similarly, Dr. Doris Rapp had a young boy patient who developed severe tics from foods to which he was allergic. She said that his facial muscles twitched so much that he couldn't eat and wasn't even able to walk. She found that his problem stemmed from molds and certain foods.

DIABETES AND OTHER CARBOHYDRATE-METABOLISM DISORDERS

According to Dr. Philpott, allergies may also be linked to diabetes. He discovered this connection, much to his surprise, while monitoring mental patients for chemical disturbances. He was checking blood-sugar levels of patients before and after they ate particular foods, and some of the patients just happened to be diabetic. Unexpectedly, he found that when he eliminated the substances to which they reacted and enhanced their nutrients, not only did their mental states improve but their diabetes often disappeared as well.

A large percentage of the patients who took insulin no longer needed the medication. These patients had developed maturity-onset diabetes, the type of diabetes that strikes later in life. With this form of the disease, the patient has enough insulin but it is not doing its job. The same was not true, however, for juvenile diabetes. In this case, the pancreas is severely injured and no longer produces adequate insulin.

Dr. Philpott discovered that in cases of maturity-onset diabetes, chemical food reactions cause the tissues and the cells themselves to swell. When the cells are swollen, the insulin cannot perform its function of carrying glucose from the blood into the cells. This failure is called insulin resistance.

Similarly, Dr. John Potts has shown diabetes to be caused by reactions to foods and chemicals. His findings were published in the official journal of the American Diabetic Association, *The Journal of Diabetes.* Once the cause of the reaction was removed, the patients' insulin resistance disappeared. About two-thirds of the patients could be taken off of insulin. The remainder had to continue taking the drug, but they needed only one-third as much insulin once they had removed the foods from their diets that caused allergies.

Dr. Potts also found that while fat was an important stressor in the development of maturity-onset diabetes—80 percent of its victims are overweight—it was not the cause of the disorder. He came to this conclusion after patients who did not lose a single pound were cleared of the disease.

Dr. Philpott sees a definite connection between diabetes and most other diseases. That connection is an abnormal blood-sugar level after a meal. In a sense, he says, all degenerative diseases represent early-stage diabetes. For that reason, it would be helpful for doctors to classify diseases in two phases: diabetes stage one to describe a carbohydrate disorder, and diabetes stage two to describe a chronic state in which the blood sugar remains elevated all the time.

According to Dr. Philpott, schizophrenic and diabetic patients not only have a disordered carbohydrate metabolism (which is related to the citric acid cycle, a process of oxidation that eventually allows useful energy to be released) but also have disordered ammonia processing (which is related to the urea cycle). Ammonia, a by-product of protein metabolism, is mildly toxic, and it must be tied up very quickly in the urea cycle and released through the urine as a nontoxic substance called urea. But people who are deficient in certain substances, such as manganese or arginine, do not process ammonia correctly. Every emergency room doctor knows this fact, so one of the first things to do for unconscious patients is to test their blood ammonia to detect a diabetic coma. The high level of ammonia begins to kill off neurons in the brain and spinal cord; the mental state begins to deteriorate and the muscles start to waste away from lack of innervation.

ALS, a Form of Diabetes

Amyotrophic lateral sclerosis (ALS), also known as Lou Gehrig's disease, is similar to amyotrophy, or the wasting away of muscles. Dr. Philpott says that all patients suffering from this disease are diabetic, even though modern medicine has failed to recognize this connection. Epidemiologically, many of the same reactions occur with both conditions, he says. Much like diabetes, ALS is caused by an abundance of ammonia in the body. And ALS patients use insulin, as do those with maturity-onset diabetes.

Dr. Philpott says he has been able to reverse ALS in patients, just as he has done with diabetes, by eliminating certain allergy-causing foods and other substances. This is an extraordinary breakthrough when you consider that traditional medicine calls ALS an irreversible condition and that the majority of patients die within ten years from the time of their diagnosis.

Alzheimer's Disease

Dr. Philpott also claims that Alzheimer's disease is connected to high levels of ammonia in the system. This belief was confirmed by a study conducted in Canada and published in *The Journal of Psychiatry*.

More commonly, Alzheimer's disease is thought to be caused in part by high amounts of heavy-metal poisoning, especially aluminum poisoning. These findings, however, do not hold true in all cases of Alzheimer's, while high levels of ammonia exist most of the time.

So the common thread between diabetes, ALS, and Alzheimer's appears to be a reaction to foods and chemicals resulting in high levels of ammonia and in elevated blood sugar.

IRRITABLE BOWEL SYNDROME

Gastrointestinal disturbances, such as diarrhea, constipation, bloating, and flatulence, are often loosely assigned the term *irritable bowel syndrome.* The typical gastroenterologist treats these problems with medicines designed to calm down the stomach and intestines. But the only way to get to the root of the disturbance is to examine your diet carefully, since the gastrointestinal system is directly linked to what you put in your mouth.

Commonly, people with gastrointestinal disturbances react severely to milk. It is a major culprit because as we grow older, we lose the enzyme that breaks it down; then, as the milk putrifies, one gets gas. Gluten sensitivity is also common in people with gastrointestinal symptoms such as bloating and mild intestinal discomfort. Gluten is a component of wheat and other grains, the name for which is derived from the Latin for glue, since it is an insoluble protein with binding qualities.

PREMENSTRUAL SYNDROME (PMS)

According to Dr. Robbins, women with PMS often are allergic to their own progesterone hormone. An environmental doctor can make an allergy vaccine to counter this. Women with PMS also need to build themselves up nutritionally. This can be done with magnesium (400 to 800 mg), vitamin B_6 (approximately 50 mg), and vitamin E (200–400 IU). It's best to take these nutrients during the second half of the menstrual cycle.

In addition, you can help to lessen the effects of PMS by paying particular attention to your diet and by participating in an aerobic exercise, such as jogging, bicycling, or swimming. Following these various approaches, many former PMS sufferers will find they have fewer symptoms and improved immune- and nervous-system function during the premenstrual time frame.

YEAST INFECTIONS

Like candida, yeasts are normal inhabitants of the skin, mouth, genital tract, and gastrointestinal tract. Many people have a mistaken image of their bodies as sterile, germ-free vessels, but that is simply not the reality. A healthy body contains millions, and possibly billions, of different microorganisms that have essential biological functions. Some of these functions include synthesizing vitamin K, facilitating vitamin B_{12}, and maintaining a physiological pH of the mucous membranes they inhabit. These healthful microorganisms also prevent the overgrowth of pathogenic microorganisms by using the space and food the harmful ones would otherwise take. And some of these favorable bacteria, like lactobacillus and bifidobacter, even make their own antibiotics to fight the harmful bacteria. Therefore, candida and other microbes perform many important functions to help keep you well. They will only harm you when your body gets out of balance, which allows one or more of these organisms to grow beyond a healthy threshold.

Unfortunately, more people suffer from an overgrowth of candida and from other yeast infections today than ever before. This prevalence is due to the widespread use of substances like antibiotics, sugar, oral contraceptives, and steroids. In fact, Dr. William Crook of Jackson, Tennessee, has estimated that upwards of 60 million Americans suffer from candida in any given year.

The most common cause of candida is the oral antibiotic, the "panacea" of modern medicine. While antibiotics kill the offending bacteria, they also kill many of the helpful bacteria of the colon. Yet, they do not kill off candida, since this form of yeast has a totally different makeup from that of a bacteria. As a result, the candida has more food to eat and more space to grow, and it rapidly proliferates. This growth then upsets the chemistry of the colon walls and causes local inflammation. Some of the sugars and carbohydrates normally present there also begin to ferment, causing gas, pain, and diarrhea or constipation. The resulting condition can be termed a candida colitis.

Most doctors choose to ignore the inherent dangers of antibiotics by calling these symptoms typical side effects of the medications. The *Physician's Desk Reference* (PDR) or the package insert of almost any antibiotic will tell you, in effect, that the accepted side effects of the drug include gas, intestinal upset, diarrhea, and constipation. But it's dangerous to view these symptoms as acceptable because you may not take any corrective action when they occur, figuring that once you finish taking the antibiotic the symptoms will go away. You may even take multiple rounds of antibiotics because you do not recognize their potentially devastating effects.

Yeast infections also may be caused by dietary indiscretion and stress. If you eat sugar in excess, for example, it will feed the yeast and upset the normal balance in your system. Likewise, yeast overgrowth can be caused by exposures to poisons such as mercury, by birth control pills, which can change the chemistry of your body, or by molds and mold spores.

Once women have an overgrowth of yeast in their colon, it can easily inoculate the genital tract and produce postantibiotic vaginitis. At that point, you might try a vaginal suppository or cream, which will probably offer temporary relief by killing the local infection of the yeast in the vagina. However, 80 percent of these infections recur because of the large reservoir of candida still living in the colon. The most popular of these preparations is Nystatin, which can actually worsen the condition by increasing permeability and allowing more undigested macromolecules to pass through your intestines. At this point, you probably have an impairment in your immune system as well, which would ordinarily arrest the development of the yeast. This impairment is, in fact, caused by the yeast itself.

Eventually, this overgrowth can spread to other parts of the body and cause any number of symptoms. While candida usually begins in the colon and spreads to the genital organs, it can show up in the mouth or gastrointestinal tract as well. Some of its symptoms include the following: hyperactivity, depression, anxiety, premenstrual syndrome, disorientation, colitis, irritable bowel, intestinal gas, diarrhea, constipation, cystitis, loss of menstrual periods, painful menstruation (dysmenorrhea), classical and recalcitrant vaginitis, dizziness, poor memory, impaired intellect, headache, weight gain, cold extremities, fatigue, acne, arthritis, rapid heartbeat, and irregular pulse. Thyroiditis, an inflammation of the thyroid gland often related to the body's immune system's attacking itself with the thyroid the target, results in diminished thyroid function.

The theory that candida can create multisystemic illness is not new. It was first set forth more than thirteen years ago by Dr. Orion Truss. But mainstream medicine, for the most part, has not accepted the theory, and part of that resistance may stem from the medical community's reluctance to accept the fact that a yeast infection can affect any organ from the skin and mouth to the brain and bladder. On the surface, it may indeed seem unlikely that candida can affect the entire body. But when you look closely at the actual mechanisms of the disease, its ability to do so becomes more clear.

How Candida Can Harm You

Candida can cause problems throughout the body in four ways: (1) through suppression of the immune system; (2) through the production of acetaldehyde, which is a harmful intermediate as the yeast ferments carbohydrate; (3) through the direct allergic properties of the yeast; and (4) by interfering with the female hormones. Below, we explore each of these areas.

1. Immune-System Impairment Candida affects the immune system in two ways because the latter consists of two subsystems: the cellular immune system and the humoral immune system. The cellular system is composed of white blood cells and other cells throughout the body. The T cells (thymus-mediated) direct the B cells (bone-marrow mediated), which produce antibodies. These antibodies, in turn, become part of and give directions to the humoral system. The immune-related cells directly attack bacteria, fungi, viruses, tumor cells, and human *Candida albicans*—yeast cells. While the mechanical action of the cells is fighting off foreign substances, the humoral mechanism has biochemical mediators—such as the aforementioned antibodies—that also attack these invaders. Unfortunately, human *Candida albicans,* when growing in excess, burdens the cellular system as well as the humoral system. Both the cellular and humoral systems must work in harmony and balance; otherwise, the body may overreact, part of which is the process of allergy formation.

Two mechanisms allow candida to suppress cellular immunity. First, candida itself makes a toxin that weakens cellular immunity. And second, the presence of yeast in the system for a long time causes the immune system to develop a tolerance to it so that it does not attack the candida. Once this happens, the yeast can proliferate without challenge.

Since the cellular immune system helps to control viruses, the suppression of this system will make you more susceptible to viruses like Epstein-Barr, herpes, cytomegalovirus, and possibly even the HIV virus. A correlation exists between HIV activity and candida infection, which is most possibly due to the suppression of cellular immunity.

In the case of candida, the humoral immunity reacts by attempting to compensate for the depressed cellular immunity. That means you will show high levels of antibodies to candida on a blood test, but this does not indicate a resolution or a cure. It simply means that the humoral immune system is trying to compensate for the cellular immune system's inability to do its job.

Another problem arises from the suppression of the cellular immune system: The immune system loses its control mechanisms, and you can then develop antibodies against the body's own organs. In this way, yeast infections can lead to autoimmune complexes such as thyroiditis and antiovarian antibodies. Immune-system impairment also causes fatigue and, as mentioned earlier, secondary allergies to foods and to environmental chemicals. This dysfunction also explains how you can get symptoms such as arthritis, cystitis, ovarian failure, lack of menstruation, and even acne, since you upset the skin's immunity.

2. Acetaldehyde Production Candida produces acetaldehyde as a by-product of its fermentation of carbohydate in the human digestive system. The acetaldehyde directly poisons the immune system and also inhibits coenzyme A, which is part of the citric-acid-production cycle of energy.

Acetaldehyde also impairs the detoxification process, making it difficult to excrete toxic environmental substances and other metabolic poisons. It hinders this process by blocking and competing with these substances for breakdown and excretion. Once acetaldehyde blocks the degradation of environmental and metabolic poisons, you may find yourself more sensitive to chemicals. You may become sick when you get your clothes dry-cleaned or when your house gets painted, more so than if you did not have the yeast allergy.

Acetaldehyde can wreak havoc in other ways as well. It impairs the normal degradation of epinephrine and norepinephrine, for example. Persistently high levels of these hormones can cause anxiety, fear, heart palpitations, irregular heartbeat, and tachycardia (rapid heartbeat). Acetaldehyde also acts as a hapten, which means that it binds onto body proteins and makes them appear foreign to the immune system. This, in turn, sets off an autoimmune cascade.

The acetaldehyde produced in the body from the fermentation of carbohydrate is a neurotoxin that can cause the dizziness and disorientation experienced by candida patients. In one research study, Japanese scientist Dr. Iwata studied a gentleman who was accused of drunk driving when, in fact, his yeast fermentation, which created the acetaldehyde (alcohollike toxin) in his blood, was causing the drunken sensation.

In addition, acetaldehyde blocks free fatty-acid synthesis. This process causes the red blood cells produced by the body to have stiff membranes, resulting in impaired circulation. This can explain the cold hands, cold feet, and restless leg syndrome experienced by some candida patients.

By poisoning enzymes, acetaldehyde synthesizes cholesterol and steroid sex hormones. This disorder can account for premenstrual syndrome, the lack of fertility, the loss of libido, and the disruption of menstrual cycles in those infected with candida.

3. Direct Allergic Properties of Yeast In addition to acetaldehyde, candida gives off other toxins as well that can create an autoimmune disorder and induce secondary allergies to various foods and chemicals. Dr. Christopher Calapai, an osteopath practicing in New York City, has attempted to identify the specific immune toxins candida produces, but all of these toxins have not yet been identified. At this point, candida is known to consist of approximately seventy-nine known chemicals that have been isolated through immunological methods, but there are probably many more.

4. Interference with Female Hormones Candida appears to interfere with normal female hormone components by blocking progesterone and possibly estrogen. It can induce antiovarian antibodies by mimicking some of the antigens of a normal ovary, which then induce an immune reaction against your own ovaries. This can cause premenstrual syndrome, the loss of menstrual periods, the loss of libido, and infertility.

In one study, Dr. Truss tried to unravel the connection between candida and impaired female hormones. While the exact mechanism of this link is not entirely understood to date, the yeast most likely impairs the hormones in three ways: (1) by producing antiovarian antibodies (mentioned above); (2) by depleting folic acid, an important component of the vitamin-B-complex group involved in red blood cell formation; and (3) by producing some toxin that may block estrogens and progesterones from reaching their target organs. This last mechanism may explain why some patients have a loss of the monthly menstrual cycle following a candida infection, even though their serum estrogen and progesterone levels have remained normal. The toxin may have blocked the estrogen and progesterone from reaching the target tissues.

TREATING CANDIDA AND OTHER YEAST DISORDERS

When treating a yeast disorder, you need to pay close attention to your diet. It's especially important to eliminate sugar, since it serves as a major source of food for the yeast and allows it to thrive. Sugar also suppresses the immune system by diverting the body's zinc and B-complex vitamins for the requirements of metabolizing sugar for energy. Zinc and B complex are also important components of the immune system.

Another dietary strategy is to eliminate fermented or yeast-containing products, such as MSG, hydrolyzed (chemically processed) vegetable protein, tea, pickles, miso, tempeh, and related foods, until the excess yeast can be controlled and eliminated. And since yeasts can induce allergies, it's wise to eliminate foods to which you are allergic and rotate the other foods in your diet to lessen your allergic burden.

Neutralizing injections of candida extract also may prove helpful. Dr. Albert Robbins says that when these allergies are corrected through allergy vaccines, affected individuals can feel dramatically better.

Some doctors give yeast injections to build up your tolerance to yeast progressively, an acceptable but slightly different approach from that of neutralization therapy. In the first instance you try to induce an immunity to yeast; in the second you attempt to immediately eliminate the crippling effect of the yeast on T-cell function. The thymus-directed T cells are critical to the immune system since they direct the B cells, which produce the antibodies.

According to Dr. Robbins, the *American Journal of Obstetrics and Gynecology* reported in September 1990 that women with candida organisms such as *Candida albicans* (the common white-colored infection) or *Candida tropicalis* (a less-common yeast form) can gain complete relief from their symptoms by undergoing candida immunotherapy and by avoiding chemical exposures to such things as fragrances and polyester clothing. The chemicals in fragrances and man-made polyester cloth seem to provoke candida imbalance.

Dr. Marjorie Siebert says that some specific preparations can be used to help kill and eliminate the yeast. One of her remedies is an herbal tannate that mimics the active compounds in tea. It works by agglutinating (combining into a mass) yeast cells, removing them from the mucosal wall, and making it easier for the body to eliminate them. Another compound for killing yeast is garlic, especially in the bulb form. Garlic both kills the yeast and inhibits its adherence to mucosal walls. The Chinese use garlic intravenously, in fact, but in America it is only available orally.

Other remedies for eliminating yeast include citrus seed extract from grapefruits. In addition, you might try goldenseal or berberine, an herbal product that has antiyeast, antiparasitic, and antibacterial properties.

To resolve yeast infestation, you also need to get the aldehyde metabolite under control using the following two preparations. First, make sure you get enough of the mineral molybdenum, an essential trace mineral, which plays a vital role in the breakdown of aldehydes. The recommended dose is 50 to 150 mcg per day with meals. In some cases, an injection of molybdenum may be needed to facilitate absorption. As a hexavalent (meaning it has a +6 charge), molybdenum is not an easy mineral to absorb, especially if candida in the intestine are hampering absorption. A second product useful in helping to control aldehyde buildup is pantetheine, which enhances acetaldehyde degradation. Pantetheine is a precursor to coenzyme A, so you will be replenishing some of the coenzyme A that the acetaldehyde has depleted and inactivated.

Zinc also stimulates the immune system and helps to build the integrity of the mucous membranes. Zinc is best taken with vitamin A and copper, which also help to rebuild the immune system. Vitamin C and echinacea are important antiallergy compounds and immune stimulants as well. And you may want to try 1,000 to 2,000 mcg of biotin, which appears to help treat yeast infections. Conversely, you should avoid cysteine preparations because they appear to increase the growth of candida.

Omega-3 and omega-6 fatty acids, which help to fluidize red cell membranes and improve circulation, also have an immune-modulating effect in which they temper the overactive humoral immune system. This is an important function, since, as mentioned earlier, the humoral immunity overcompensates for the malfunctioning cell-mediated immunity when candida suppresses it. The omega-3 and -6, through their positive effects on lymphocytes, will help to balance out this dysregulation.

Magnesium is also important because it serves as a cofactor in many detoxification reactions. It also helps to counter fatigue, especially when given with potassium as an aspartate. An injection usually provides the most rapid results.

People with candida have been found to have low levels of folic acid as well. Folic acid is a proestrogen so a deficiency of it may contribute to problems with the female reproductive and hormonal system.

Case Studies of Candida Patients

Dr. Siebert offers two examples of candida patients who were successfully treated with the methods described above. In the first instance, a young man had developed candida after long-term usage of antibiotics, which were prescribed by his doctor for an acne condition and an ear infection. "I had him take some homeopathic remedy, drink a lot of water to try to loosen up and make soluble the mucous in his ear, increase his vitamin C, and take a little extra zinc. I also gave him a tannate preparation and acidophillus. After that, he no longer needed the antibiotics and he has continually been getting better."[11]

In another instance, Dr. Siebert was able to help a woman who came to her complaining mostly of depression, phobia, and headaches that became worse prior to her menstrual periods. Due to the woman's limited financial means, Dr. Siebert treated her empirically with a neutralizing dose of yeast. Once she found the correct dosage, the patient went into a complete remission.

In one less-successful example, a woman who came to Dr. Siebert with multiple sclerosis and an extremely high level of candida antibodies in her blood responded well initially to treatments but then stopped everything at once.

> A woman came to see me who wanted another opinion on how to cure her multiple sclerosis. She wanted to see what could be done other than physical therapy and being told she just had to live with it. I tested her and found her to have a six hundred titre to candida, which is one of the highest I have seen in my three years of practice.

I wanted to treat her with neutralization but she was afraid, and rightfully so, that this might cause an exacerbation of her multiple sclerosis if we did, in fact, provoke her symptoms and could not neutralize them. She was also afraid to take antiyeast medications, once again fearing a reaction would exacerbate her multiple sclerosis. But she did agree to intravenous vitamin C. She also ingested acidophilus, pantetheine, and a multiple vitamin and mineral supplement. We tried all that and the patient did much better. She was even able to take on three part-time jobs.

Then some terrible things happened. She had a flood in her apartment, her parents decided to move away, and she had some relationship problems. She started getting numbness in her legs and her internist insisted on putting her into the hospital. Once there, they cut off all of her vitamins, and unfortunately, she deteriorated very rapidly.

I believe the problem resulted from this woman going from taking 6 to 10 grams of vitamin C a day to taking the RDA of 30 mg a day. This caused her to develop a rebound scurvy because the small amounts of vitamin C that were present were going to the most essential functions.[12]

4

Childhood Allergies

It is particularly disheartening when doctors misdiagnose children who have a food allergy or a chemical sensitivity and then place them on Ritalin or some other psychoactive drug. Parents who seek out the real causes of their children's problems deserve a lot of credit because they must do some hard work, usually without the support of their family or pediatrician. If anything, says Dr. Dorothy Calabrese, of San Clemente, California, the traditional approach to treatment gets support. So these children continue to take Ritalin and enter expensive programs that are huge tax burdens.

Dr. Doris Rapp, a pediatrician and allergist, says that a drug may be necessary on occasion, but it is generally not the answer. "If you have a nail in your shoe causing a sore on your foot, the answer is not to put a Band-Aid on the sore but to take out the nail," she says. "The answer is to explore what is making your child ill because only you can know the body of your child."[1]

HOW ALLERGIES DEVELOP AND MANIFEST IN CHILDREN OF DIFFERENT AGES

Allergies Before Birth

Some children are born with allergies because their mothers have food allergies and chemical sensitivities while the fetuses are in the womb. Dr. Rapp explains, "During pregnancy your baby may kick so hard that you become bruised from the inside. If you ask yourself what you just ate, it might be the milk, or the dairy products, or the banana or chocolate cannolis you just binged on that is causing your baby to suddenly send you a message, 'Hey mom, you're eating the wrong thing.' "[2]

Allergies During Infancy

During infancy, babies often develop allergies when they begin to drink formulas, which may even lead to severe colic. This usually points to a milk problem, but the allergy also may stem from a soy formula or from the corn in the milk.

Dr. Rapp recommends formulas with no dextrose, or corn syrup, because the corn can cause chronic problems. Some of these babies are so smart, she says, that they actually push away their bottle but eat their food vigorously, which tells you that they are sensitive to something in the bottle.

She also says that breast-fed children usually have fewer problems than those who drink formulas. However, if a mother who breast-feeds binges on a lot of cheese or milk, it can enter the breast milk and affect the child, causing irritability, an inability to sleep, prolonged crying episodes, excessive drool, and perspiration.

Infants who suffer from allergies are those who must be

walked and bounced constantly. You can't cuddle them quietly in your arms because they will throw their heads back. Sometimes they begin to get ear infections, one after another, from a buildup of fluid behind their eardrums. In most instances, the problem stems from an allergy to milk and dairy products. Some of these children end up having surgery before they are even a year old.

When mothers stop breast-feeding, children frequently begin to develop allergies. They can develop nasal congestion and bronchiolitis, which is an early form of asthma. The infant's lungs go into spasm and you hear wheezing sounds. And once a baby has bronchiolitis, he or she has a 66 percent chance of developing asthma later in life. These babies also have a lot of nose mucus from allergies in the nose. And a noisy chest may indicate that the chest has allergies.

Allergies in Toddlers

By the time an allergic child reaches the "terrible twos," there will be an explosion every time you say no to the child. To a certain degree this is normal, but the toddler with allergies generally acts out aggressions more than other children do.

Be sure to look for physical signs of an allergy as well. If your child has dark eye circles, red ear lobes, wiggly legs, and a spacey look to his eyes, especially after he eats a meal, enters a dusty room, or the like, you have to wonder if these factors also are causing the sudden explosive episodes.

Foods, dust, molds, pollens, and chemicals usually start to cause trouble by the time children are two, three, and four years old. If they get worse in the summer, pollen or other things outside could be the cause. If they are worse in the house, dust or mold may be the culprit. And if the symptoms remain the same year-round, indoors and out, the child may be allergic to a food. If your child has a chemical sensitivity, you may notice that he or she frequently smells chemicals before anyone else or gets sick when riding in cars.

Allergies in Older Children

As allergic children pass the toddler stage, they may cough when they start to run, laugh, or exercise. Again, consider this to be an early warning sign that they may be developing asthma.

In addition, use the following procedure to check their breathing: Put your ear next to your child's chest and ask him or her to breathe deeply with an open mouth. If all you hear is breathing, your child is fine. But if you hear a squeak and whistle sound along with the breathing, asthma may be developing.

During the school years, children may begin to develop behavioral and learning problems if an allergy affects the brain. One day they get *A*'s and the next day *F*'s in the same subject. Nobody understands their Dr. Jekyll/Mr. Hyde personalities. In the most severe instances, they are perfect angels one minute and highly explosive the next—hitting, kicking, or spitting. Dr. Rapp notes that these personality changes also can be related to hypoglycemia. In some cases, the blood-sugar problems will disappear when the allergy is treated.

The aggressive behaviors can carry over into adulthood as the allergies lead people to lose control. As, for example, men who become violent, punching or knocking things over in a bar or restaurant after having a beer made from corn. If the beer had been made from rice, they might not have acted so violently.

According to Dr. Francis Waickman, some children may even exhibit bizarre personality changes from allergies. They may appear to have schizoid personalities, even though they are not schizophrenic in the true psychiatric sense.

Some children with allergies will go to the opposite extreme and become withdrawn. They may crawl under the furniture, refrain from being touched, and say things like "I wish I were dead" and "Nobody loves me." These children are experiencing allergic fatigue, a condition first written about in the 1930s. Dr. Doris Rapp has videotaped some children who experienced suicidal depression after she put a drop of tree pollen, ragweed pollen, or mold on their arms. She shows how they become bright eyed and cheerful again just seven or eight minutes after they receive the correct neutralizing dilution.

Allergies can cause some children's bladders to spasm. Many times, these children wet their beds every night after the age of five because of the milk or fruit juice they drink at bedtime. Some of the juices that can cause a problem include orange, apple, grapefruit, pineapple, and grape. These drinks can cause their bladders to spasm in the daytime, too. The children dribble in their pants or have to race like mad to get to the toilet.

Another physical symptom in children (as well as adults) from food allergies is bloating, which causes them to belch or pass gas rectally. This occurs when the stomach separates the foods that cause trouble from those that don't. If your child can taste peanut butter when he or she belches, the body is saying that the rest of the food can pass through the intestines but that the peanut butter must be slowed up because it is causing an allergic reaction.

These reactions usually occur fifteen minutes to an hour after the food is eaten. The immediate reactions from milk, for example, can include headaches, bellyaches, or leg aches. Other reactions may be delayed, such as colitis, bed wetting, eczema, or rashes in the creases of the arms and legs.

Allergies in school-aged children may be worsened by the foods they eat at school or by unhealthy chemical exposures in the building. (More about that will be discussed later in this chapter under "Allergies and Schools.")

Allergies in Adolescents

During adolescence, boys seem to have less trouble with allergies than do girls. Girls begin to crave the foods to which they are allergic just before menses. If they were to write down their five favorite foods, in fact, they would be apt to find the very offenders that cause their chronic health problems. They begin to complain of headaches, fatigue, irritability, and depression. These symptoms remain with many women into adulthood.

As time passes, many of these symptoms begin to generalize. As a result, an allergic teenager may become depressed, rather than develop hay fever or asthma, when the grass needs to be cut or when he or she encounters weeds or molds.

As the allergies become progressively worse, people begin to get other symptoms, including bloating, gas, diarrhea, constipation, or belching. These types of symptoms usually indicate a milk allergy and a lactose intolerance. Recurrent earaches, recurrent leg aches, congestion, and noises related to mucus or irritation in the throat causing a throaty sound or even a clucking noise all point to a milk allergy as well.

END-STAGE SYMPTOMS OF ALLERGIES

What type of long-term effects can allergies produce if not addressed in childhood? When you ignore the early warning signs, the problems you experience later on can be quite serious. You may start to pass a little blood, for example, leading your doctor to diagnose a problem such as irritable bowel, Crohn's disease, or ulcerative colitis. Dr. Doris Rapp says that your bowels talk to you, but that few people pay attention. The problem gradually gets worse until, forty years later, you end up with a serious bowel problem. As a result, an allergy that starts in the childhood years can lead to the types of symptoms we now see in the older generation.

In addition to affecting the bladder, untreated allergies can affect the blood vessels and result in high blood pressure, an irregular heartbeat, or arteriosclerosis, which is a thickening and hardening of the arterial wall with loss of elasticity. They can also cause arthritis and many of the other symptoms mentioned in chapter three.

ALLERGIES AND SCHOOL

Sick Schools

Children who become sensitized to massive chemical exposures, such as a gas leak in the house, easily become ultrasensitive to every little thing in their environment, including chemicals, waxes, sprays, and disinfectants used in their schools. They develop what is known as a spreading phenomenon, in which they cannot tolerate substances that did not bother them before the exposure. These may include chemicals on paper and in marking pencils, the smell of fabric softeners, and the perfumes that people around them use. In some cases, the chemical overload is so great that an affected child cannot attend school at all. These children experience a personality change and right away some doctor wants to put them on Ritalin.

Dr. William Rea offers this case history of a patient who would get an allergic form of arthritis every time she attended school:

> This girl came down with chronic arthritis and was in bed for three years. She had been to all the famous medical centers in New York and nobody could find out what triggered it. But we found that there were several chemical pollutants, like formaldehyde and phenols, that caused her problems.
>
> We got her well and sent her back but her problem returned upon going back to school. In fact, she would get so ill that she would become nonfunctional. She had been an outstanding gymnast, and therefore was aware of her body's functions. Of course, when her joints got bad, she couldn't do any of the gymnastic things.
>
> Now she is in a less-polluted building. She can do her gymnastics again but when she is in a polluted building in the school area she can't. It's quite clear how she needs a relatively clean environment to not have problems.[3]

Another account comes from Dr. Francis Waickman, who says that one of his child patients had major emotional problems in a particular classroom, which was located next to a swimming pool that gave off a heavy odor of chlorine.

Once transferred to a different school, the child had no problems whatsoever. He has noted similar personality changes in children who have trouble in school on Monday morning because of the cleaning chemicals used over the weekend but are fine on Friday.

Dr. Albert Robbins believes that every child with behavioral problems should be thoroughly examined for allergies by an environmental physician because allergies often target the nervous system. This approach can be quite successful with children. "School teachers write me letters saying, I don't know what you did with this kid but he is doing so much better in school now that you have corrected his allergies. It's like a miracle."[4] He adds that certain nutritional supplements, like magnesium, vitamin B_6, and zinc, can be tremendously beneficial for these children.

Clean Classrooms

In Waterloo, Canada, "clean classrooms" have proven to be quite successful. In addition to having the floor, walls, and windows physically cleaned, administrators installed a purifying system that cleaned the air of dust, mold, and the like. Also, chemicals were not allowed in the classroom.

The children who attended the clean classrooms had fewer infections than most other children. Children who could only attend schools 64 percent of the time now attend 84 percent of the time. Previously, these children were taught at home, at the cost of $100 per day, 180 days per year. Therefore, cleaning up the classroom saved that school $18,000 a year. Also, their schoolchildren's academic performance improved.

Allergies and IQ Changes in Children

Dr. Francis Waickman has a number of patients who were unable to reach their intellectual potential until they were diagnosed and treated for food allergies. His most severe case was a seven-year-old girl who had been told by many physicians that she had no allergies. A psychologist had tested her IQ and reported it to be 65. Her school wanted to put her in a class for emotionally and mentally retarded children. However, her mother realized that at two years of age the girl had been using pronouns correctly. Therefore, she believed her daughter's low IQ was caused by something other than retardation.

Dr. Waickman explored the girl's history and discovered that she had had severe colic during her first nine months. Her formula also was changed multiple times. By twelve months of age she had eczema, by eighteen months she had repeated ear infections, and by two years of age she had started going downhill intellectually.

Through testing, she was shown to be allergic to eleven foods. She was treated for these allergies and then given the same IQ tests by the same psychologist eleven months later. This time, she scored 129 and was placed in an advanced class.

Dr. William Rea tells another story of a little girl who was failing in school because of multiple sensitivities she had developed. He found that she was sensitive to four or five different types of foods, as well as to molds and formaldehyde. She also was found to be sensitive to the copy paper on which she took her exams. When she took oral exams or was tested on handwriting paper, she could get *A*'s. But the moment she had to take a test from copy paper, she wasn't able to think at all.

5

Allergy-Provoking Substances

POLLUTED PLACES

Some of the worst concentrations of contaminants can be found in our modern homes and public buildings.

Sick Buildings

Beginning in the 1970s, public buildings were made tighter to increase energy efficiency. Builders wanted to keep the cold out in the northern climates and the heat out in the southern climates. To that end, they created buildings with no windows and thus no ventilation, in which all the air would come through a central air system. These systems have proven to be quite toxic because they can spew out unclean air that's filled with molds and chemicals. The tightly sealed buildings are also filled with chemicals that outgas, or slowly leak into the air.

We become most affected by these poisons indoors because the amounts are highly concentrated, especially when the building cannot be aired out because there are no windows. At present, certain states have passed laws requiring owners to heat up the buildings before people can move in so that the substances can leak, or outgas more rapidly, which helps. Some of the more common chemicals found indoors are mentioned later in this chapter.

Sick Houses

Suppose that you go to bed and wake up in the middle of the night wheezing. It could be from what you ate just before bedtime, or it could be due to sleeping between permanent-press sheets that contain formadehyde. Maybe you feel sick because your mattress contains formaldehyde as a flame retardant or your pillow is made from a synthetic material. Perhaps it could be the plastic mattress cover that gives off a smell. Or maybe your nightclothes weren't completely dry when you went to bed and the moldy smell is giving you trouble. As you can see, any number of things in your home may be responsible for making you sick.

In her book, *Is This Your Child?*, Dr. Doris Rapp made a list of all the chemicals a person might be exposed to on a typical day. The list actually frightened her. Just in the bathroom alone there are chemicals in the toilet paper, the mouthwash, and the toothpaste. More can be found in the soap you use, in your washcloth, and in your towels because of the cleaning solutions you use. And even when you take a shower, the chlorine in the water forms chloroform that can actually hurt you, especially if you take long showers. By the end of one day, she says, you would be surprised to find that you were exposed to hundreds and hundreds of chemicals that, for the most part, have not been tested for their effects once inside your body.

New homes are known to be particularly toxic. People often become sick from the formaldehyde found in the pressboard material and from the new paint and rugs that outgas for a time. Some people become so severely ill from these homes that they are forced to move out. Dr. Robbins offers an example:

> A woman came to me after having moved into a new home and developed a flulike illness that never went away. I ultimately found that her home had been insulated with a urea formaldehyde foam insulation. As a result, she developed asthma and a muscle and joint syndrome that appeared to be a classical arthritis. We measured the formaldehyde levels and found them to be higher than normal. Also, the pressboard in the kitchen cabinets and in her closets were outgassing formaldehyde, which she was breathing in. The gasses were causing changes in her immune system and detoxification system until her body was no longer capable of dealing with chemical exposures. Eventually she had to move out.[1]

Cars and Other Vehicles

Some children and adults feel fine until they get in the car or school bus in the morning. Then the many chemicals that can outgas from vehicles begin to make them sick. These include the smell of gasoline, the smell of auto exhaust, and the smell of synthetic leather or plastic seats. All of these things can make you fatigued by the time you reach work or school.

Airplanes

When you are inside an airplane and pulling onto the runway, high levels of jet fuel fumes come right into the cabin and can make you very ill. Once the plane ascends several thousand feet, you can have problems with ozone. And if smoking is permitted on board, it can make matters worse.

Fumes can outgas from the seats as well. In first and business class, especially, a lot of formaldehyde comes from the type of seats used. By contrast, the tourist class has fabric seats that generally are less offensive.

On international and other long flights, people sometimes become sensitive to the foam in their seats. You can prevent this problem by taking along some aluminum foil, some leather, or a fabric seat to use. Newspapers and magazines also can outgas fumes and create problems. And during landing, jet fuel fumes enter the cabin once again.

While drinking alcohol during the flight can make you feel worse, drinking plenty of spring water might help to flush out a bit of the toxins. Taking vitamin C before arriving at the airport can help to counter a lot of these substances too since it is a powerful antioxidant that protects tissues from chemical injury. High doses of vitamin C, such as 8 or 12 grams (8,000 or 12,000 mg), spread out over an entire 24 hour period, neutralize some toxins in general and free radicals in particular.

LESS-TOXIC PLACES TO LIVE

Dr. William Rea states that environmental contamination is a worldwide problem. Even places like the Arizona desert have become pollen-filled from the growing of nonnative plants. Fortunately, some recent laws have been created to stop the growing of these plants.

Still, some places are safer to live in than others, says Dr. Rea. Some of the cleaner areas can be found in northern Arizona, near Prescott and Sedona, and along the Grand Canyon up into the Taos area, in New Mexico and in Sante

Fe. He also says some areas in western Texas are better for people with environmental sensitivities.

INDOOR POLLUTANTS

For decades, we have been led to believe that the numerous chemicals in our environment are harmless. But we can now see that these chemicals make people sick, even when they exist at levels way below those officially considered dangerous. And the number of chemically laden products in our immediate vicinity is staggering. In our homes we can find such poisons as pesticides, mothballs, room deodorizers, particleboard, carpeting, adhesives, house cleansers, detergents, chemically fragranced fabric softeners, volatile oils from dry-cleaned clothing, and even toxic personal-care products. To those we can add the possibility of radon or asbestos particles.

In industry, exposures to solvents has become a primary source of illness. All these poisons accumulate in our bodies and can ultimately take our immune systems on a downward spiral. Added to that, your body is being zapped by computers, video-display terminals, and copy and fax machines, all of which give off heavy doses of electromagnetic radiation. The invisible energies in the electromagnetic spectrum are man-made energies; our bodies have not adapted to these artificial waves.

Some of the chemicals we may encounter in our homes and public buildings are discussed below:

Animal Danders

Pets in the home cause allergic reactions in many people. Dr. Michael Galante says that many children come to him with rashes, chronic ear infections, and even emotional problems that are caused by allergies to their pets. While it's best to give these animals up, many people because of an emotional attachment find it difficult to do so.

Asbestos

At this point, everyone knows that asbestos is extremely dangerous. Although it is no longer used in new buildings, it is still present to a large degree. When you are exposed to these microscopic fibers, they can enter your lungs and remain there forever. Even a single asbestos fiber can cause a tumor over time. The type of cancer they can cause is one of the worst forms of lung cancer.

Carbon Monoxide

An estimated 4.5 million people are exposed to indoor levels of carbon monoxide that exceed the federal safety limits—and these limits may be far too high from the start. Significant amounts of carbon monoxide can come from space heaters, gas, coal, kerosene appliances, furnaces, and stoves.

Many portable space heaters can cause serious problems when they are not vented outdoors. A study at Yale Medical School found that some of these heaters polluted the air of an average-size ventilated room to a level of about 12 ppm (parts per million) of carbon monoxide. A day spent in a room with a heater of this type can produce nervous-system symptoms by raising the brain's carboxyhemoglobin level. This makes you more susceptible to chronic fatigue syndrome and brain fog. About two hundred people a year die from carbon monoxide poisoning from space heaters alone.

Deodorizers

Commercial deodorizers only add more toxic fumes to our air. They often contain carcinogenic ingredients found in pesticides, and some of them work by deadening the nerve endings in our noses. They are easily absorbed through the skin and can damage the central nervous system.

Electromagnetic Radiation (EMR)

EMR is emitted from modern electronic appliances, including television sets, electric blankets, digital clocks, heated waterbeds, microwave ovens, and video-display terminals. Since this contamination is invisible, it's easy to believe that it doesn't exist and that the modern conveniences to which we have become accustomed are totally safe.

The contrary has proven to be true, however, and the twenty-four-hour-a-day bombardment from EMR has been correlated with an increase in leukemia and an acceleration in the growth of cancer cells up to thirty times. It has also been associated with abortions, miscarriages, and birth defects. Since EMR interferes with the body's revitalization processes it may create other conditions as well. These include sleep disorders like insomnia, chronic fatigue, mood swings, irritability, and loss of energy.

According to studies, wiring in our homes that carries alternating current emits a harmful electromagnetic field. Long-term exposure to this field, which switches direction sixty times per second, causes the chromosomes within the cells to vibrate in resonance to it. After a while, the cells lose their ability to fight that disturbance and they may actually fracture.

Fluorescent Lighting

Fluorescent lighting, found in all commercial buildings and in more and more homes today, may contribute to many types of health problems. For starters, the common fluorescent tube light does not contain the full spectrum found in natural sunlight. This deficiency has been associated with depression and decreased productivity in the workplace. And in children it has been correlated with hyperactivity as well.

The flicker produced by fluorescent lights causes other problems. These small pulses of energy, which are too quick to be consciously observed, nevertheless register in the brain. They can result in fatigue, eyestrain, and eventual damage to the central nervous system.

Also, the cathode ends (far ends) of the tube give off X rays. They also emit radio-frequency disturbances as they get older and are about to burn out.

Fluoride

Fluoride is one of many toxins that come through our water supply. Its advocates tell us that fluoride helps to prevent cavities in teeth, but many people are unaware of the damage it may be doing to their defense system. In one study, Dr. John Yomiyanis found that regularly drinking water with just 1 ppm of fluoride was enough to cause an adverse immune reaction.

Formaldehyde

Formaldehyde is a ubiquitous toxin found throughout the home and workplace, particularly in pressed-wood products, particleboard, plywood paneling, and most medium-density fiberboards. Some 80 percent of the furniture people have in their homes probably outgasses formaldehyde. Additionally, formaldehyde is contained in everything from carpets, upholstery, and permanent-press fabric to paper products and cosmetics. In fact, nail polish and eye makeup may contain up to 55 percent formaldehyde. It is a primary ingredient in urea-formaldehyde foam insulation as well.

Formaldehyde is a potent irritant that can affect your nose, eyes, throat, and brain, thereby causing fatigue and respiratory problems. Formaldehyde poisoning has been linked to systemic lupus, a disease thought to be of the autoimmune category, wherein the body produces antibodies that attack its own tissues, especially skin and connective tissues. This process is simulated in the laboratory when the antibodies attack cell nuclei in the test tube. A similar illness wherein a positive antinuclear reaction occurs is rheumatoid arthritis.

Formaldehyde can harm us when it is absorbed or inhaled through the skin and attaches to body proteins and their configurations. A circulating white cell will see a protein with formaldehyde stuck to the end of it and say, in essence, "Wait a second. This doesn't look right. We've got to attack this." That's one way people end up developing antibodies to their own tissues.

Whether or not you will have a noticeable reaction to formaldehyde may depend upon your nutritional status. In particular, a lack of the essential metallic element molybdenum has been associated with formaldehyde poisoning because the enzyme that clears formaldehyde from the system depends upon this mineral. When you have a molybdenum deficiency, you will not expel your formaldehyde as quickly as if you had a full complement of the element. People who are exposed to mercury tend to lose their molybdenum. This makes them all the more susceptible to this kind of poisoning.

PESTICIDES

Pesticides have long been known to be extremely toxic to bugs and foliage and they present a major problem both in and out of doors. Their use is widespread, particularly in rural areas where people use these chemicals to maintain their lawns. They can easily travel to urban areas in the winds.

The pesticide industry has been kidding itself—and the public—about the serious consequences of using chemicals such as parathion, malathion, and dichlor compounds. These chemicals get into the groundwater and poison those living nearby. Dr. William Rea tells of one such case in which an electric company sprayed herbicides underneath a power line to kill weeds. The chemicals got into a nearby well and caused serious long-term consequences to an entire family and its pets:

> After the chemicals got into their drinking water the dog died from it and the horse had a colt with a condition called hydrocephalus where part of the brain is blocked off. Then the little girl developed diabetes from which she almost died and the other child became swollen and very ill. Later on, another baby was born who developed hydrocephalus, just like the horse. When tested, we found high levels of herbicide in the baby's blood.[2]

How do pesticides harm us? Like other chemical toxins, most pesticides are absorbed by the fat tissue in the body.

The pesticide often goes to the myelin sheath, which is a fatty coating protecting the nervous system, and to the dura mater, which is a fatty sheath covering the brain. This is one reason why pesticides cause a lot of neurological disorders. High concentrations of pesticides can also be found in the kidneys and liver, which attempt to rid the body of them.

Some experts have theorized that certain people with multiple sclerosis may owe their condition partially or completely to pesticide poisoning. Some even say the condition is not multiple sclerosis at all, but rather a manifestation of pesticide poisoning.

Radon

Radon is a naturally occurring, odorless, and invisible gas that results from the breakdown of the uranium contained in almost all soil. Radon is usually found in the basement of a home. If you spend a prolonged amount of time in such a home, the radon may contribute to the development of lung cancer.

Fortunately, radon is easy to detect and eliminate. A number of moderately priced home-detection kits can help you to discover if radon is collecting in your home. And since radon dissipates quickly when mixed with air, the situation can be completely remedied by installing fans and vents to the outside.

Volatile Organic Chemicals

Volatile organic chemicals can be found in fabric-care products, disinfectants, paint products, furniture polishes, and waxes. Fabric-care products, like spot removers and dry-cleaning solvents, contain the carcinogens benzene, one of the environment's most dangerous chemicals, and tuoline. And methylene chloride and trichloroethylene often are used in shoe dyes, polishes, and cleansers.

Organic solvents are used in dry cleaning as well. They can have toxic effects on the kidneys, heart, liver, and respiratory system. Dr. William Rea reports that 80 percent of his patients have dry-cleaning fluid in their blood and that most of this is absorbed because the dry-cleaned clothes go into a closet near people's beds.

A similar problem can occur with vinyl chloride, which is the substance plastic car-seat covers leach out. This chemical can get deposited in the joints and kidneys as well as in other parts of the body. When it accumulates in the joints, you can end up with rheumatoid arthritis.

OTHER POLLUTANTS

Antibiotics

The use of antibiotics was introduced to the population at large in the early 1940s. Now, fifty years later, their use is more widespread than ever. Not only are antibiotics given in medications, but they also are routinely injected into animals and even into the seeds from which our foods are grown.

While antibiotics are potent killers of bacteria, the problem is that they only know how to destroy. They literally kill bacteria throughout our bodies, making us more susceptible to the overgrowth of fungi, yeasts, and viruses. Since our food chain has been so inundated with antibiotics, they are no doubt responsible, in large part, for weakening our systems.

Dr. I-Tsu Chao gives this example of how antibiotics can

cause side effects that lead to serious complications in a patient:

> I had one patient who was very sensitive to wheat and rice. She would always get a violent reaction and an infection from it. Before coming to see me, she saw another doctor who gave her antibiotics for these infections. The antibiotic caused her to get a yeast infection and then a urinary infection. One day she could not even pass urine.[3]

He concludes that the only way to get rid of any disease effectively is to address the cause. Then the symptoms will disappear automatically.

Chlorine

The safety of the chlorine that's added to our drinking water has raised serious questions. While the chlorine is meant to destroy germs, it does not kill them all. And although we add chemicals like chlorine to the water, we don't take any other chemicals out. So if the factory down the street puts chemicals into the water supply, those chemicals still end up in your drinking water. If you use a lawn spray or if there is aerial spraying in your area, these chemicals go into the ground, get into the water table, and eventually come out through your faucet. Then you will be drinking these chemicals in addition to the chlorine.

Chlorinated drinking water can cause bladder conditions. People with these problems experience burning or chronic frequency of urination. In most cases, doctors cannot determine what is wrong with these patients.

The problem can be solved by drinking nonchlorinated spring water from glass bottles. But it's important to ask your bottled-water supplier whether or not the water has ever been chlorinated, since most state rules and regulations forbid water from being transported in bulk across their state lines unless it is chlorinated. Many bottled-water companies ship chlorinated water in big tank trucks, take it to their local bottling plant, run it through filters to dechlorinate it, and then bottle and sell it. This causes the water to form trihalomethanes, which are organic chemicals with chlorine attached to them. Many of these are carcinogenic unless the manufacturer runs the water through a large series of filters. Again, the solution is to buy water that has never been chlorinated. Of course, some mineral waters are not shipped in bulk and thus have no chlorine.

Heavy Metals

Some of the most notable environmental contaminants are the naturally occurring heavy metals that have become misplaced as a result of human intervention. These metals, including lead, cadmium, and mercury, accumulate in the body and weaken enzyme systems by poisoning them. Once that occurs, people have a tendency to become more allergic to foods. And the heavy metals have other inherent dangers as well. For example, a recent *Time* magazine article reported that one in six children may be exposed to levels of lead high enough to actually stunt their development. The dangers of one heavy metal—mercury—are detailed at length below.

Mercury

Mercury is one of the most insidious toxins in the environment today. The dental amalgams being placed in people's mouths, for example, consist of 50 percent mercury. Some of these particles get into the body and can cause a myriad of problems within six months to five years in people who are susceptible to mercury.

Dr. Alfred Zamm explains what makes a person prone to mercury poisoning:

> The problem as I see it is not so much whether it's a poison, but why everyone doesn't get sick from it. . . . The answer is a twofold problem. It is the nature of the mercury and the intrinsic nature of the person. To give a blatant example, not everyone who eats strawberries gets hives, but some people will. There is nothing genetically wrong with the strawberry. It is a genetic inability to handle a normal substance. With mercury we have a genetic inability to handle an abnormal substance, which we call xenobionic, or foreign to the natural state of the body.[4]

According to the traditional classical medical text, Goodman and Gilman's *The Pharmacological Basis of Therapeutics,* adds Dr. Zamm, the symptoms of mercury poisoning are so varied and so difficult to prove that they often go undiagnosed unless they are acute. Chronic low-grade mercury poisoning can cause symptoms to occur from the top of the head down to the toes.

Some of mercury poisoning's symptoms are related to a sugar intolerance. This occurs because a critical group of the acetyl coenzyme A enzyme, called the SH group, is poisoned. The SH group helps you to burn up the substances you need for energy. Affected people crave sugar because they need it. Yet they can't handle it. Eating it gives them a temporary sugar high followed by a two- to three-day low. They will mistakenly think they are hypoglycemic.

In reality, their Krebs cycle, which handles carbohydrates, is poisoned. They become carbohydrate intolerant, and this can cause tiredness, headaches, and all kinds of central-nervous-system disorders. They may experience a lack of concentration, distorted thought processes, emotional disturbances, hearing distortions, blurred vision, a less-acute sense of taste and smell, cardiac irregularities, an irregular pulse, food intolerance, and asthma. The list goes on and on. The reason for such varied symptoms is that the problem manifests in the weakest part of the body's makeup. Indeed, many specialists may see cases of mercury poisoning and call it something else.

People with any of the above symptoms are candidates for mercury poisoning, but they do not necessarily have it. These people can take several steps on their own to detect its presence. One such test consists of taking 50 mcg of selenium daily for a week or two to see if it helps you to feel better. If it does, that may be an indication of mercury poisoning because selenium neutralizes the mercury and prevents it from poisoning enzymes. Some people feel better when they combine 15 mg of zinc twice a day with the selenium. And thiamin (vitamin B_1) taken twice a day in a 50 mg tablet helps some people to feel miraculously better.

These methods don't necessarily prove that you have mercury poisoning, of course. But if you have unexplained health problems that no one can solve, it may be a good idea to have the mercury removed from your mouth to see if it resolves your problems. Dr. Zamm tells of one such patient who was third in command at one of the largest companies in the world until a virus combined with mercury poisoning made his immune system so dysfunctional that he could no longer work. Nine months after having his mercury fillings removed, he was traveling all over the world again.

Two alternative types of fillings can be used in place of mercury. Plastic is an inexpensive choice, but be sure to have a small test filling placed in your front tooth for three weeks to see if any problems arise. If it cannot be tolerated, then gold with zinc oxiphosphoric acid cement must be used instead. Be careful using ugenol, which many people cannot tolerate. And do not have many fillings placed in your mouth at one time.

Dr. Marjorie Siebert notes that while dental amalgams have gotten a lot of attention for their role in mercury poisoning, they are not the only source of this immune-crippling agent. Mercury poisoning also can come from fish, including the popular varieties such as tuna fish. The larger the fish, she says, the greater your chances of getting mercury. When the waters get polluted, the plankton and one-celled organisms absorb the mercury and change it to methylmercury, a more absorbable and much more toxic form of the substance. One fish eats the plankton, a bigger fish eats that fish, and so on, all the while concentrating the mercury right up through the food chain. Shellfish are a big source of mercury as well, since these scavengers and bottom feeders tend to get more of the mercury that goes into the ocean.

The vegetables you eat also may have mercury because the fungicides used on them contain mercury. This mercury concentrates right onto the vegetables; and in some cases, such as with carrots, right into them. Indeed, many people who drink carrot juice to bolster their immunity get a big dose of mercury in addition to their vitamins and minerals. Also, fungicides used on wheat and other grains may have a bearing on grain allergies.

Other sources of mercury include hair dyes, mascara, contact lens solutions that are preserved with thimerosal, contraceptive gels, and the felt that children use in school projects. And until recently, indoor paint was allowed to contain mercury. In addition, some air-conditioner filters are treated with mercury. This means that on a hot day, when you close your windows and turn on your air conditioner, you get some mercury atomizing out of your air-conditioner fluid.

Microbiological Organisms

In *Chemicals in the Human Food Chain,* Carl Winter states that food safety is an issue of great concern for the American public and that microbiological concerns are the number one safety priority, as indicated by the Food and Drug Administration as well as the World Health Organization's Center for Disease Control. The presence of bacteria, fungi, algae, and various types of microbes in food present some very significant risks to large percentages of the population. For example, it has been estimated that this country alone has millions of cases of food poisoning each year, resulting in thousands of deaths. This is especially unfortunate, since food poisoning theoretically can be prevented easily by keeping things warm when they should be warm and refrigerated when they should be cold.

Molds

In many localities, such as Manhattan and Long Island, the rain volume and surrounding waters create big problems with high mold counts in the air. Molds can also grow if you have a leaky pipe or faucet in your house. They are potent immune suppressors and can cause you to become ill.

Parasites

Many people are walking around today with amoebas and other parasites. According to Dr. Francis Waickman, anyone with chronic gastrointestinal symptoms probably has them. While the parasites themselves may not cause environmental illness, they increase your susceptibility to them by weakening your systems and lowering your overall threshold. Parasites can cause wide swings in blood-sugar levels and increase overall body toxicity. An excessive toxic load can lessen your natural resistance to disease, causing symptoms of memory confusion, impaired motivation, and lack of concentration. Then secondary bacterial infections can occur, and you may end up with additional infections such as *Candida albicans* overgrowth, Epstein-Barr viral resurgence, or that of cytomegalovirus, the virus causing infectious mononucleosis. Most people have these viruses in check. It is only when the viruses swing out of control that the problems begin.

Preservatives

Dr. Doris Rapp says that today's convenience foods contain dangerous chemical preservatives and that inadequate studies are being performed to prove their safety:

> Some of the chemicals put in foods have been checked—but not all of them—for safety. And even when they check, they feed them to rats and other animals. If the animal's organs look all right they say that the chemical is all right. But what if that rat starts to eat the other rats and becomes otherwise aggressive? In other words, are there other things not being investigated when they do these studies to say a certain thing is safe?[5]

She says that Dr. Dennis Remington's book, *The Bitter Truth about Artificial Sweeteners,* reveals the politics behind the release of aspartame, an artificial sweetener, in this country. Each time an official from the EPA was about to release information on the artificial sweetener, there was foot dragging and extended delays. When the report finally came out, it revealed that the sweetener caused brain problems in experimental animals. Even when these chemicals are found to be suspect, it seems they may be deemed acceptable for use by the general public.

VIRUSES

In the 1960s, a lot of research got underway on DNA, genetic gene splicing, cross species, and the like. We have since seen a myriad of viral conditions including many new strains such as AIDS, Epstein-Barr, and chronic fatigue syndrome.

We have always assumed that vaccines were safe and that they protected our immune systems, not weakened them. But could we have been wrong in our thinking? Is it possible that we have released a mutated viral strain into our vaccines and food, viruses that will work in ways we do not yet understand to undermine the very foundation of our immune system? And is it possible that these viral strains can cause sensitivities to things that we could previously tolerate? Some immunologists and virologists believe this is so. And if this theory is right, environmental medicine had best start looking at viruses to determine how they relate to illness.

Some environmental practitioners already recognize this problem, especially as it concerns the cross virus. Dr. Lockyer says, "Cross viruses—that is, viruses being transmitted from one species to another or crossing from one country to another—are fairly recent. These alone, if given to a foreign population, can tear the immune system down in the same way that many other environmental factors have done."[6] And Dr. Alan Levin who specializes in pathology and immunology adds, "The measles virus in a Caucasian female causes a self-limiting disease process in most cases. In native Polynesians, however, it causes a devastating disease, avasculitis, which destroys these people."[7] He further explains that a virus may be benevolent to one population and deadly to another because the host, and not the virus, causes the illness:

> In order to get sick you have to have the appropriate receptors, the appropriate transport mechanisms, and you have to be able to intercolate the genome of the virus into your own genome. For instance, the Epstein-Barr virus enters through a specific receptor on the cell. Then it is transported into the nucleus and then it is intercolated into the cell with your own proteins. You do it yourself.[8]

In addition, Dr. Levin points out that viruses are not bad in and of themselves. "Viruses can also be really good, as they are vectors of genetic information and vectors of evolution," he says. "We've got to recognize that we don't have to treat all viruses as diseases, since diseases are not necessarily caused by them. Diseases are caused by individuals not being able to respond appropriately to that virus."[9]

6

Testing for and Treating Food Allergies and Chemical Sensitivities

TESTING YOURSELF

How do you identify the foods and chemicals to which you are sensitive? According to Dr. Francis Waickman, you must learn to listen to your body and recognize when you are not feeling well. Then you must be able to connect that feeling with the foods and other substances to which you have been exposed. Dr. Doris Rapp adds that people with a chronic and undiagnosed illness should ask themselves if they can figure out the cause of the problem. One way to do this is to ask yourself: What did I eat, touch, or smell before I suddenly felt worse?

Another tactic is to note the time of day during which these reactions occur. For example, your child may be making poor progress in school in the afternoon but doing well in the morning. Perhaps he has a short attention span and appears to be lethargic or hyperactive at this time. You should immediately wonder if the problem could be due to something he ate at lunchtime or to a chemical exposure at this time of the day.

Be sure to consider whether your reactions get worse indoors or out of doors as well. If you feel worse in the house, the culprit may be house dust, mites, danders from animals, and molds. Moisture causes molds, which exist in cloth or wadding, to grow and multiply. You also need to ask: Am I better in one room than in another? If you always get sick right after you leave the bathroom, the problem may be scouring powder, chlorine, your after-shave, the soap you use, or mold.

If you feel fine in the house but get sick on the street, think about the reason why. Are they laying asphalt on the street? Or did they just do aerial spraying and contaminate the whole neighborhood with some chemical? Do you get sick every time the lawn-spray truck comes down the street, or do your children suddenly complain of dizziness, headaches, weakness, or an inability to think at this very time?

Meanwhile, if your symptoms get worse outside in the spring or fall, you have to think of molds and pollens. The essential difference between these two sensitivities is that pollens almost always cause itching of the eyes or nose, while molds produce a slight burning of the eyelid. However, the same runny or stuffy nose, postnasal drainage, or coughing can occur from a sensitivity to either molds or pollens. If you start to think of cause-and-effect relationships, some answers will begin to come to you.

Another factor to consider is the difference in the way you feel before and after a meal. This distinction can make it particularly easy to detect allergy-producing foods in children, says Dr. Rapp. For example, you could have your child draw a picture or write his or her name before eating and then again fifteen minutes after eating. If the child is having an allergic reaction, he or she won't be able to color within the lines or write. By testing for foods individually, you can determine the cause of the problem. In her books, Dr. Rapp says the most highly allergenic foods for children are milk, dairy products, wheat, baked goods, eggs, chocolate, corn, sugar, food dyes, preservatives, and orange juice.

We can also determine which foods we are allergic to by identifying those we crave the most. Dr. Rapp says that sometimes we eat that food in a disguised form:

> Many people tell me, I hate milk but I love cheese and ice cream and yogurt. That is what is making them sick. The clue is they hate the milk. If you love a food and crave it, that frequently is the thing that is causing you trouble. If you can't live without your cup of coffee, or your cheese, that could very well be the cause of your problem.[1]

KEEPING A JOURNAL

One excellent way to isolate the foods and chemicals that make you ill is to keep a journal. Your mind simply is not a good enough computer to make these connections on its own. For instance, if you suddenly notice you have a headache, you would write "headache" on a page and then write down what you ate, touched, or smelled at that time. The next time this occurs, you open to the same page and repeat the process. After two or three times, you may notice that you only get headaches when you eat cinnamon or when you eat mushrooms, and you've made the connection.

In some cases, you'll need to analyze the situation a bit further. If you suspect the common denominator is bread, for example, then you must determine whether the wheat, yeast, or sugar in the bread is responsible. To do so, eat another food that does not contain two of the ingredients but has the third to see if that upsets you. You have to explore these things like a detective.

CHALLENGING YOURSELF WITH FOODS

To further test for allergies, eliminate the food that you suspect is causing problems from your diet for four days. On the fifth day, eat that food alone. If you suspect wheat, for example, omit all forms of wheat for this time period and then eat wheat by itself on the fifth day. A bowl of cracked-wheat cereal made with plain water would suit the purpose fine.

The majority of these reactions can be seen immediately. Eighty percent of people who are allergic to wheat will have some problems within one hour of eating the wheat alone, and 99 percent of people will have trouble within the first two hours. Other reactions take longer to see. Even though the reactions begin to occur immediately, you may not perceive them for several hours. That is where an environmentally trained physician can be helpful in pinpointing the problem.

PULSE TESTING

Another good indicator of food allergies is your pulse rate before and after a meal. To take your pulse, place the palm of one hand under the wrist of the other and fold your fingers over the top of the wrist. If you touch very gently with your second and third fingers, you will feel the pulse.

Count the beats for one full minute. Ordinarily, the pulse will beat seventy or eighty times a minute before eating. If the food you eat disagrees with you, however, your pulse may increase by twenty, thirty, or even forty beats within ten minutes. It's as if your body has sent out a silent alarm saying, "What did you put inside me now?"

If you have high blood pressure, you may get a rise in blood pressure rather than a more rapid pulse after eating a food to which you are allergic. In this instance, you might want to get a blood pressure cuff to check your pressure after eating. And if you have asthma, you should check your breathing before and after eating.

In addition, note whether these changes occur when you travel through a polluted part of town or when you are near a certain chemical in your house.

WHAT AN ENVIRONMENTAL DOCTOR CAN DO FOR YOU

Unmasking

Doctors use several methods to determine which specific chemicals are causing a chronic illness, whether it be arthritis, asthma, or another condition. Dr. Albert Robbins, for example, puts his patients through a process of unmasking:

> The first thing I do is have my patients avoid all scented items. I start with soaps, shampoos, conditioners, hair sprays, underarm deodorants, and fabric softeners. The second thing I do that is extremely important is to place them on a low-allergy diet; that is, a diet without common allergy-producing foods, like milk. This should be a clean

> diet without preservatives and without processed foods. In addition, I have them avoid all alcoholic beverages and I advise people who smoke to stop smoking immediately. From this environmental approach I can see whether their symptoms are getting better or worse. If they get somewhat better, I know I am on the right track.[2]

Neutralization Immunotherapy

After unmasking the patient, Dr. Robbins uses blood tests to check for defects in the immune system. He also uses blood tests and skin tests to further check for allergies to a wide range of substances—foods, chemicals, pollens, dusts, molds, etc. When he discovers which items his patients are allergic to, he then places them on allergy vaccines.

This type of vaccine, generally referred to as low-dose immunotherapy or neutralization immunotherapy, differs from the classical allergist's method of treatment. The classical method tends to start most patients at similar doses of the antigen to which they are allergic and to increase the dose on a preset uniform schedule. On the other hand, most environmental doctors determine a specific dilution, or low dose, of each antigen and custom mix a treatment vial with the specific low-dose dilution of each tested antigen. The low-dose method usually achieves a more effective correction of the allergy over a shorter time.

Dr. Joseph S. Wojcik of Bronxville, New York, who specializes in allergies and practices environmental medicine, explains why this procedure is so effective:

> We continue to test our patients until their skin reactions disappear; then we make up a vaccine and give them a dose in the amount that we find, during testing, stops their

> symptoms from appearing. When we give injections in that amount, the body will make blocking antibodies against allergens. For example, if the person is allergic to a certain food, blocking antibodies will prevent the reaction from happening.[3]

Dr. Wojcik adds that the reactions sometimes stop completely unless the patient has become overloaded with the allergen. In the height of the pollen season, for example, they may still have some symptoms. Even so, they should be much more comfortable once they receive neutralization therapy.

Neutralization also is efficient in that the patient can administer the dilutions to him- or herself at home, either through drops under the tongue or through an injection to the arm.

BUILDING IMMUNE RESISTANCE

To restore health—and stay healthy—you must cleanse your body and rebuild your immune system. According to Dr. Martin Feldman, an environmental-medicine physician experienced in allergy, six steps must be taken when attempting to build and balance immune function. They are: (1) Test for adequacy of basic immune-system nutrients and restore those deficient; (2) Reduce exposure to known and unknown allergenic substances; (3) Test for environmental and food allergens to determine your specific profile of reactivity and treat selected antigen sensitivity by low-dose neutralization therapy; (4) Test for function of immune system and the anatomical organs (thymus, spleen, bone marrow, and lymphatic system) and rebalance the dysfunctional parts; (5) Test for the immune pathogens—parasites, yeast, "unfriendly" bacteria—and assist the body in controlling these; (6) Test for the possibility of digestive malabsorption state and delineate which aspect(s) of the digestion process are inefficient, and assist the underactive part(s).

THE BASIC IMMUNE-SYSTEM NUTRIENTS

The basic immune nutrients are: vitamin A, zinc, vitamin C, bioflavonoids, GLA (gamma linoleic acid), EFA (essential fatty acids), the B complex vitamins, vitamin E, and selenium. The specific practical aspects of using these building blocks are described in detail in part three, pages 293–301. These building blocks are critical since, when present, they will assist the weakened immune system to build up its strength and nourish the overactive or poorly modulated immune system to rebalance toward normal function.

One can provide the body with nutrients in absorbable form by eating and drinking organically grown live foods, which also contain the most absorbable form of energy. "When you drink some of these raw juices, it's like drinking sunshine," says Dr. Michael Galante. He believes that paying attention to the diet is essential in the treatment of any allergy condition.[4]

TESTING FOR EXPOSURE TO KNOWN OR UNKNOWN ALLERGENS

The more you assault your immune system, the greater your allergic burden becomes. This can be compared to a rising score in a pinball machine. The more you are exposed to different allergens, the more your allergic score rises. For this reason, limiting your exposure before big trouble occurs should be a priority. Some allergens, such as dust or molds or animal dander, may be avoided or removed from that part of the environment over which you can exert control, such as your home. Identifying most inhalant or environmental allergens is simple via a blood sample that is analyzed for IgE antibody levels to specific substances. The IgE levels correlate well with the body's sensitivities to inhalants since this type of reactivity is, in fact, IgE mediated. Some environmental allergens, such as odors, scents, chemicals in the workplace, newsprint, and substances in the water supply, may require detective work.

Whereas basic inhalant allergens can be determined with straightforward blood tests measuring IgE antibody levels, most food sensitivities require other testing methods: for example, eliminating and reintroducing possible food culprits to check for allergy symptoms, testing the blood for IgG levels, examining under a microscope how cells react to toxins, or intradermal (between the layers of skin) testing. Many allergic persons can then avoid the offending foods with good results. Other persons may manage by rotating their foods so that they do not eat the same food more than once every four days.

A lot depends upon the total sensitivity score to both inhalants and foods. If the total sensitivity is moderate to severe, then the program may require the contemporary low-dose immunotherapy, also called neutralization. Again, depending on the total number and severity of allergens, a corrective dose or doses may be administered to diminish sensitivity to selected foods as well as selected inhalants.

TREATING THE ANATOMICAL COMPONENTS OF YOUR IMMUNE SYSTEM

As mentioned, the four parts of the anatomy directly related to immune system functioning are the bone marrow, the thymus gland, the spleen, and the lymphatic system. The immune system has antibodies and lymphocytes (the cellular mediators of immunity) circulating throughout the entire bloodstream as well, but these four anatomical areas should be examined closely when checking for underlying causes of an underactive or overactive immunity.

At this time we do not know how to enhance the bone marrow directly through nutritional intervention. However, nourishment of the other three areas may help in bringing the bone marrow into proper function.

The thymus directs the T cells, which in turn communicate instructions to the B cells, which then produce specific antibodies. An example of a severe malfunction of T-cell production is the paucity of such cells in those patients with HIV antibodies who develop infections as a result of their lack of total T cells, especially T helper cells.

When you become allergic, your thymus gland often does not work up to par because an enormous amount of immune-system function is thymus related.

If the thymus is found to be malfunctioning, how can it be rebalanced? First, the body can be balanced with the general immune-enhancing nutrients mentioned earlier. Then other nutrients more directly related to thymus repair can be of use. Some of these include echinacea, astragalus, and osha root. Homeopathic remedies, which are extremely diluted and highly energized substances, also may prove helpful. One such solution made specifically for the thymus gland is animal thymus diluted and seccussed to 5X, which is a dilution of one part to one hundred thousand, or to 6X, which is one part to one million. Animal thymus tablets are available, as well; their effectiveness ranges from superior to average to substandard.

Most allergic persons do respond to nutritional thymus rebalancing, but there is a subgroup of persons who do not achieve thymus balance. In this resistant group, it has been Dr. Feldman's clinical experience that a common denominator is a problem with the neck region. Although there is no obvious anatomical relationship, nevertheless, many persons with a tendency toward stiffness, tension, pain, or misalignment of the neck vertebrae are much more resistant to thymus correction.

In some cases, a sluggish spleen may hinder immune functioning, although this problem is less common than an imbalanced thymus. The spleen is not necessarily diseased—just out of balance. If this is the case, spleen function can also be optimized with nutrients basic for the immune system plus herbs, homeopathics, and actual animal spleen.

Lymphatics prove to be a bit more complicated to optimize or rebalance than either the thymus or the spleen because they comprise a flow system throughout the body. In a sense, the lymphatic system works much like the blood circulation, only it's more directly related to immune function. The best ways to work with the lymphatic system include massages, herbal preparations, or some combination of the two methods.

THE PRESENCE OF IMMUNE-WEAKENING PATHOGENS

Whereas all humans harbor *Candida albicans* within their lower digestive system, these pathogens may overgrow and then stress the immune mechanism. Very often, the digestive system becomes excessively alkaline, which promotes the proliferation of the otherwise benevolent yeasts. Very often the digestive problem precedes the yeast problem. Many other pathogens may inhabit the gut, such as *Giardia lamblia* and *Endamoeba histolytica.* These are not benevolent and are invaders; the two most common parasites, they seem to weaken the body's overall metabolism as well as stressing the immune system.

Newer laboratory technologies are available from specialized laboratories whereby a stool sample or swab of the rectal area is stained via markers that demonstrate even fragments of the specific parasites. This is a new and promising development in diagnosing pathogenic conditions. Those physicians who take the effort to seek out these advanced laboratories make available a whole new area of immune-system repair. In addition to the presence of the parasite villains, it is also possible to analyze the stool for the component of friendly bacteria species that normally inhabit the gut. Nutritionally oriented physicians with this information can then recommend eating specific concentrated products that contain literally billions of *Lactobacillus acidophilus* or the Bifido strain to rebalance the gut. Although many pharmaceuticals are available to kill the pathogenic parasites, there are also gentler natural antagonists, such as grapefruit seed extract, artemisia annua, black walnut, and garlic.

ABSORBING NUTRIENTS EFFICIENTLY FROM YOUR FOODS

Many persons with even mild digestive symptoms, such as indigestion, heartburn, belching, burping, flatulence, diarrhea, and constipation, have less-than-optimal digestion efficiency. If the process of assimilating your food does not provide the basic nutrients for your immune system, then the system is more likely to become under- or overactive. The steps of digestion include: (1) stomach acid production; (2) pancreas enzyme production; (3) bile secretion by the gall bladder; and (4) assimilation through the walls of the small intestine. An attentive physician can isolate and analyze each of these steps and prescribe natural therapies to correct the weak link along the path of digestion.

CLEANSING AND BUILDING THE IMMUNE SYSTEM WITH HERBS

Most holistic physicians recognize the value of herbs in enhancing the immune system. Specifically, herbs help to diminish viral activity and to detoxify and strengthen the entire system. Many herbs have been successfully used throughout history for this purpose. Herbal medicine has been used in places like China and India for over five thousand years and is a mainstay of those countries' medical practices today.

In recent years, Western medicine has begun to test some of these herbs in the hopes of finding ways to treat the immune-crippling diseases of modern times. The results are impressive. In one study conducted a few years ago by a group of doctors, pharmacologists, and pharmacognostists (pharmacologists of natural products) who went to China, it was found that most of the properties attributed to the herbs of traditional Chinese medicine could be well supported by modern scientific research in which the plant's chemical composition was evaluated. Approximately 80 percent of the time, the long-term trial-and-error methodology used by the ancient practitioners to produce a materia medica was accurate, rational, and well used.

It may come as a surprise to most Americans that 80 percent of the world's population still relies on these kinds of traditional remedies rather than on the kind of medicine accepted by the modern American and European model, according to the World Health Organization.

Rob McCaleb is director of the nonprofit Herb Research Foundation in Boulder, Colorado. This center houses one of the largest repositories of herbal research in the world, with thirty-five to forty thousand scientific studies on herbs and other nutrients from which to draw information.

The last ten years have seen a tremendous improvement in the quality of herbs in the marketplace, according to Rob McCaleb. Previously, most available herbs were encapsulated in a powdered form. Now you can find concentrated powdered extracts of herbs in which nothing has been eliminated from them other than some of the bulk and cellulose.

In some cases, the sellers enhance the extracts using only a specific part of the plant that has more active properties. With ginseng, for example, much evidence concludes that the ginsenicides are the most active ingredient. Therefore, you get a more active ginseng product by strengthening the content of ginsenicides in the formula without eliminating any of the other components. (See part three,

Basic Immune-Building Nutrients and Herbs, for a description of some of these herbs.)

OTHER HELPFUL TREATMENTS

Homeopathic Remedies

The exact mechanisms of homeopathic remedies generally are not well understood. Nevertheless, they do seem to help with recovery from food allergies and chemical sensitivities and many people use them for this purpose. Dr. Michael Galante says, "The wonderful thing about homeopathy is that it is very simple to understand because you can't understand it."[5] Indeed, despite the theories that try to explain it, no one really understands how it works. But Dr. Galante says that his main interest is in using what does work, whether or not he understands the process involved. Even Dr. Samuel Hahnemann, the founder of homeopathy, emphasized that the function of a doctor was to heal patients in a humble and very serious way. He was adamant in his belief that doctors should not try to look like big shots and expound great theories about healing.

Homeopathy is best understood when examined from an energetic, rather than a mechanistic, point of view. In essence, this means looking at the same thing seen in a different light because, as Einstein said, energy and matter are interchangeable. As Dr. Galante explains, you dilute homeopathic remedies by taking a pinhead of the substance, putting it in alcohol, and then shaking it over and over until there is no more physical substance—only the essence of it. Therefore, homeopathic treatment works on a subtler level than the physical. He continues, "Hahnemann, who was a real conservative German, didn't want to talk about spiritual things until his last book, where he mentioned a spiritlike vital force. That was the only way he could explain how homeopathy worked."[6] This vital force has an innate intelligence and exists within every person to control all the bodily functions. Dr. Galante continues:

> It is an integrated, animating spiritlike force. It is for this reason that homeopathy acts in such a complete way. When the vibration of your constitutional remedy resonates with the vibration of your vital force, you will stimulate that force, which will then help you to unblock your energies. These are energies that have been blocked either by previous illnesses, present illness, or inherited weakness. So, you can actually undo inherited weakness with homeopathy.[7]

Dr. Schachter believes homeopathics can help to correct underlying problems with the immune system. "We find that the state of the immune system can affect how people respond to various foods. If you correct the problem, suddenly you can eat a much wider range of foods."[8] Homeopathic remedies play a role in correcting such problems by helping you to raise you reaction threshold. They may even increase your tolerance of the highly nutritional foods to which you were overreacting. As a result, you can obtain the much-needed vitamins, minerals, and enzymes in which you have become deficient.

Two systems of homeopathic treatment are being administered today: classical and complex. Both systems operate on the philosophy of "like curing like." According to this philosophy, if you receive the same substance that has made you sick in very minute quantities, it will help you to get well again.

With classical homeopathy, the practitioner learns as much as possible about you, including your fears, likes, dislikes, physical and emotional symptoms, and history. He or she then comes up with a single remedy that will best help to balance your system.

Complex homeopathy, on the other hand, uses an electric machine to measure energy flows throughout your body. On the basis of that reading, the practitioner chooses a series of homeopathic remedies to balance out different parts of your body. In addition, this machine can identify specific factors that are blocking your ability to heal, such as dental amalgams, impacted wisdom teeth, or the need for a chiropractic adjustment.

Dr. Galante, who used to treat patients with complex homeopathy, now prefers the classical method of treatment because he believes the single remedy that's determined to be best for your constitution will correct all other imbalances in your system as well. This approach, along with modifications in diet, has proven to be highly successful with his environmentally ill patients.

The modern medicine establishment, which is basically allopathic, meaning that it focuses on treating symptoms, shuns the idea of homeopathy. But if you think about it, the use of vaccinations and immunizations works on homeopathic principles—in an attempt to prevent or antidote a virus or flu, vaccines administer a substance that is similar in nature. Vaccines are actually a perversion of homeopathic principles, however, and homeopathy works just as well, without the risk of side effects that vaccines present. Numerous reports from Hahnemann bear out this claim. During epidemics of disease, he would travel from town to town administering homeopathic doses of the illness to people. The townspeople who received them experienced little or no occurrence of the disease, which in Hahnemann's time was cholera.

MAGNETS

Sometimes, as with one of Dr. Philpott's patients, magnets can provide relief after all else has failed. The patient's mother reports:

> When she stayed in her clean environment she thrived, but in the outside world she destabilized. That was not the kind of quality of life I wanted for her. Finally, I saw Dr. Philpott, who introduced me to magnetic therapy, and this made the difference. Now she was able to do all the things other teenagers did, including being able to work with computers for a time, going to the mall, to the movie theater, to a bowling alley. All these places would have been unthinkable years ago.[9]

Magnetic instruments, when properly used, may help to relieve symptoms at a faster rate. The two types include solid-state magnets and magnets with a pulsating frequency, which merely add another dimension to which the body will respond. Different kinds of magnets also can be combined to produce similar effects.

A solid-state magnet can achieve excellent results if the gauss strength, which is the unit of magnetic force, is high enough and the placement of the magnet is correct. If you place the negative pole of the magnet over an inflamed area, for example, it will help to reduce the inflammation if the magnetic field is strong enough to penetrate the area deeply.

Dr. Philpott says that magnets can even help with brain allergies. One patient of his had become psychotic from various foods and chemicals. She would curl up in the fetal position and suck her thumb. But when Dr. Philpott treated her with solid-state magnets, nutrition and oxygen therapy, she totally recovered and became fully functional.

Stress-Management Techniques

The brain can modify its own neurochemistry through various relaxation, stress management, and suggestion techniques, such as biofeedback, visual imagery, and self-hypnosis. These methods have proved to help people with environmental illness about 50 percent of the time. According to Dr. Richard Podell of New Providence, New Jersey, people with environmental illness have been able, in effect, to "turn down" the volume of their illness, but not completely cure themselves of it, with the use of these techniques. However, the kinds of things that have severely aggravated them before treatment become only minor annoyances after five or six sessions.

When treating diseases that have multiple causes, he says, different things seem to help different people. "Some do well on neutralization shots; some do well with extra selenium and other minerals; and some do well with hypnosis. We haven't yet gotten to the point where we can predict who's who."[10]

Exercise

Exercise can help you to sweat out many toxins, but it can be a double-edged sword if you have environmental sensitivities. Since running requires greater energy, the body must also inhale a greater volume of air—and everything in it. If you run by busy roads, for example, you may be absorbing as many pollutants as you are casting off. Likewise, swimming in chlorinated pools can increase your chemical intake. Breathing in these different toxins becomes even more harmful when you are not receiving the proper nutrients.

Even running in a seemingly nonpolluted area can pose problems. Parks and woods may have been sprayed with herbicides, and even pine and cedar forests can give off odors that irritate you. Dusts, molds, and pollens can create problems as well, so you must take the necessary precautions when exercising. A face mask may filter out some of these irritants, but will be only moderately effective.

DETOXIFYING THE HOME

You can make your home allergy free without spending a fortune by taking some basic steps. In the bedroom, for instance, you can get rid of the dusty, moldy carpet. Use the plain wooden floor instead with a washable, cotton throw rug next to the bed. You can use aluminum foil to cover your mattress instead of plastic, and then use 100 percent cotton sheets and blankets to avoid the chemicals in the permanent-press fabrics. And wool blankets can be sandwiched in the center of nonwool blankets so that you don't breathe in the wool fibers. Some other things you can do are mentioned below in more detail.

Air Filters and Negative Ionizers

The first step to improving air quality is to find out exactly what pollutants you are breathing in by having the air in your home and office tested for molds, bacteria, and other particles. You would do well to seek out the services of an environmental-medicine physician who has access to appropriate laboratories and can interpret the data obtained.

Then, the air can be vastly improved with a filtration system. Many such units are on the market, but the best ones combine air purifiers with negative ionizers. The filter will collect positively charged particles, like molds, dust, and danders, and the negative ionizer will help to neutralize the pollutants by bonding to the contaminants before they fall to the ground.

If you place your air purifier directly into a window and seal the sides around it, you will limit the amount of pollutants coming into the room even more. Many people mistakenly place their unit three to four feet away from a window, which prevents most of the incoming air from being drawn into the system.

Dr. Doris Rapp notes that some air purifiers may even take germs out of the air. She has spoken to a few mothers who put these units into their children's classrooms at school. The teachers reported that the children in these classrooms had fewer infections.

However, Dr. William Rea suggests that air filters should not be kept running all the time, since a lot of people become sensitive to the charcoal in the filters. You could run the filters when you are not at home or put them in certain rooms where you do not spend a lot of time.

Another system, called the ozonator, can be used if it has been tested and shown not to put any nitrous oxide gas into the air. By requesting specifications from the manufacturers, you can find out this information.

In addition, you might try some natural filters, which can do a great job of absorbing pollution. These include spider plants, Brazilian palms, wide-leafed wandering Jews, and marigolds.

Lessening Exposure to Electromagnetic Radiation

You can lessen your exposure to electromagnetic radiation in several ways. Following are some precautions you can take:

1. Move appliances away from the areas where you spend a lot of your time. Remember that a wall is not a barrier, so be aware of your proximity to major appliances in other rooms.
2. If you own a digital clock, move it away from the bed or, better yet, replace it with a battery-operated or wind-up clock.
3. If you use an electric blanket, be sure to turn it off and unplug it before you go to sleep. Simply turning off the device will not stop it from emitting electromagnetic fields.
4. Stay six to eight feet away from your television set.
5. When cooking with a microwave, never stand directly in front of it. Its magnetic field extends from eight to twelve feet into the environment at a level of 3 milligauss or higher, which exceeds the body's tolerance level. The milligauss is a unit of electrical measure.

You can also buy devices that check the amount of electromagnetic radiation (EMR) being emitted. Most green books and magazines advertise them. They range in price from about $120 to thousands of dollars, depending upon their sophistication.

A meter on the machine registers the amount of EMR to which you are being exposed. If the meter reads .01 before you turn on the television set and 5.0 afterwards, you are being exposed to dangerously high levels. If you step back six feet from the screen, the number may drop to .05. And if you step back ten feet, there may be no radiation affecting you at all. When using such a device, it's important to remember that the fields are directional. As a result, measurement may be low in one direction and high in another. Also, some companies will come into your home and measure these fields, including some power companies.

If you work with a computer, you can test its effect on you by taking your resting pulse rate for sixty seconds before you sit down at the video display terminal. Take your pulse again after the machine has been turned on, and then one more time after working on it for twenty minutes. A higher pulse rate indicates you are having a reaction.

Chemically Free Personal-Care Products

Whenever possible, buy hand and body soaps that do not contain artificial scents or colors. Many inexpensive herbal soaps that fit this description can be found in health-food stores.

You can use one of these natural soaps in place of shaving cream, which often contains ammonium and ethanol, both of which may cause sensitivities. It's not the shaving cream itself that allows for a good shave, but the heating of the area first with a hot, wet towel to soften the hair and allow for a better cut.

Shampoo can be made out of one cup of liquid castile soap and a half cup of distilled water or olive or avocado oil. Sesame oil can be used as a hair conditioner.

You can make an inexpensive, natural toothpaste by mixing peppermint extract, available at health-food stores, with baking soda. A deodorant made from equal parts baking soda and cornstarch will prove effective as well. Cornstarch can also be used in place of talcum powder, which may contain asbestos fibers because it is mined in the same area.

Sesame-seed oil contains vitamin E, which also makes it a good moisturizer to use in place of commercial ones. A natural facial scrub can be made from vegetable oil and applied with a soft loofah to remove epidermal skin. And to remove grease from your hands, butter is much safer than the organic solvents available on the market.

Women should look for natural cosmetics that do not contain harmful ingredients commonly found in cosmetics, such as coal-tar dyes, turpentine, and formaldehyde.

Natural Room Deodorizers

Harmful room deodorizers can be replaced with healthier alternatives, such as baking soda, lemon juice, and vinegar. Boiling peppermint will act as a natural room deodorizer as well. Ventilating your rooms by opening windows and using an exhaust fan is a simple solution for stale smells.

Alternatives to Pesticides

In place of insect sprays, which contain neurotoxic substances, use the nontoxic ones now available on the market, such as the nonodorizing diatomaceous varieties. Indoors, boric acid is a safe way to get rid of cockroaches and ants. And to prevent them from returning, simply apply a borderline of garlic extract around the room. The garlic exudes an odor that tends to repel many insects.

In the garden, you can use a product called Safer Insecticidal Soap on your fruits and vegetables. This product, a nontoxic insecticide made with naturally occurring fatty acids, will kill most garden pests without harming the beneficial bugs. You can also purchase by mail order beneficial insects such as ladybugs and praying mantises that will help to keep pesky bug populations under control.

When landscaping, consider using an alternative ground cover in place of a grass lawn. This will both conserve water and reduce your need to use a chemical fertilizer.

Less-Toxic Housepaints

When painting your house, be sure to buy water-based latex house paint because it releases fewer toxins into the air than do the oil-based ones. In addition, check the labels for volatile organic compounds and buy the one that has the least amount.

Safer Cleaning Products

Commercial cleaning products are laden with harmful chemicals. Fortunately, some healthy alternatives are available that work just as effectively.

In lieu of products made with ammonia, use three tablespoons of vinegar to one quart of water in a spray bottle to clean glass. Baking powder can be used instead of scouring powder as an abrasive cleanser in the bathroom and kitchen. And borax mixed with water serves as an excellent all-purpose cleanser.

To clean clothes, you can use washing soda mixed with soap in place of commercial laundry detergents. Wash your clothes once with pure washing soda to eliminate any residue from detergents; then add the mixture. You can also add one cup of vinegar to the final rinse cycle as a fabric softener. In addition, some natural soaps and detergents can now be obtained that are less chlorinated and less toxic than most commercial brands on the market. Some good detergents to use include washing soda, as mentioned above, and borax or Bon Ami.

If your clothes must be dry-cleaned, either soak them in cold water afterwards to remove some of the chemicals or hang them outside for a while, preferably in a place that has a breeze. Placing them in an area heated by the sun also will volatilize most of the dry-cleaning fluid and remove it.

CLEANING UP THE NEIGHBORHOOD

If an outside agency, such as a utility company, wants to spray pesticides near your home or in a state park, is there anything you can do to prevent it from happening?

According to Mary LaMiele, Director of the National Center for Environmental Health Strategies in New Jersey, there are certain steps that an individual or a consumer action group can take to stop harmful pollution and promote the use of safer alternatives.

In the above example, the first course of action is to gather current information on the dangers of pesticides. From the general accounting office, you can get copies of reports issued over the years that substantiate the fact that these substances, which are mostly untested, are known to be neurotoxic.

Armed with this information, you can then approach the utility company or parks department and show them the impact pesticides are likely to have on people, pets, and wildlife. At the same time, it's a good idea to present them with information on the less-toxic choices available. One such option might be a manual type of weed control—literally cutting down on undergrowth where harmful bugs thrive—that can be used in place of pesticides.

The reception you receive at this point will determine

whether or not you need to take the next step of encouraging the agency to contact other organizations with expertise in this area.

In the worst-case scenario, you will be faced with an agency that is truly stubborn in its desire to use toxic substances. In that case, you will need to defend your rights and your environment, be it through some type of legal means or another type of advocacy.[11]

Do not become discouraged and give up the cause before you even begin. You may see everything in sight becoming polluted and throw up your hands and say, how can I change the world? But by taking small steps yourself, such as buying foods that do not have preservatives and buying drinks in glass rather than plastic containers, you can set an example for others to follow.

7

The Traditional vs. the Environmental Approaches to Allergy Medicine

Dr. John Boyles traces the split in approaches to allergy medicine to the discovery of penicillin:

> I think philosophically, perhaps, the division started many years ago when a scientist in England left the cover off of his petri dish and a little mold settled on the colony. It wiped out (the colony) and he discovered penicillin. That discovery of antibiotics forever changed the way doctors approached medicine.
>
> Prior to that discovery, specialists in medicine in this country tried to find out why a patient was allergic or why he had symptoms. After penicillin, it was such a tremendous leap forward in our ability to control infectious disease that this magic bullet was given to the internist. The internist then decided he would find a magic bullet for every disease.[1]

Unfortunately, he says, there is no such magic bullet for allergies because they are chronic problems that do not respond to drug therapy in the long run.

Herbalist Rob McCaleb agrees with that assessment. He adds:

> Our medical system is based almost entirely on the protection and treatment of disease, and this has really hurt our ability to look at a wider and more benign approach to working with the body and its own systems in building health, rather than just fight a specific disease condition. In fact, it strikes me that the modern, Western medical system is almost a militaristic idea. We talk about the therapeutic arsenal and we take toxins to kill a cancer, to kill a bacteria, to kill a virus, and so on.
>
> Herbs don't work in this way, and it is possible that this is why many of them have been overlooked for so long by our scientists. They have always been looking for something that they could put in a petri dish that would kill something. Well, echinacea won't do that and neither will astragalus because they work by stimulating the immune system to do its job better. They work with the body, which is always a better approach than working against it.
>
> This is not to say that there is no place for antibiotics within health care. There certainly is. But this is different. Here we are talking about good, safe dietary supplements from natural sources with a long and ancient safety record and a history of use by humans, which gives them a better incidence of safety than the limited kinds of rodent experiments that the FDA seems to focus on when they are looking at safety information.[2]

According to Dr. John Trowbridge, the difference between the environmental doctor and the more traditional one shows in their timing and their treatment. Traditional doctors usually do not recognize, label, or treat a problem until years after its inception. Their treatment, as mentioned, consists largely of drug therapy for the control of symptoms. Environmental doctors, on the other hand, examine their patients closely from the start to determine what factors are setting off adverse reactions. They then work to eliminate the causes of the problems, not just the symptoms. Dr. Trowbridge, who was trained in both approaches to medicine, further explains the limitations and possible dangers of the conventional approach to diagnosis and treatment:

> Traditional practitioners stop asking questions too early. For instance, if a patient comes in with joint pains, the average delay from the onset of pain to actually being told that an arthritic condition exists is about four years. At that point, patients are usually prescribed antiinflammatory medications, which, incidentally, are not harmless. One man who came to me too late died from a bleeding ulcer brought on by his arthritis medicine.[3]

By contrast, the doctor of environmental medicine will approach patients holistically and spend a great deal of time with them to ask lots of questions, listen to their complaints, and get a broad history base from which patterns of reaction may be found. "People need individualized treatments for their specific problems," Dr. Trowbridge says. "A large part of the failure of American medicine is in treating diseases, not patients."[4]

The cause-and-effect relationship between exposure to a substance and a reaction to it may not be obvious. The environmental doctor will work closely with patients to backtrack to an earlier time where the condition may have originally begun. For example, one of Dr. Wojcik's patients came to him because chlorine caused him to lose consciousness. They were able to retrace his sensitivity to a dusty, moldy library:

> He first came to me complaining of a reaction to chlorine whereby he would actually have brownouts, fainting, or loss of consciousness spells. This all started in the service. One time the ship he was on stopped in Mexico, where overchlorinated water was brought on to make sure germs in the water would not get on board. They were drinking it and showering in it. This caused him to become sensitive to chlorine and to start to actually lose consciousness upon exposure to it.
>
> In coming here we tried to backtrack, which we always do, to an earlier age, when this type of central nervous system reaction might have begun. We found that when he was in college he would study in the dusty, moldy, library, which would make him fall asleep. In other words, he had central nervous system reactions at that earlier time too.[5]

According to Dr. Wojcik, the backtracking process often involves so much detective work that the results cannot be proven easily through the double-blind study that the current medical paradigm considers to be the true proof of cause and effect. "It is difficult to make the link between an exposure to a chemical, virus, or other contaminant, and a person's illness," he says. "This link, to me, is most important and I believe insurance companies and the public must begin to look at this serious phenomenon."[6]

Sometimes more extensive measures must be taken to identify and resolve the cause of the problem. Dr. Trowbridge tells of one such patient, who had had a heart attack in his forties and anginalike pains in his chest afterwards. He underwent some very specific environmental testing after a standard environmental evaluation did not get to the root of his problem. "He was placed in a vapor box and exposed to a variety of fumes and vapors. His chest pain came on with a number of common chemicals found in the air. They found that upon breathing in certain chemicals, his arteries would spasm and cause chest pains from a restriction of blood flow to his heart.[7]

Once the causes of his problem were found, he was placed on an intensive detoxification program, which included chelation therapy, an intravenous treatment to remove metals from the body and to improve circulation. He also took high doses of vitamins C and E, which are antioxidants, as well as beta carotene, zinc, and other important nutrients that he lacked. In addition, it was necessary to send him away from the city for two years.

As you can see, environmental medicine uses a thorough approach to diagnosis and tries to consider all the possibilities. "Very often it is like peeling back an onion," says Dr. Richard Podell. "You may find a person is sensitive to formaldehyde and also sensitive to certain foods and many other things. Most doctors don't have the time or patience for this and it is really quick and easy for them to say, sorry, there is nothing wrong with you, when it is not true."[8]

The environmental doctor also learns to listen closely to what his patients have to say, while the traditional doctor, for the most part, ignores them. Dr. Marshall Mandell of Norwalk, Connecticut, comments:

> This is what bothers me so much about the medical profession. They stand off like gods. They make pronouncements but they won't get in there and do a little work, and they won't pay any attention to intelligent patients who tell them that when I eat this or go there or get exposed to this, I don't feel good. They are not being listened to. The doctors don't realize that their patients are just as smart as they are: They just didn't go to medical school.[9]

Traditional diagnostic techniques no longer work for modern afflictions, such as chronic fatigue syndrome, Epstein-Barr, and candida, because the methods look for too few possible causal factors. Dr. Christopher Calapai comments: "Unfortunately, many physicians are trying to deal with chronic fatigue by narrowing the diagnosis down to one or two possible causes. By doing this they may be missing any number of other things that may actually be contributing to the situation."[10]

He says another mistake these doctors make is to confuse the antibodies to a virus with the actual illness itself:

> When the Epstein-Barr virus came out initially, there was only one blood test that was drawn to diagnose whether or not the patient had it, an IgG blood test. Now the IgG, when elevated, only means that you have been exposed to that virus somewhere in your past. It doesn't tell whether you are actively having a problem with it now. So many people were incorrectly diagnosed with Epstein-Barr virus syndrome and they were told that it was the cause of their fatigue when it actually may not have been.[11]

Still another limitation of blood testing is that it does not recognize the normal range for an individual; it simply lets you know if you are within a standard normal range. Dr. Calapai gives this example of how the tests can be inaccurate in diagnosing hypothyroidism:

> If your blood is drawn at any point and you are within the normal range, even if you are at the low end of normal, you are told that everything is okay. But you really need to compare your thyroid blood test to a previous one to find out what is normal for you. Let's say you were at the eightieth percentile of normal and now you are down to

> the twentieth percentile. That's a very big drop. There is a much bigger difference between a drop from the eightieth to the twentieth percentile than from the twentieth to below the normal level, so you have to take that into consideration.[12]

Contrary to what many people believe, environmental medicine is not a radically new approach to treatment but an ultraconservative one. Dr. Alfred Zamm explains:

> I am a traditional physician, a conservative doctor, but in my extreme conservatism I may appear to be nontraditional. When I say "conservative" I mean I don't trust anything until proven scientifically so I don't want my patients to take anything unless I can prove that it will not harm them. And I carry this to such an extreme that I don't want my patients to take colored vitamin pills when they are pregnant because it hasn't been proven that these color dyes are safe to the developing fetus. I try to protect my patients.[13]

Dr. Boyles also favors this approach:

> Things that have been around for a long time are the ones you want to investigate. Nobody talks about laetrile as a cancer cure anymore because it didn't work, but homeopathy, vitamins properly given—these kinds of things have been around for a long time. And there is nothing new about food allergy. It was first described in the 1920s very accurately.[14]

Doctors who choose to practice in this way usually do so because it gives them a sense of personal satisfaction to help patients who, for the most part, are considered to be hopeless by the medical mainstream. For example, Dr.

Michael Schachter, who received his graduate medical training at one of the finest medical schools in the country, Columbia College of Physicians and Surgeons in New York, says that he chooses to practice environmental medicine despite his formal background, which downgraded and ridiculed the very techniques he now uses to treat patients. "I personally have found that this has made all the difference in terms of practicing with patients," he says. "I get satisfaction from really being able to help patients who have not been helped by traditional means."[15]

WHY ENVIRONMENTAL MEDICINE IS NOT WIDELY PRACTICED

Most Doctors Are in the Dark

Despite its effectiveness, environmental medicine has not grown in popularity for several reasons. One such factor is that doctors have remained ignorant of environmental practice because of the limitations of their medical school training. Dr. Alan Levin comments:

> Even today in the medical schools, preventive medicine and nutrition are very, very minor courses. Everybody laughs at them. The people who teach them are second-class citizens. The important things are pharmacology, internal medicine, surgery, and how to deal with a disease once it happens. They are not concerned with altering people's diets or environments so that they don't develop a disease.[16]

Dr. Doris Rapp says that her involvement with environmental medicine had nothing to do with her medical training. Rather, she became involved through a fortunate circumstance that took place after she was already a doctor:

> I think my education in medicine was not correct because, although almost everything I talk about today was written in medical literature in the thirties by Dr. Rowe, in the forties by Drs. Rinkel and Randolph, and in the fifties by Dr. Speer, when I studied medicine I was told these men were not right. If I hadn't gone to the right medical meeting in 1975, I wouldn't know what I know now. If a doctor isn't as fortunate as I was he will have a hard time finding out about these things.[17]

Although this meeting was a turning point in Dr. Rapp's career, she was not easily convinced of the merits of environmental medicine at the start. The environmental doctors at the meeting said they rarely used drugs, even cortisone, which she did not believe. This prompted her to set out to disprove these doctors:

> I was skeptical and negative at that point so I went to a couple of their offices to expose them. They said they could put a drop of a standard allergy extract on somebody's arm and make them have symptoms. They could produce a headache, muscle ache, hyperactivity, belly ache, etc., and then with a weaker dilution of the same allergy extract make that patient's symptoms go away. I felt this was all nonsense.
>
> Then I tried it, and I was absolutely flabbergasted to find that I could produce and eliminate symptoms by using progressively weaker dilutions of allergy extract. The concept was totally foreign to everything I had been taught.
>
> It doesn't make sense logically and I can't explain why it works, but there are many children and adults today who are suffering and who can't wait for another twenty or

thirty years until someone explains to them why it helps them when they can be helped right now.[18]

Dr. Gary Oberg, the current president of the American Academy of Environmental Medicine, believes that practicing physicians generally are doing the best they can with the knowledge they have:

> Physicians are human beings who are often put in life and death situations. In order for them to be able to function without going under from stress, they have to have a great deal of confidence in the way they see things working. What they are going to recommend [as far as they know] is actually in the best interest of the patient and reflects science as accurately as the state-of-the-art and the current situation allows. If they were presented with the environmental medicine paradigm, which significantly questions the accuracy and efficacy of what they are using in these situations, it would cause a great deal of anxiety and fear and would undercut the confidence that a physician needs to deal with these life and death situations.[19]

The Five Misconceptions of Traditional Physicians

Dr. Oberg says that physicians labor under five major misconceptions. Because they have no knowledge of the field other than these five precepts, they generally see no reason to explore the role the environment plays in health and disease. These misconceptions include the following:

1. It Is Not Widely Recognized. They do not consider environmental medicine to be a valid approach to treatment because it is not a recognized specialty and it is not taught in any recognized medical school. In actuality, this is not a legitimate criticism for several reasons. First of all, environmental medicine is based upon a holistic philosophy. As such, it does not contain a unique body of facts that would allow it to be practiced independently from any other specialty.

Indeed, the more accepted notion of treatment, in which the body is artificially divided into isolated systems that are jealously guarded as the provinces of separate specialties, actually defies the true nature of the way the body works. This particular perspective depreciates the true nature of chronic and degenerative disease and provides one of the main stumbling blocks to the acceptance of environmental medicine today.

It would be much more appropriate for physicians to view this discipline not as a separate entity (as many other specialties look upon themselves) but as a new and improved orientation that more accurately recognizes and accommodates the environment's ability to affect the body's complex biological mechanisms. Environmental medicine takes into account the dynamic interactions that occur between biological systems. It also reveals the absurdity of isolating the biologic dysfunctions in one organ or system during treatment because of a particular limited specialty.

Environmental medicine should not be downgraded as a separate discipline since it is relevant to all branches of medicine. It is much more natural to look upon it as an approach that augments and improves the effectiveness of all specialties in treating disease. It is nonsense to try to isolate certain laws of biology to accommodate any one particular specialty.

In addition, it's inaccurate to invalidate environmental medicine simply because medical schools and residency programs do not teach it. While it may not be formally taught as a separate specialty, many astute teachers in medical training appreciate this new discipline and teach it to their students as the most practical and effective way of dealing with certain diseases. And the fact that the entire model is not routinely taught in medical school does not reflect an inadequacy of the model itself. Rather, it reflects just how far medical education in this country has to go before all practitioners routinely learn the concepts that currently offer the most effective way of dealing with the types of afflictions so prevalent in our society.

2. It Has No Scientific Basis. Doctors believe that other specialists have evaluated environmental medicine and found it to have no scientific basis. But this criticism has two major flaws. First, it mistakenly assumes that environmental medicine is a separate specialty. And second, it fails to recognize that doctors in other specialties evaluating environmental medicine have absolutely no training or experience in the discipline's concepts and, for the most part, refuse to have any meaningful dialogue with anyone who does. Therefore, these doctors are not in the position to judge a discipline as complex as environmental medicine, and they may come to many distorted conclusions.

The naysayers also like to claim that nothing in the scientific literature supports environmental medicine's concepts and the diagnostic and treatment methods they encompass. To the contrary, there is extensive literature to support these concepts and treatment techniques. Just because the articles do not get into the prestigious medical journals does not mean the studies do not exist.

Dr. Doris Rapp says that a practicing environmental physician has a tough time getting work published. She describes one frustrating experience she had in trying to do so:

> I'm a clinical doctor in practice, but the ones who decide what goes into the journals are the academic physicians. These doctors are doing full-time research in hospitals. Many times they research with new drugs and become the world's expert on some medication. When you're a world expert on some medicine, you hardly want somebody to come along and say use a simple one-week elimination diet to get rid of your problems instead.
>
> In order for me to write an article and get it into an allergy journal, it must first be read over by a group of these academic allergists. I have received articles back [to which a doctor said], I do not believe what was written and if this is published in this journal, I will resign from the editorial board. This was on a simple double-blind study I performed on a youngster who became hyperactive if he ate certain foods.[20]

She notes that many published studies also are biased because of the people sponsoring them. For example, one study that proved food dyes do not cause hyperactivity was paid for by the food industry. And when Dr. Rapp wrote a letter to the magazine criticizing the study, she was unable to get it published. Since doctors read the initial articles but never get to see criticisms of them, they will have a hard time discovering alternative approaches to treatment. "Our journals are strictly edited," she says, "so you don't know everything that is going on in medicine."[21]

3. The Causes of Environmental Illnesses Can't Be Proven. The third misconception is that environmentally treated illnesses are not acceptable because the mechanisms that explain them are not entirely known. This is an extremely hypocritical criticism, but doctors make it rather frequently. In reality, conventional medicine is replete with empirical and descriptive diagnoses and treatments where the mechanisms that cause the disease are unknown. In fact, many times physicians will give a name to patients' diseases just to label them, but then tell the patients that they don't know why they have the disease. Or they don't know how a drug works but will use it anyway.

The real issue is not whether the phenomenon has been accurately observed or whether it can be immediately explained, but whether the treatments can be proven effective by objective means. Effective treatments are those that can correct or improve the function of a biologic mechanism that does not work correctly, regardless of whether the full nature of the mechanism is known and understood—you don't have to be able to take apart an automobile in order to drive it.

4. Environmental Illnesses Are Psychosomatic. The fourth misconception is that patients who complain of environmentally triggered illnesses require psychiatric diagnoses. The opponents of environmental medicine would like us to believe that these patients have diseases that do not exist and that environmental doctors treat the imaginary ailments with techniques that do not work. This is one of the most popular concepts being put forth by skeptics of the discipline. They say that the correct way to deal with these patients is simply to pat them on the head and hope that they will, through the confidence of hearing that nothing is really wrong with them, snap out of it. In reality, this is quite patronizing and unfair.

These doctors assume that if a patient's symptoms seem to fit a known psychiatric diagnosis, then the possibility of a valid medical reason for the problem is automatically eliminated. They seem to forget that psychiatric diagnoses are mainly descriptive and generally have no biochemical markers to prove their presence or even their existence. Therefore, a psychiatric diagnosis should be made only after an appropriate and adequate medical evaluation has found no other reason for the symptoms.

To make a presumptive psychiatric diagnosis before ruling out a medical one is not only pejorative but also a disservice to the patient, especially if that diagnosis is based on an ignorance of how to rule out an environmentally caused illness to the central nervous system. Some patients have psychoneurological complaints with bona fide medical symptoms, and any type of chronic illness, especially if it is disabling, can produce real psychological consequences. These must be appropriately recognized and treated. There are patients, of course, who have legitimate psychiatric diseases that are not environmentally related. But it is a physician's professional responsibility to make an appropriate and adequate assessment in each and every case. If they do not know how to do that, then they must refer the patient to someone who does.

5. Environmental Medicine Involves Impractical Treatments. The fifth common misperception is that environmental illnesses require bizarre treatment methods that turn patients into environmental cripples. Granted, a small percentage of people with severe problems for multiple chemical sensitivities must initially follow severe life-style restrictions to remain well. It's important to realize, however, that such patients comprise only a small percentage of the population with environmentally triggered illnesses. Also, the severe life-style alterations that may be necessary for the minority usually are temporary measures that last only until the patients become tolerant enough to resume more normal activities.

According to Dr. William Philpott, many doctors do not practice environmental medicine today simply because they are closed minded by nature. He says that according to psychological studies the types of people who choose to become doctors generally have obsessive-compulsive personalities. These people tend to latch onto something strongly and become comfortable with that fixed idea. They are uncomfortable with change, even to the point that it overrides their ability to make an intellectual assessment of its values. In medical school, the doctor learns a certain set of rules and gets rewarded for following them. Therefore, he feels no desire to change. Dr. Philpott believes that unless doctors get the experience needed to test patients with environmental medicine, they will form their judgments according to the set of rules they have learned to follow, rather than from firsthand experience.

To begin to change this mind-set, Dr. Dorothy Calabrese believes doctors who practice environmental medicine must go back to their alma maters and try to influence the direction of medical education:

> The saddest thing about my medical education at Columbia is a lack of creativity about teaching medicine. That is because there is so much to be taught. I think they are looking for suggestions now, and I will try to work with them. We all need to go back to our alumni associations

> and speak with our deans and say, we need to look at medical education from a creative standpoint, not just learn all the facts but to look at problems in new ways.[22]

POLITICAL AND ECONOMIC REASONS

According to Dr. Oberg, the medical paradigm upon which physicians perceive health and disease is complicated by political and economic vested interests. Indeed, all but the most naïve would have to acknowledge that these interests have a powerful influence on the way science and medicine are practiced.

Dr. Levin holds similar beliefs but also feels that medicine will undergo positive changes in the coming years as patients begin to mobilize and demand more effective treatments from their health-care providers. "The people with breast cancer are beginning to recognize that what the gay community has done is very positive and now they are beginning to mobilize as well," he says. Dr. Levin also encourages physicians to take control of their practice so that ". . . they, along with the patients, will make a force that will control American medicine and American culture."[23]

Additionally, most patients do not know of environmental medicine's benefits because their primary-care physicians provide unscientific misinformation about it. These physicians believe they must compete for patients and, therefore, try to discourage their clients from seeing someone else who might help them. For example, Dr. Doris Rapp saw one patient who was referred to her by another doctor. Some time later the doctor called to ask her why she had stolen his patient. When she said that she didn't steal him, the doctor replied that the patient hadn't returned to him in six months. She said the patient hadn't been to *her* in six months either. The referring doctor, it seems, wasn't used to the idea that patients could be helped and might not need to run back to him all the time.

Other doctors may avoid the practice of environmental medicine for financial reasons. It is a time-consuming discipline, and time is money in the medicine field. It takes time to figure out answers and to educate people. They have to read books, study, and take some responsibility for their own medical care. While the doctor who treats patients in this way will be rewarded because the patients feel better, she probably will have to work harder to earn less money. In addition, she may need more assistants in the office to help teach people about why they are sick. This will cost her more money as well. The result: Relatively few doctors are anxious to learn environmental medicine.

Dr. John Boyles says that allergists in this country are internists with a lot of academic power. They use their influence to gain a monopoly on the allergy field that allows them to survive financially. These allergists have tried to legislate a monopoly in allergy by opposing those allergists who take an alternate approach that incorporates a healthy life-style and diagnostic techniques. In doing so, they are trying to put environmental doctors out of business so that patients must be treated by general allergists.

These same physicians also can persuade the insurance industry not to cover the costs of alternative treatments, which has a great political and economic impact on the state of environmental medicine today. They tell the insurance companies that the environmental approaches are experimental or unscientific and therefore should not be covered by insurance premiums. Since the insurance industry likes to collect your premiums and deny your claims, they will listen to anyone who tells them they should not cover certain types of care. This is a shortsighted strategy, since the treatment of causes rather than symptoms would, in the long term, save insurance companies a great deal of money.

In addition, if simple solutions to major illnesses were recognized, they would cut into fund-raising revenues of some special-interest groups. Dr. Marshall Mandell comments:

> I cannot cure multiple sclerosis, but I can make a big difference in these people with better nutrition. And cerebral palsy can be aggravated by allergies. I've videotaped it. But doctors just continue to run telethons to collect money and ignore these things. This is what is so frustrating. The same is true for the Arthritis Foundation. We can turn arthritis on and off. Many times the Arthritis Foundation tells people to beware of quacks. We certainly would interfere with their fund-raising telethons if patients realized that diet might be affecting their joints.[24]

According to Dr. Oberg, the chemical companies also work to keep environmental medicine down because they realize that many of their products contribute significantly to the causes of these diseases and they do not want to take responsibility for it. They fear that if environmental medicine were better known, lawyers would be upon them like a pack of vultures and that they might even end up in bankruptcy because of the legal costs.

Dr. Boyles notes that the hundred or so chemical companies in the United States, whose sole business is to produce chemicals, actively use their tremendous power and financial resources to fight against cleaning up the environment:

> Chemical manufacturing associations in the U.S. have twenty full-time lobbies in Washington. . . . They are lobbying against laws for clean air, clean water, and clean lifestyles, and the money that is spent to this end is just unbelievable. The smallest company in this association pays yearly dues of seven thousand dollars, and the biggest companies probably spend millions.
>
> They understand what environmental medicine is about quite accurately. They put out position papers which they give to all their members. These papers precisely describe what we in environmental medicine are trying to do to help our patients. And they even coach people on how to be against it without attracting attention. It is really hard to believe, but this is what is happening in the U.S.[25]

According to Dr. Boyles, the chemical companies say that doctors of environmental medicine are quacks and that diseases produced by multiple chemical sensitivities do not exist. If anything, they say, these are psychological diseases. With this tactic, they can try to deny people Workers' Compensation when they have been contaminated by chemicals on the job. But if these interests succeed in wiping out the concept of chemical allergy, the results will be disastrous as more and more people become poisoned by horrible chemicals.

Huge profits also motivate the multibillion-dollar pharmaceutical industry to keep environmental medicine out of the picture. These companies earn their money by creating palliative treatments—i.e., those that reduce the violence of a disease—for ongoing chronic problems. Dr. Calapai comments, "When you can create a medication, whether it be a cream, a lotion, or a tablet, it becomes a very profitable situation and the drug manufacturers try to capitalize on it."[26] Dr. William Rea adds,

> Today in the United States, a physician who's doing a very good job of helping people and doing no harm whatsoever is a liability to this six-hundred-billion-dollar-a-year industry. Because if people began to realize that the air they breathe, the beverages they drink, and the food they eat all have an impact upon their immune systems, and hence upon their sensitivity tolerance, resulting in irritable bowel syndrome, migraine headaches, tachycardia, and a lot of other conditions that traditional medicine says are simply of unknown origin, people would not be so chronically dependent upon prescription medications.[27]

Dr. John Boyles explains how the drug industry encourages doctors to perpetuate the myth that food and chemical allergy do not exist:

> Throughout the years, internists have said that food and chemical allergy do not exist. By doing so, they were painting themselves into a corner and they don't know how to get out from there. So they continue this line and the pharmaceutical companies, which have tremendous power and vast monetary resources, back them. One company alone spends twenty million dollars a year to entertain physicians and teach them how to use their drugs. . . .
>
> Environmental medicine is something that pharmaceutical companies don't want to see exist because if a patient can remove foods from his diet and control his colitis or his ulcers, then he won't have to take these expensive medicines for the rest of his life.[28]

Dr. Oberg concludes that it would be naïve to assume that environmental medicine will prevail just because it has been proven effective, since science does not progress in a vacuum. Rather, it is strongly influenced by the political, economic, and social ramifications of a particular model of science going forward or being rejected. The only way for environmental medicine to become more widely accepted, he believes, is for people with the best interests of humanity and the planet at heart to form coalitions and to work together:

> These interrelationships should be based on good scholarship, good science, honesty, and integrity. I think once this is done we will be able to move forward, and I am quite confident that in the long run the concepts of environmental medicine, with the preventive aspects of strengthening the human body and of keeping the environment and the diet clean, will be seen as the only way to go for humanity.[29]

THE OVERSELLING OF SCIENCE

Carl Winter, author of *Chemicals in the Human Food Chain*, states in his book that science has really been oversold for the past few decades. Our society fervently believes that science has all the answers, when in reality it has a long way to go.

In particular, science falls way short of understanding all the chemicals being used in society today. Toxicological testing is extremely difficult, especially when accessing combinations of chemicals. You can only make decisions about the dangerous effects of chemicals based upon the information you have at the moment, and often it takes time to see these effects. In many instances, that which is believed true at one stage is later proven false.

Toxicology also is problematic because you cannot

prove safety. Indeed, *safety* is not a scientific term but a societal definition of what we believe to be an acceptable risk. Exposures to low levels of chemicals do not immediately affect the body. Cancer, for example, may show up years after low-level exposures take place, making it difficult to discern the relationship. Therefore, we may be able to say that an exposure to a certain amount of a chemical for a certain length of time may cause a given effect, but we cannot say with scientific certainty that an exposure has no effect.

Dr. Michael Galante says that from a homeopathic point of view, there is no safe dosage of a toxin. "Something which is one part per million or one part per billion is active and therefore not harmless. So substances such as those found in pesticides, like parathion, malathion, dichlor, and the vast numbers of other chemicals in use today are, in my opinion, extremely toxic."[30]

The only way to make progress with science, according to Dr. Gary Oberg, is to adopt Thomas Huxley's attitude when he said, "When you are doing scientific inquiry, sit down before mother nature as a small child. Be prepared to cast aside all preconceived notions and to follow her into whatever abyss she leads or you shall learn nothing."[31]

THE IMPORTANCE OF ENVIRONMENTAL MEDICINE TODAY

Inevitably, environmental medicine will be accepted by our society because it is the only approach that addresses the causes of modern disease. Dr. James Miller explains: "For every illness there must be some cause. If mainstream doctors would really search and try to eliminate the cause, which is what we try to do in environmental medicine, they would probably be able to eliminate the problem."[32]

Diseases today differ from those of the past because they stem from environmental factors that stress people's immune systems beyond normal tolerance levels. Once that occurs, the person never quite feels the same unless he or she can identify the cause of the problem, eliminate it, and then rebuild the immune system. Dr. Richard Podell comments, "This is no doubt a population of people who are very ill, and if you look at what most of these people were like beforehand, you will find they were fine until they got sprayed with pesticides or had a really bad viral infection. After that, they weren't the same."[33]

In addition, the types of diseases seen today involve multiple systems of the body and result from multiple factors. By detoxifying the body and enhancing the immune system in general, environmental medicine can effectively eliminate these multiple symptoms. Dr. Dorothy Calabrese says:

> It has a wonderful impact on multiple symptoms. Many people come in with neurological, intestinal, respiratory, psychiatric, and skin disorders, and just by getting the immune system on course, these people will do extremely well. Many, if not all, symptoms go away. It's not like you are targeting one area. You are helping the whole person, and that's more exciting than anything I've seen in medicine.[34]

In addition, the techniques used to eliminate toxins from the system can help to slow down the aging process and retain health in later years. Dr. John Trowbridge explains how environmental medicine can help you to age more comfortably:

> We're not out to absolutely reverse everything so that you live forever, but we try to stop the acceleration of injury patterns happening within your system. We simply want to create a healthy balance within your body so that it can handle what it is supposed to handle at the right rate. Then you are going to age comfortably because you will not have problems like blockages in your blood vessels, arthritis, or jumpy muscles. When we have done that, we have done our job.[35]

Dr. Levin says that today's patients with environmental contamination are the "canaries of society" warning us of an imminent danger:

> A hundred years ago miners would take a canary with them into the coal mines to warn them of coal gas which was invisible, colorless, odorless, and tasteless. It just killed people. Canaries were taken in because if they fell off their perches and died this would give the miners, who were not as sensitive, a chance to rush out and be saved.
>
> Similarly, people seeing clinical ecologists today, and suffering from the twenty-first century disease of supersensitivity to chemicals, are the canaries of our society. They are warning us that the sixty thousand chemicals being introduced each year into our environment, which have never been here before, are not fit to breathe, drink, wear, and spray on as perfume. We have to start listening to these canaries or we are all going to succumb.[36]

Environmental medicine may also help to create a healthier society. Dr. Doris Rapp says that foods and chemicals may be responsible for allergy-prone children turning into societal delinquents. She cites several studies that show this relationship. For example, *Teens, Crime and Delinquency*, by Barbara Reed, studies delinquents in holding centers, probation centers, and prisons. The study shows unequivocally that certain individuals, after eating certain foods, have total personality changes and become more aggressive, belligerent, negative, and irritable. They act out in ways that are unacceptable by society.

Dr. Gary Oberg believes that the American medical bill, which has passed the $800-billion-a-year mark, will finally sway society to accept environmental medicine. This bill surpasses the total cost of running the government, the national defense, and the public educational system combined. According to Dr. Oberg, people are beginning to realize that we cannot control this problem long term by taking potshots at isolated chemicals or pesticides. Rather, we must teach the entire population a whole new paradigm of how the environment and the human organism interact to create either health or disease.

He believes that both science and our perceptions of the world progress when our old systems fail. A particular scientific or political paradigm rules until it cannot address or treat some of the fundamental problems and questions in society. This builds up like a pressure cooker until more and more failures with the conventional approach occur, such as the crisis we face today with our health-care system. Finally, there is an explosive, rather than a gradual change. One belief system is discarded and another is taken up.

Inevitably, we will discard the paradigm that believes most illnesses in this country can be treated with drugs. You go to a physician with a headache and he gives you a headache pill. You go to a physician with asthma and he gives you an asthma pill. Truly this is absurd, and it does not begin to answer the health challenges we face today.

The new paradigm must be the one that understands the interaction between environmental stresses and the individual. Ultimately, the public will seek out this new model and force government, industry, and insurance companies to adopt policies that help us to stay healthy rather than support our sickness.

8

Personal Testimonials

Healing Allergies with Wheat Grass

WOMAN:

I had allergies to cats and to dust that would give me itchy hives all over my body. I would have trouble breathing and I would cough pretty badly too.

Then one day, a friend of mine recommended that I try wheat grass juice. I began drinking it twice a day, an ounce in the morning and an ounce in the evening. After three weeks I doubled the amount. Before long, my allergies went away. After a week on the wheat grass, I could go near cats without getting the itchy hives.[1]

Tracing an Environmental Illness to Childhood

WOMAN:

I suffer from environmental illness, which I have traced to my childhood when I would go to shopping malls with my mother. I remember feeling lethargic; my feet would drag and I would barely be able to hold myself up before even one hour went by. I used to think I reacted that way just because we were shopping.

Now as an adult if I become overloaded with toxicity I can easily get these same symptoms. I have found that by cleaning up my environment to keep it as toxin free as possible and by eating the right kinds of foods I can get relief from my symptoms.[2]

Respiratory Illness from Indoor Air Pollution

MAN:

I found a lot of indoor pollution in my apartment. I live in a church and the area partitioned off for my living space had asbestos ceiling tiles and fluorescent lights. After moving in, I started to get frequent upper respiratory infections. At first I thought it was just due to the place being drafty, but after visiting an environmental doctor I learned that my problem might be from the asbestos.

Since the owners weren't about to replace the ceiling tiles, I decided to do the job myself. That cleared up most of my problem. Then I put in a large air purifier and a negative ionizer near the window, which really made a difference. All of a sudden, I wasn't going to the doctor every two months with another bout of bronchitis.[3]

The Benefits of Exercise and Nutrition

KEVIN:

Before my involvement in sports, I was troubled with a variety of physical ailments. I had hay fever throughout most of the early and late growing season and I was a cold-weather asthmatic as well. At the time I wasn't paying close attention to what I was eating. I was a junk-food junkie.

After I started training, however, my body demanded

better food: unprocessed food, fruits, vegetables, and a lot more salads. I also cut back on red meat.

I received a lot of benefit from the combination of exercise and good nutrition. Recently, I have even been able to train in the cold weather because I am no longer suffering from asthma. I am sleeping a lot better too.[4]

Nutrition Instead of Drugs for a Hyperactive Child

WOMAN:

I am a psychotherapist for children. I was working with a hyperactive boy who was on medication through our clinic.

As I am not generally for drug therapy, I had a talk with his mother about what he eats, how he starts his day, and that kind of thing. I learned that he would begin each day by having a cup of black coffee with his mother. Then he would go to his special-education class and act bonkers.

I asked his mother to please stop the coffee, and I talked to her about possible reactions he might be having to dairy as well. Fortunately, she did stop feeding her son coffee and dairy. As a result, he was doing great in school in the mornings.

After lunch, however, he still would have problems. We talked about this and decided that his behavior was probably a reaction to the school lunchroom food. Maybe there was something in what he was eating—preservatives, colorings, sugar, and that kind of thing—that was affecting him.

I suggested that instead of eating the food from school she give him food to bring from home. She followed my advice and as a result her son has been able to get off of his medication.

He has had the best school year ever. There have been no behavior problems and he is excelling in his schoolwork. She is so grateful to see this turnaround in her son whom everybody had disliked. I think it is amazing to see [someone's] behavior and ability to concentrate improve so through a change in diet.[5]

Overcoming Asthma with Diet and Chelation

JAMES HOWARD:

Back in the eighties I started getting allergies. I kept going to doctors for my condition, about ten in all, but they never were able to help me. My condition worsened and turned into asthma, and I was on six medications, including prednisone.

Then one day I talked to someone in a health store who recommended I see Dr. Trowbridge. I went to him and he found that I had a yeast syndrome and multiple food allergies.

He put me on a strict caveman's diet, which cut out practically all sweets. I didn't eat anything but fresh foods. This helped me somewhat but I was still having some problems so I decided to try chelation therapy.

During my workup, the doctor found that I had an iron-storage abnormality which stimulated free radicals to attack my system and bring on asthma and allergies. I also was found to have a very high concentration of lead and cadmium in my system.

The chelation therapy combined with nutrients made the difference. I began to feel remarkably better within only six or seven treatments. Everybody says when you have asthma you have it for life, but that isn't true. In fact, I haven't taken any asthma medications for close to five years now. So, there must be a connection between what I have done and how I am feeling.[6]

Overcoming Chronic Fatigue

JIM:

I was chronically fatigued to the point of not being able to play ball with my son after coming home from teaching. I had to lie down. The only way I could keep working was with a lot of coffee.

Looking back, I had a lot of symptoms. For one, my eyes were blurry a lot. I went to a doctor for that about ten years ago and he said it was from old age. At the time I was thirty-five years old.

Finally I found a doctor of environmental medicine, Dr. Schachter, who diagnosed me as having multiple allergies. Before that I never thought of myself as allergic because I didn't have classic hay-fever symptoms. So if you would have asked me five years ago if I was allergic I would have said no, when in reality I was allergic to just about everything.

I was given electronic acupuncture testing, which found that I had layer upon layer of problems that needed to be cleared away over a period of two to three years. The tests found many blockages to healing, like an appendectomy scar from when I was two years old that was affecting my digestion. The adrenals and pancreas were pretty well worn out too, and I had hypoglycemia and a couple of other problems.

Through a combination of nutrients and homeopathic treatments I have gotten much, much better. In fact, it is remarkable how far I've come. But it didn't all happen right away. Before I got better I got worse. It's like an alcoholic getting off alcohol and realizing he has cirrhosis of the liver. As I started to clear out I actually started to get worse because the things I had been using to mask my symptoms—like nicotine, caffeine, and alcohol—weren't there anymore. I wanted to quit dozens of times. The only thing that kept me going was that I had so much time and money invested in what I was doing. The most important thing I learned from this is to stick with a program because it takes a while to get better.

I have learned to support people like Dr. Schachter who are exploring new holistic methods in medicine. The people who are benefiting the most are the ones who have exhausted all the traditional approaches. That's what happened to me. I was so allergic to everything I couldn't be treated in the usual way. The fact that I have gotten better shows that what you are doing can make a difference in people's lives.[7]

Healing Through Homeopathy and the Removal of Dental Amalgams

BARBARA:

I became ill after repeated exposures to chemicals at work. I worked in a testing laboratory where they sprayed with insecticides, and in another place where they had fumes from printing inks. I also had extensive exposure to tobacco both at home and in the workplace.

I was experiencing a variety of symptoms: headaches, anxiety, and light-headedness. I also developed food allergies at this time and a tightness in the chest. Probably the most frustrating thing about environmental sensitivity is that people don't understand that you are ill since your symptoms aren't visible. There is even a lack of understanding amongst family and friends. At times I had hoped I would get hives so that people would understand by seeing the symptoms.

My treatment has basically consisted of homeopathy, the removal of dental amalgams, a rotation diet, and some other things like exercise and supplements. I started with some homeopathic remedies, both the classical and complex, and gradually I began to see changes. The first thing I noticed was that the hypoglycemia I had experienced for a number of years, where I had been waking up in the middle of the night and raiding the refrigerator, started to disappear. Gradually, some of the chemical sensitivities also started to become less prominent. Then my amalgams were removed and I think this enhanced my benefits from the homeopathic remedies even more.

Overall, I had a dramatic recovery. Whereas before it was impossible for me to do things a normal young woman would do, like wear nail polish, color my hair, read the newspaper, wear perfume, and that kind of thing, following treatment I am now able to do things like read the newspaper without putting a plastic bag over it. Although I try to avoid things that may be toxic, at least I have a choice as to what I do.

Now I am an example to others. It doesn't work to get on the soapbox and preach, but when people see that your health has improved they begin to come to you and ask questions. Then you have an opportunity to explain to them about environmental medicine and how it can help. So my healing has been a wonderful learning experience for myself and for others as well.[8]

Overcoming Asthma and Food Allergies

LINDA:

I have had asthma from the time I was thirteen until recently, and I am in my mid-forties now. It was so bad that I used to sleep with my head between my legs in order to breathe.

Up until a couple a years ago, I would go to a doctor who religiously every week would give me the shots you get in the hospital, Adrenalin and whatever, just to be able to breathe. I went to other doctors too but all they did was prescribe medication, and that would only give me temporary relief. I also tried these atomizer things which were time released, but when the time was up I was back with the same condition.

I became addicted to these treatments, even though I never really wanted to do this kind of thing because I felt it was not right for my body. It went against my grain.

I had terrible food allergies. I would open the refrigerator door and almost want to cry because this would make me sleepy, this would make me feel confused, and this would make me this and that.

My reactions to food were so bad at times that I would become nonfunctional to the point of being unable to do anything but lie in bed. I couldn't move or breathe. My ribs hurt so badly that I felt as if I had been hit by a baseball bat. I just ached throughout my whole body.

Then, through the grace of God, I met someone who told me about Dr. Schachter. He diagnosed me with the electronic acupuncture device which is truly phenomenal. It shows where you are weak from toxicity. The meter showed that I had mercury poisoning and that may explain why I was feeling really depressed. I was only in my mid-forties and this lack of energy was getting me down more and more. Next I was given measured homeopathic remedies to build up my strength. It really worked. My asthma went away in one year.

I feel like a new person. During the winter I can now run races with my kids, which in the past was unheard of. A couple of steps in the cold weather used to make me need an oxygen mask. And last week when the weather was horrendously hot, I was able to stay outside gardening.

Also, I had my son see Dr. Schachter. My son was put on Ritalin at times because he had a problem with his schoolwork. I was very much against this because I had heard of its drastic side effects. The electric acupuncture machine diagnosed him as having parasites which nobody else ever found. By getting rid of these parasites he was able to calm down and do his schoolwork better without medication. Now he is the person he was meant to be before all these problems interfered with his natural state of being.[9]

Healing with Magnets

IRENE:

It started when we moved from the polluted city into the "clean" suburbs. Three weeks later, my daughter, who had never had an ear infection in her life, developed fluid in the ears. I took her to a pediatrician who gave her the standard antibiotics, even though she did not have an ear infection. That started a spiral that ended with her being on theophylline and on broad-spectrum antibiotics continually for almost a year. At the end of the year we were told that the only way to alleviate the problem was to take out her adenoids and put tubes in her ears.

Being holistically oriented, I felt that conventional medicine had had its chance and that I would try an alternative approach. I put her on vitamins A, C, E, and zinc, and within a month she was holding stable. However, shortly thereafter her health began to deteriorate again from the broad-spectrum antibiotics she had been taking and from the "clean" suburbs, which turned out to be extremely toxic. Our neighbors continually sprayed their lawns, and our house, which looked wonderful with its vinyl wallpaper, linoleum, and wall-to-wall carpeting, was making her even more sick.

We made the decision to build and move into an environmentally safe home. We even drilled a three-hundred-foot well for clean water, which we test regularly, and we did not allow plastics and formaldehydes into the home.

She started getting somewhat better. However, the chemical sensitivities which were brought on from all the other medications she had been on, or from a genetic predisposition which made her react to chemicals, never subsided no matter what we did. We tried acupuncture and homeopathy, which would keep her stable for only short periods of time.

It got to the point where she could no longer go to her class because her school had a photo lab next to her room. She had to stay home and get a home tutor for a year. Basically, she was now a prisoner of her own home. When she stayed in her clean environment she thrived, but when she went into the outside world she destabilized. That was not the quality of life I wanted for her.

Finally, I saw Dr. Philpott, in Manhattan, who introduced me to magnetic therapy, and this is what made the difference. Now she was able to do the things other teenagers did. Not that magnetic therapy alone was a cure-all. Dr. Philpott put her on a full rotation diet and on certain supplements as well. But magnetic therapy did make a major difference for my child, who has been classified as having magnetic deficiency syndrome.[10]

Asthma and Arthritis from Food Allergies

GLEN:

As a teenager, I began developing allergies. My symptoms began as chronic sneezing and coughing and later evolved into a severe case of asthma. I would also experience aches and pains throughout my body, which I later learned to be symptoms of arthritis.

I went to some so-called allergy specialists who put me on a series of allergy medications. Even though years went by and I never got any better, I was always warned not to stop taking the injections because the benefits were cumulative. I was told that if I stopped taking the injections all my years spent getting them would have been wasted. So I never stopped, figuring I would only get worse, even though I never got any better.

I was very fortunate when in my early twenties a colleague of mine referred me to Dr. Chao. Dr. Chao started from scratch. He made me maintain a food diary and we began to see a correlation between what I was eating and what I was experiencing as allergy, arthritis, and asthma.

Over the years, more and more foods and airborne particles were identified and my symptoms became less and less severe. He identified over four dozen different foods that were causing me trouble.

The side effects from the medications I had been taking were causing severe reactions in me as well. The asthma medications caused my heart to beat a mile a minute. It made me feel as though I had been kicked in the back of my head by a mule, and it never did anything to cure my symptoms because I was still chronically asthmatic.

Gradually, as these different foods and drugs were eliminated from my diet I got better. I have now been off all my medications for many years, and during this time I have had no asthmatic symptoms whatsoever, no joint pains, no symptoms of arthritis. I am in the best shape I have ever been in my life.

Here's an interesting anecdote. Once when I was visiting someone in a hospital I overheard a doctor counseling a young girl and her parents. The parents said that the girl seemed to have terrible problems whenever she went horseback riding, and asked if any connection between the horses and her asthma existed. The doctor said none existed and that it was just a coincidence. Well, they told me the same thing regarding my asthma, which really became severe whenever I was exposed to animals.

Doctors need to rethink allergy medicine because their understanding of it is back in the Stone Age. They are very quick to prescribe all types of medications to treat symptoms while untreated causes exacerbate. My untreated coughing as a kid exacerbated into asthma because it wasn't corrected.[11]

Ulcers from Food Allergies

LILLIAN:

I always thought I had a cast-iron stomach. I never even had a stomachache. Then one day I found I had a perforated ulcer. I never even knew I had an ulcer before that. I was given an operation for it and resolved to never have another ulcer again if I could help it.

I believed ulcers to be psychosomatic in nature so I went to an analyst. He told me to resign from all my committees. I listened to him but still got another bleeding ulcer. Now I was really upset because they wanted to operate and take out a good part of my stomach to prevent me from producing too much acid.

As I was in the hospital bed thinking about it, I could not understand the logic. I was a chemistry teacher and I couldn't see why, if I was producing too much acid, I couldn't neutralize it. Why did I have to go through surgery? I started to think about what I could do.

I called my internist and asked, why couldn't I neutralize the acid? He hesitated before saying that we could try to neutralize it and then went on to say that even if I had the surgery it was no guarantee that I wouldn't get another ulcer. When I heard that I thought, what have I got to lose if I try something else?

I called a friend of mine who had treated arthritis with a simple diet and I called someone else who had treated a neurological disease with diet. It occurred to me that since I was producing too much acid that maybe the problem was a chemical one. Being a chemistry teacher, it made a lot of sense to me that since foods are chemicals they might have something to do with my condition. My existing doctors did not think anything of my theory.

Then I called Dr. Chao, though I had never seen him before, because he was helping a friend of mine. I told him that I had a bleeding ulcer on the verge of perforating and asked if he could help me. He said yes and I told the doctor to cancel my surgery.

I went straight from the hospital to Dr. Chao's office and he simply told me to do the following: He said to keep a diary while eating whatever my internist told me to have. This was the first time I had kept records like these. The internist had put me on a milk diet, which was traditional for ulcer patients, and I could tell by the fifth day that any time I drank milk the pain would get worse. By the time I got to Dr. Chao's I was worried my ulcer might perforate again and he confirmed the fact that it was the milk. I was so relieved to hear that. I felt I had a new lease on life and that I wasn't going to die, which had been my biggest fear.

That's how it all started. Dr. Chao removed the milk, and cane sugar too, which he said was usually a problem. Then lots of things changed. I used to be depressed so often that I thought it was my nature, but now I was no longer depressed. I had taken a leave of absence from my job because of my illness and I had been worried that not having a structure in my life would get me depressed. Instead I was so happy that strangers would come up to me in the street and talk. My face must have had a very nice expression. I couldn't get over it. It was just a wonderful turnaround.

From there I asked if there was anything else I was sensitive to. I found the reason I was tired all the time wasn't because of age: I wasn't even fifty then. It was because of wheat. And I found the reason I would get leg cramps every day was from apples. As these different foods were removed from my diet, my skin, which had been sallow, changed to a better color. I haven't gotten a cold in a very long time either. Overall, it has been wonderful and it has changed my whole life.[12]

Multiple Allergies

KATIE

I thought I was a fairly healthy kid even though I had what I now know to be childhood allergies. Basically, I had constant headaches, severe postnasal drip, and a runny nose all the time.

As I grew older other problems developed. In my teens I had problems taking normal medications. In my twenties when I went on the pill, I had violent mood swings. That was the first time I knew something was wrong. In my thirties I became very depressed. I went into therapy and was put on antidepressants. I had many problems after that: severe PMS, horrible migraines that lasted for up to four weeks, and a terrific weight gain that I couldn't even control with diet.

I went from doctor to doctor to doctor saying, look at me. I don't look right. My skin color is off. I don't feel good. There is something wrong. Help me. All they would say was, we'll run some tests, and that would infuriate me. I was a basket case and I ended up in a psychiatric hospital for three days where I only got worse. No one could reach me or talk to me. It was just horrible.

I checked myself out against my doctor's orders and went to stay with my sister in San Clemente. She had found out about Dr. Calabrese and I went to see her thinking I had nothing to lose.

I will never forget the first day I saw her. She took one look at me and said, I know what is wrong with you. No one had ever said that to me and it made a strong impact on me. I even get a little choked up now thinking about it because it was so unbelievable. Here was someone who could give me hope. I was looking terrible then, as I had lost a lot of hair and I was bloated and so overweight.

I talked to her and we began to put the pieces together. I realized that not only had my thyroid gone out several years earlier, and not only did I have allergies that had never before been addressed, but I was also having reactions to pesticides that I was spraying in my home for bugs, not realizing that that was triggering off reactions. And I had plants to the point of my house looking like a conservatory, not realizing that the molds and dirt were also doing me in.

I began to change my life-style and within four weeks was feeling like I was a teenager again. My depression lifted almost immediately, my weight started coming down, and I felt fabulous. This was the first time someone actually connected the plants, the foods, the pesticides, all those things which in combination were doing me in. Suddenly having them removed from my life, everything turned around. It was phenomenal.

My other physicians still think I should be locked up. They say there is no correlation between illness and food. I had to switch doctors because these physicians were not able to help me and were not willing to listen and understand that if you look hard enough you can put two and two together and get four.[13]

Infant with Multiple Allergies

MELODY:

As an infant, my son, who is now five, was very, very fussy, which a lot of mothers can identify with. He was diagnosed as having colic.

He wouldn't put on weight and he wouldn't eat foods. He was eventually labeled mentally retarded, which was very disturbing. During infancy, he wouldn't lie down flat, so I would sleep on the rocking chair with him and hold him upright so that he could breathe and get some sleep. And he had a multitude of rashes. Our general practitioner was sympathetic to this and said that my son must have allergies, which he would treat with medication. As far as foods were concerned, however, he felt that there was no relationship there. So we just kept dealing with it in that way. Soon, however, he began having bloody stools.

I began keeping a diary to see if there was some correlation between what he ate and what was happening. I also put him on a rotation diet and noticed some improvement from that, but as he became older new problems developed. We noticed that whenever he was around plastics, like soft plastic toys, he began having a real raspy sound to his cry, so we eliminated plastic from our environment, which is no small task in this day and age. He did better after we did these types of things but he was still bleeding. The doctors wanted to treat him with medication to cover up the symptoms but do nothing to find out the cause of his problem.

I began reading a lot of books on allergy that kept referring to environmental problems, and I searched that avenue more and more. I began to notice how he would get worse during crop-dusting time. We live in a cotton area and whenever we would have him out in the car while they were crop dusting he would have an extremely difficult time breathing. In fact, he did stop breathing a couple of times. When this would happen I would bring him to the hospital and the doctors would label him [as having] SIDS [Sudden Infant Death Syndrome]. We were feeling a lot of frustration and getting no answers from the medical profession.

Finally I heard of Dr. Calabrese and went to see her. I found that he had an underlying thyroid problem as well as more food allergies than I had originally thought, and environmental allergies too.

Since that time he is a changed child. His behavior problems have considerably decreased. He has normal intelligence and he is developing normally physically. He is able to ride a bike, which the doctors told me he would never do. And he is tolerating a wider variety of foods, which is wonderful. He is still on a rotation diet but we can go out to eat once in a while and he does not get sick, which is just absolutely amazing to us. Also, he sleeps through the night now lying flat, and he can tolerate some plastic in his environment. We feel he is a different child.[14]

Multiple Allergies

JOHN:

I used to have multiple allergies from inhalants, foods, and chemicals. During the really severe weather in the summer and winter, and during the change of seasons, I would not only have problems with a stuffed-up head or runny nose but I would also have digestive problems where I would get diarrhea. I would also get headaches, weakness, and fatigue.

Now I am receiving shots weekly for inhalants. I take food drops and chemical drops on a daily basis, which have helped me to eliminate a number of my problems. For instance, I used to get lesions on my hands for a number of years. They would break out and start bleeding and there was no way to control it. I went to people who treat skin problems but all they could do was treat symptoms. The minute I stopped using the creams or doing whatever they told me to do, I would break out again.

Since I started taking food and chemical drops these symptoms have become nonexistent. They have gone away complete.[15]

Multiple Allergies in Children

MRS. MINOR:

My daughter has suffered from multiple allergies since she was a little girl. We discovered this early on when we found she couldn't eat pistachio nuts and some other classic food-allergy producers. She began taking shots for inhalant allergies since she was three for a severe eczema condition that she had all over her body.

After several different trips to various doctors we were recommended to Dr. Calapei, who tested her for inhalants and food. She has been seeing him for about four years with great results. Her skin has cleared up almost all the way. She is on a rotation diet, which seems to keep everything pretty much under control.[16]

Food Allergies

SARAH:

I went to Dr. Seibert a couple of months ago for tests and my liver test came back very bad. I was very concerned. I told her I ate a lot of whole wheat bread that I baked myself from organic sources where no pesticides were used. She insisted that since I was hypoglycemic and had some trace mineral deficiencies that I could not handle refined grains. So, I stopped eating the bread and started eating brown rice and kasha instead. Also, I took out my juicer and started making juices and blending salads.

Six weeks later I went for a blood test, which was completely normal. All this happened just because I omitted the flour and drank lots of juice and water and blended salads. I am feeling much better now, thank God. I sleep much better too.[17]

General Malaise

MARIA:

I am in my sixties and in the last twenty years I have gone to eight doctors for a condition of general malaise. They all said I was fine and that there was nothing wrong with me. One doctor even suggested I see a psychiatrist. I felt like a hypochondriac so I went to a psychiatrist who said there was nothing wrong with me in that department either. At that point I gave up and was feeling very depressed.

Then last year I got the address of Dr. Seibert from a health-food store. I didn't feel hopeful but I went. She took a lot of tests and found out that I had various ailments, like a candida condition, borderline Epstein-Barr, and a thyroid that was not functioning right. She gave me some supplements, a thyroid treatment, and put me on a very strict diet. I have followed my diet religiously and am feeling better than I have felt in the last thirty years.[18]

Vitamin Therapy for Asthma and Candida

CHARLOTTE:

I had been hospitalized three times for two weeks at a time, and I was on steroids and all kinds of drugs. I was almost crazy from the high doses of steroids and my heart was racing all the time. I couldn't function.

I found Dr. Levin, who put me on IV vitamin therapy and cleared up my diet. I found out that I was lactose intolerant. Before, I had been taking my pills with milk and with ice cream and my doctor had said that that was fine.

About three weeks into my new diet I just cleared up. I started to lose weight, feel better, breathe again, and function like a normal human being. It was almost miraculous and I couldn't believe it.

Now I have two jobs. I run around and I feel great. I am no longer experiencing the asthma or the candida, which came on from the steroids and from all the other medications I had been taking. I haven't been hospitalized in five years since going to Dr. Levin. I am functioning like a normal human being and I love it.[19]

Allergies

LISA:

I had a lot of symptoms, mostly stemming from allergies and problems I was having with my digestive system. I had severe migraine headaches, constant laryngitis, and eczema. I was tired all the time and I had sore muscles and joints. I also had chronic diarrhea, intestinal cramps, and acid indigestion. All this basically started when I was ten years old and I am thirty now.

I had been misdiagnosed for my allergies and treated for many years with antibiotics, which only made my allergies a lot worse by suppressing my immune system. I had been to a lot of internal-medicine specialists for my digestive problems but the diarrhea was getting worse and worse. By the time I saw Dr. Levin, five years ago, I was pretty much emaciated and I really couldn't keep any food down. My allergy symptoms were horrible.

Dr. Levin taught me about proper nutrition. He taught me to eat whole foods with no preservatives and to use a rotation diet to control the different food allergies I had. Basically, he taught me to take care of myself through proper nutrition, exercise, and the elimination of a lot of the chemical household cleaning products and personal-care products I had been using that were making me ill. Today, five years later, I am healthy and happy and a completely different person.[20]

Schizophrenia from Brain Allergies

JENNIFER'S FATHER:

As a baby, Jennifer had severe allergies and asthma. When she was in bed at night breathing, you could hear her all the way down the hall.

When Jennifer was fourteen, she tried to commit suicide so we took her to a local hospital. They held her there for about two weeks, during which time they ran all kinds of tests and had several different doctors look at her. They diagnosed her as having schizophrenia for which she was given various drugs. But the drugs made her get progressively worse.

She could only stay in a local hospital for so long so they shipped her to a state hospital. The state hospital didn't seem to do much for her. They said she seemed to be schizophrenic but that it was peculiar. So they shipped her to yet another hospital which also didn't do anything for her.

Soon after that we brought Jennifer home. She got a little better and then worse again. Soon she got really bad so we took her back to the local hospital. We asked the doctor where we could have her diagnosed and he recommended a well-known mental hospital. We took her there, in Connecticut, and they said they were going to try to help her without drugs. But she got out of hand and they gave her drugs. She was there for six months getting worse all the time.

I was listening to a TV talk show one day and heard a doctor talking about allergies. I called her on the phone and she put me in contact with Dr. Mandell, who tested Jennifer and found her to be allergic to dairy products, wheat, and yellow food dyes. Now my daughter is on a rotation diet and doing absolutely fine. She is working and living a perfectly normal life.

Before Dr. Mandell got her, the doctors with degrees at this hospital took me aside and told me that Jennifer was borderline retarded with a severe mental illness. They said that she probably was going to be on medication for the rest of her life and in and out of institutions. But my daughter is doing wonderfully today.

There is a lot more to mental illness than the psychiatric profession knows about. They never even look at the allergies. My daughter loved milk and used to gulp it down at the hospital. They made chocolate-chip cookies and she would eat the whole batch. And she loved potato chips. All this stuff was what was causing her problem and keeping her sick. I tried going back to tell the doctors about my daughter but they didn't even want to discuss it.

Another thing, she was on Haldol, Cogentin, and Pamelor. When I would go visit her the saliva would run out of her mouth, she could hardly walk, and she would shake terribly. Once she started the drugs she never had her period and her bowel movements were all screwed up. It was all from these medicines, none of which had anything to do with the problem.[21]

Multiple Sclerosis

PATTY BRANDT:

I was diagnosed with multiple sclerosis about fifteen years ago. During that time, I had a chronic progressive form of the disease where my symptoms would get worse and worse. My symptoms were basically fatigue and loss of motor control in my arms and legs.

Conventional medicine would treat me by giving me a walker, a cane, some braces. They would treat what was happening with equipment. No one would ever stop and look at what was actually causing my illness.

I noticed over the years that some foods bothered me in different ways so I tried staying off of them but I really didn't have much information to go by. Then I heard about Dr. Mandell and went to be tested by him. He said, I can't promise you a cure or that we can do anything, but we will certainly look into it and try to help you as much as possible. This was more than any doctor had ever said to me before.

He did the testing in his office and I was amazed to see how my symptoms would come and go from different foods I was being tested for. With lamb, lettuce, wheat, tuna, and salmon, I would become very tired and unable to lift my head. When the test was over I would be right back to where I was before the test, which was much better. Other tests were given to me where I could not lift my arms off the table or off my chair, and this repeatedly happened. After the testing was all over I went home and found I could control my symptoms with foods. I could make myself much better just by watching what I ate.

Without Dr. Mandell's help, I certainly would be a lot more tired. I would not be able to get up and do the things I do. I have an eleven-year-old daughter and I keep up with her as much as possible around the house. Now I can stand up in the shower, and at times I wash my own hair. These are things I hadn't been able to do for years. I can also climb steps and walk distances in my house. I'm sure that at this point, if it were not for the changes I have made in my diet, I would be much more debilitated.[22]

Multiple Sclerosis

PAT BYRNES:

I used to eat the same foods almost every day. I would get up every morning, drink apple juice, and have chicken four to five times a week. After being tested, these proved to be foods I was very allergic to. Isolated, chicken would even make my hand immobile.

I have continued to rotate chicken as a food in my diet and have become very conscious of how often I eat apples and some other foods. As Dr. Mandell said, while this certainly is not going to be a cure for multiple sclerosis I can feel better if I watch my diet carefully.

I also want to point out that my internist recently put me on an antibiotic for facial acne. I had never had skin problems in my life and it was during a time when my diet was very bad since I had been on vacation and traveling, which made it very difficult for me to watch my diet. So he put me on these antibiotics. The antibiotics, I feel, made it more difficult to walk. I went off of them and watched my diet, avoiding wheat with yeast, and the acne went away. I didn't need the antibiotics. But if I were to start eating those foods again the acne would come back.[23]

Asthma

CHERYL:

When my son, Michael, was about three he developed an asthma condition so severe that he couldn't go outside or even across a room without having an attack. He was also diagnosed as hyperactive and all the doctors told me the two often go hand in hand.

Michael was on 750 mg of theophylline a day and a syrup full of red food coloring. He was also on Ritalin. Michael was at the hospital emergency room every weekend to get shots of Adrenalin to help him breathe. But as soon as we would get him home he would have another asthma attack. It was rough on him.

When Michael was five we took him to Philadelphia to the Spitz clinic. Dr. Ballacatto told us about Dr. Mandell and suggested we take Michael there. Michael was tested and found to be allergic to just about everything that he loved [to eat].

Now he is eleven and a half going into middle school this fall. He is no longer on any asthma medication. He rides his bike, swims, and is on the swim team. He does everything a normal healthy boy does, and has no asthma attacks anymore. We are really pleased with how Dr. Mandell was able to help Michael. He is a totally different child.[24]

Severe Headaches and Food Allergies

CATHY:

My son, Joey, started having very severe headaches when he was ten. We went through the standard procedures with our regular doctor, who sent him for a CAT scan since he would wake up in the middle of the night with severe headaches. That was very frightening to me as a parent and very frightening to my ten-year-old. Fortunately, there was nothing there. Then he went to a neurologist and to a dentist to see if he had temporomandibular syndrome—pain where the jaw meets the skull.

Michael was at the point of being up all night, every night, from coughing. He had lost weight and could not attend school. I finally decided to take him to an allergist and chose a traditional one. He started getting some treatment and we were thrilled to find him allergic to anything.

The treatment worked for a while but he still had "allergy eyes." They were red, irritated, and itchy with dark circles under them. Then the headaches and cough came back. And he couldn't sleep again. Before long, he had every symptom come back that was previously there. He became so fatigued that he could not get off the sofa for very long periods of time. It was an effort for him just to get up to eat or to live the life that a child should live. He had earaches and every symptom imaginable including digestive problems.

At that point I was told that Michael was a very depressed child who should go to a psychiatrist. This was after a period of two to three years of going from doctor to doctor to doctor. We went to a psychiatrist even though I felt that there was nothing mentally wrong with him. After a period of time I was very dissatisfied with that because he still couldn't attend school and he had all these symptoms.

Then I read about Dr. Mandell in *Let's Live* magazine, where a little boy's mother had written an article about her son who had very similar symptoms to Michael's: circles under the eyes, red ears, digestive problems, and headaches. So I called up Connecticut and found out what to do.

I brought Michael for testing and they found him to be allergic to just about the world. Mostly it was wheat and red food coloring. Here is a child who lived on cereal. We're Italian and he loves pasta and pizza. But pizza would put him to sleep. Pasta, if not artichoke-flour pasta, makes him have to take a nap even now at seventeen when he is in control of his diet.

Basically, Dr. Mandell saved his life. Michael is on a rotation diet. And we have eliminated all products in the house to which he might be chemically sensitive, like cleaning products, etc. which were contributing to his headaches.

Also I had taken Michael to see an endocrinologist because of his fatigue. When I explained this to Dr. Mandell he said, let's try the basal thermometer test. Everyone else had thrown that out, including a top, top physician in a hospital here in New York City, the head of pediatric endocrinology. [Michael] was put on thyroid medication and two weeks after that he became a normal human being. He exists as any other person, goes to school, and is looking forward to college.

My advice to doctors would be to listen to patients. They are not making up stories. After testing for having perhaps some terrible illness, believe them and believe their parents. A parent lives with a child. A doctor does not, no matter how well meaning he or she may be.

My whole family has learned from this experience to eat as naturally as we can. My son has been allowed to eat outside food but he's old enough now to be in control. And when he doesn't feel well he doesn't repeat the behavior. He is as close to normal as any human being can be in this world.[25]

Migraines

ALLISON:

When I was about three I started getting bad migraine headaches and having severe pain. I would get really tired and very dizzy. It was awful. I would get very sick and incapacitated for about a week before I could get back to a normal type of life.

I went to the local children's hospital where they put me on a lot of medication. I was given a lot of tests including CAT scans and EEGs because they felt that it might be a brain tumor.

My mom thought my problem might be due to allergies and she took me around to several allergists who told her that there was really no way I could be sick from allergies because allergies didn't do this type of thing.

Then she read about Dr. Mandell and called him up. He tested me and it turned out that I was allergic to almost everything there is. I was put on a rotation diet and told to stay away from certain things like grains and milk products. This made me much better.

I still have headaches but they are less frequent, and much less painful. They only last for about a day or two. So, I'm not all the way cured but Dr. Mandell has helped me a great deal.[26]

PART TWO

The No More Allergies Diet

▲

▲

▲

As important as it is to show people the cause and effect between the environment in which they live and their physical and emotional well-being, it's equally important to take the next step, which is to provide them with a step-by-step program of change. Not everyone will be able to go to a physician for multiple tests to determine what they may be allergic to. But everyone can change their diet to some degree.

The facts are that a natural low-allergy or allergy-free diet is less expensive because it eliminates animal proteins—the most costly as well as the most polluted items that we put into our bodies. Secondly, on a diet of this type there is more variety in taste, texture, and color, resulting in foods that are more appetizing and interesting than the traditional meat and potatoes with an occasional vegetable side dish.

I have witnessed thousands of allergy sufferers, from among my radio audience, my family, and friends over the years who have rediscovered with joy that the kitchen need not be a hostile environment. The excitement of creating a dish on your own for the first time and knowing that it's a healthy dish—now that's pleasing.

I am well aware of certain taste preferences to which we have been conditioned from early on in life, such as soft and sweet, salty and crunchy. As a result, whether it's fried chicken or hamburgers with "the works," a jelly roll or ice cream, Americans eat a very limited diet that almost always contains allergy-causing foods.

As we have seen, beef, sugar, corn, wheat, and dairy are primary allergens that can rob you of essential energy. Plain old table sugar, for example, can cause a loss of chromium, zinc, magnesium, and manganese and hence weaken you making you more susceptible to allergy. Yet people are eating these foods several times a day.

I have therefore created a diet with the help of my daughter, Shelly Null, a gourmet natural foods chef, comprised of foods that are inexpensive and easy to prepare, with minimal or no allergenic activity. The eating plan is carefully constructed and designed to lessen the body's burden of toxins and help in the cleansing and revitalization processes that bring one to a state of health. Follow this dietary program and you will be obtaining complex carbohydrates, proteins, essential fatty acids, and the necessary vitamins and minerals.

Recipes

Juices

WATERCRESS CUCUMBER JUICE

2 tablespoons watercress juice (1 ounce)
1/2 cup cucumber juice (1 cucumber)
1 cup pear juice (2 pears)
1/4 cup purple cabbage juice (1/4 small head)

Combine the above ingredients in a glass, mix well, and serve.

MAKES ABOUT 2 CUPS.

KALE AND PURPLE CABBAGE JUICE

1/2 cup apple juice (2 apples)
1 cup carrot juice (2 to 3 carrots)
1/4 cup kale juice (4 leaves)
1/4 cup purple cabbage juice (1/4 small head)
1/4 cup beet juice (2 small beets)
1/2 cup celery juice (3 to 4 stalks)

Combine the above ingredients in a tall glass, mix well, and serve.

MAKES 2 3/4 CUPS.

ORANGE APRICOT JUICE

1 cup orange juice (3 oranges)
1/2 cup apricot juice (4 to 5 apricots)

Combine the above ingredients in a large glass and mix well.

MAKES 1 1/2 CUPS.

ARUGULA CUCUMBER JUICE

1 1/2 tablespoons arugula juice (1/2 ounce)
1 cup pear juice (2 pears)
3/4 cups cucumber juice (1 to 2 cucumbers)

Combine the above ingredients in a large glass, mix well, and serve.

MAKES ABOUT 2 CUPS.

ASPARAGUS CARROT JUICE

1/4 cup asparagus juice (4 to 5 stalks)
1 cup carrot juice (2 to 3 carrots)
1 cup apple juice (3 to 4 apples)

Combine the above ingredients in a large glass, mix well, and serve.

MAKES 2 1/4 CUPS.

WATERMELON BEET JUICE

1 cup watermelon juice (1/4 small watermelon)
1/4 cup beet juice (2 small beets)
1 cup cucumber juice (2 cucumbers)

Combine the above ingredients in a large glass, mix well, and serve.

MAKES 2 1/4 CUPS.

APPLE CHERRY JUICE

1 cup apple juice (3 to 4 apples)
1 1/2 tablespoons cherry juice (1/2 cup fresh or frozen cherries)
1/2 cup celery juice (3 to 4 stalks)

Combine the above ingredients in a large glass, mix well, and serve.

MAKES ABOUT 1 1/2 CUPS.

BANANA ORANGE JUICE

1 1/2 cups orange juice (4 to 5 oranges)
1/4 cup banana pulp (1/2 banana)

Combine the above ingredients in a tall glass, mix well, and serve.

MAKES 1 3/4 CUPS.

APPLE STRAWBERRY JUICE

1 3/4 cups apple juice (5 to 6 apples)
1/4 cup strawberry juice (1/2 pint)

Combine the above ingredients in a large glass, mix well, and serve.

MAKES 2 CUPS.

RASPBERRY PEAR JUICE

1 1/2 cups pear juice (3 to 4 pears)
1/4 cup raspberry juice (1 pint)

Combine the above ingredients in a large glass, mix well, and serve.

MAKES 1 3/4 CUPS.

PINEAPPLE CABBAGE JUICE

1 cup pineapple juice (1/2 pineapple)
1/4 cup purple cabbage juice (1/4 small head)
1/2 cup water

Combine the above ingredients in a large glass, mix well, and serve.

MAKES 1 3/4 CUPS.

CARROT GINGER JUICE

1 cup carrot juice (2 to 3 carrots)
1 tablespoon parsley juice (2 ounces)
1/2 cup cucumber juice (1 cucumber)
1/2 teaspoon ginger juice (1-inch slice gingerroot)

Combine the above ingredients in a large glass, mix well, and serve.

MAKES 1 3/4 CUPS.

APPLE CABBAGE JUICE

1 1/2 cups apple juice (4 to 5 apples)
1/4 cup purple cabbage juice (1/4 small head)

Combine the above ingredients in a large glass, mix well, and serve.

MAKES 1 3/4 CUPS.

CUCUMBER BLUEBERRY JUICE

1 cup cucumber juice (2 cucumbers)
1/4 cup blueberry juice (1/2 pint)
1/2 cup pear juice (1 pear)

Combine the above ingredients in a large glass, mix well, and serve.

MAKES 1 3/4 CUPS.

BOK CHOY GARLIC JUICE

2 tablespoons bok choy juice (2 leaves)
1 cup apple juice (3 to 4 apples)
1/2 teaspoon garlic juice (3 cloves)

Combine the above ingredients in a large glass, mix well, and serve.

MAKES 1 1/8 CUPS.

CAULIFLOWER LEMON JUICE

1/2 cup cauliflower juice (1/4 small head steamed for 3 minutes)
1 cup pear juice (2 pears)
1/4 cup celery juice (2 stalks)
1 1/2 tablespoons lemon juice (1 lemon)

Combine the above ingredients in a large glass, mix well, and serve.

MAKES ABOUT 1 1/2 CUPS.

KALE AND CARROT JUICE

1/4 cup kale juice (4 leaves)
3/4 cup carrot juice (2 carrots)
1/2 cup cucumber juice (1 cucumber)

Combine the above ingredients in a large glass, mix well, and serve.

MAKES 1 1/2 CUPS.

CUCUMBER PARSLEY JUICE

1 cup cucumber juice (2 cucumbers)
1 1/2 tablespoons parsley juice (1 ounce)
1/2 cup celery juice (3 stalks)

Combine the above ingredients in a large glass, mix well, and serve.

MAKES ABOUT 1 1/2 CUPS.

CRANBERRY GRAPE JUICE

3/4 cup grape juice (1/2 bunch green seedless)
2 tablespoons cranberry juice (1/4 cup cranberries)
1/2 cup cucumber juice (1 cucumber)
1/2 cup apple juice (2 apples)

Combine the above ingredients in a large glass, mix well, and serve.

MAKES ABOUT 1 3/4 CUPS.

CRANBERRY GINGER JUICE

1 cup grape juice (3/4 bunch green seedless)
1/4 cup cranberry juice (1/2 cup cranberries)
1/2 cup celery juice (3 to 4 stalks)
1/2 teaspoon ginger juice

Combine the above ingredients in a large glass, mix well, and serve.

MAKES 2 1/4 CUPS.

CRANBERRY ORANGE JUICE

2 cups orange juice (5 to 6 oranges)
1/4 cup cranberry juice (1/2 cup cranberries)

Combine the above ingredients in a large glass, mix well, and serve.

MAKES 2 1/4 CUPS.

MIXED VEGETABLE JUICE

1/4 cup celery juice (1 to 2 stalks)
1/2 cup cucumber juice (1 cucumber)
1/4 cup beet juice (2 small beets)
2 tablespoons green bell pepper juice (1/2 pepper)
1/2 cup pear juice (1 pear)
1/2 cup carrot juice (1 carrot)

Combine the above ingredients in a tall glass, mix well, and serve.

MAKES ABOUT 2 CUPS.

APRICOT LEMON JUICE

1 cup apple juice (3 to 4 apples)
1/2 cup apricot juice (8 apricots)
2 tablespoons lemon juice (1 to 2 lemons)
1 cup cucumber juice (2 cucumbers)

Combine the above ingredients in a tall glass, mix well, and serve.

MAKES ABOUT 2 1/2 CUPS.

APPLE KALE JUICE

1 1/4 cups apple juice (4 apples)
1/2 cup kale juice (4 leaves)
1/2 cup carrot juice (1 carrot)

Combine the above ingredients in a large glass, mix well, and serve.

MAKES 2 1/4 CUPS.

ORANGE BEET JUICE

1 1/2 cups orange juice (4 to 5 oranges)
1/4 cup beet juice (2 small beets)
1/2 cup celery juice (3 to 4 stalks)

Combine the above ingredients in a large glass, mix well, and serve.

MAKES 2 1/4 CUPS.

NECTARINE SPROUT JUICE

1 cup apple juice (3 to 4 apples)
1/4 cup collard green juice (4 leaves)
2 tablespoons alfalfa sprout juice (1 1/2 cups sprouts)
1/4 cup nectarine juice (1 nectarine)

Combine the above ingredients in a large glass, mix well, and serve.

MAKES ABOUT 1 1/2 CUPS.

SWISS CHARD CARROT JUICE

1 cup carrot juice (2 to 3 carrots)
1/4 cup Swiss chard juice (4 leaves)
1/2 cup cucumber juice (1 cucumber)
2 tablespoons green bell pepper juice (1/2 pepper)

Combine the above ingredients in a large glass, mix well, and serve.

MAKES ABOUT 1 3/4 CUPS.

PEACH KIWI JUICE

1 cup peach juice (3 peaches)
1/4 cup kiwi juice (3 kiwis)
1/2 cup apple juice (2 apples)
2 tablespoons alfalfa sprout juice (1 1/2 cups sprouts)

Combine the above ingredients in a large glass, mix well, and serve.

MAKES ABOUT 1 3/4 CUPS.

NECTARINE CARROT JUICE

1/2 cup apple juice (2 apples)
1/2 cup carrot juice (1 carrot)
3/4 cup nectarine juice (2 to 3 nectarines)
1/2 cup cucumber juice (1 cucumber)

Combine the above ingredients in a large glass, mix well, and serve.

MAKES 2 1/4 CUPS.

MANGO CHERRY JUICE

1 cup cucumber juice (2 cucumbers)
1/2 cup mango juice (1 mango)
2 tablespoons cherry juice (1/2 cup fresh or frozen cherries)

Combine the above ingredients in a large glass, mix well, and serve.

MAKES ABOUT 1 1/2 CUPS.

LEMON CANTALOUPE JUICE

1 1/2 tablespoons lemon juice (1 lemon)
2 cups cantaloupe juice (2 melons)

Combine the above ingredients in a large glass, mix well, and serve.

MAKES ABOUT 2 CUPS.

CUCUMBER SPROUT JUICE

1 cup cucumber juice (2 cucumbers)
1 1/2 tablespoons alfalfa sprout juice (1 cup sprouts)
1/2 cup apple juice (3 to 4 apples)

Combine the above ingredients in a large glass, mix well, and serve.

MAKES ABOUT 1 1/2 CUPS.

PLUM GRAPE JUICE

1 cup plum juice (4 to 6 sweet, peeled plums)
1/2 cup grape juice (1/3 bunch concord grapes)
1/2 cup cucumber juice (1 cucumber)

Combine the above ingredients in a large glass, mix well, and serve.

MAKES 2 CUPS.

PINEAPPLE LEMON JUICE

3/4 cups pineapple juice (1/2 pineapple)
1 1/2 tablespoons lemon juice (1 lemon)
1/2 cup water

Combine the above ingredients in a large glass, mix well, and serve.

MAKES ABOUT 1 CUP.

SWISS CHARD AND ZUCCHINI JUICE

1 cup carrot juice (2 carrots)
2 tablespoons zucchini juice (1/2 zucchini)
2 tablespoons Swiss chard juice (2 leaves)
1/4 cup tomato juice (1 tomato)
dash of cayenne pepper

Combine the above ingredients in a tall glass, mix well, and serve.

MAKES 1 1/2 CUPS.

ALFALFA SPROUT AND BEET JUICE

1 1/2 tablespoons alfalfa sprout juice (1 cup sprouts)
2 tablespoons kale juice (2 leaves)
1 cup pear juice (2 pears)
1/4 cup beet juice (2 small beets)

Combine the above ingredients in a tall glass, mix well, and serve.

MAKES ABOUT 1 1/2 CUPS.

CASABA AND PEACH JUICE

2 cups casaba melon juice (3/4 large melon)
3/4 cup peach juice (2 to 3 peaches)
1 tablespoon lemon juice (1 lemon)

Combine the above ingredients in a tall glass, mix well, and serve.

MAKES ABOUT 2 3/4 CUPS.

SPECIAL MIXED VEGETABLE SURPRISE

1 cup carrot juice (2 carrots)
1/4 cup tomato juice (1 tomato)
1 1/2 tablespoons alfalfa sprout juice (1 cup sprouts)
1/4 cup beet juice (2 small beets)
1/2 cup celery juice (4 stalks)
1 1/2 tablespoons romaine lettuce juice (2 leaves)
2 tablespoons green bell pepper juice (1/2 pepper)

Combine the above ingredients in a tall glass, mix well, and serve.

MAKES ABOUT 2 1/4 CUPS.

CARROT PLUM JUICE

1 cup carrot juice (2 carrots)
1/2 cup plum juice (2 to 3 plums)
1/2 cup apple juice (2 apples)

Combine the above ingredients in a tall glass, mix well, and serve.

MAKES 2 CUPS.

CASABA WATERMELON JUICE

1 cup casaba melon juice (1/4 to 1/2 melon)
1 1/2 cups watermelon juice (1/4 to 1/2 small watermelon)

Combine the above ingredients in a tall glass, mix well, and serve.

MAKES 2 1/2 CUPS.

CRENSHAW MELON JUICE

2 1/2 cups Crenshaw melon juice (1/2 melon)
2 tablespoon lemon juice (1 to 2 lemons)

Combine the above ingredients in a tall glass, mix well, and serve.

MAKES ABOUT 2 1/2 CUPS.

TROPICAL SURPRISE JUICE

1 1/2 cups orange juice (4 to 5 oranges)
1/2 cup banana pulp (1 banana)
1/4 cup pineapple juice (1 cup pineapple)
1 1/2 tablespoons cherry juice (1/2 cup fresh or frozen cherries)

Combine the above ingredients in a tall glass, mix well, and serve.

MAKES ABOUT 2 1/4 CUPS.

SWISS CHARD CELERY JUICE

2 tablespoons Swiss chard juice (2 leaves)
1 cup apple juice (3 to 4 apples)
1 cup celery juice (6 to 8 stalks)

Combine the above ingredients in a large glass, mix well, and serve.

MAKES ABOUT 2 CUPS.

PARSLEY KALE JUICE

1 cup apple juice (3 to 4 apples)
2 tablespoons kale juice (2 leaves)
1 1/2 tablespoons parsley juice (1 ounce)

Combine the above ingredients in a large glass, mix well, and serve.

MAKES ABOUT 1 1/4 CUPS.

Breakfast

AMARANTH WITH PEACHES AND BANANAS

2 1/2 cups water
2 cups coconut milk
1 cup amaranth
1 cup sliced peaches (fresh or frozen)
1 teaspoon pure almond extract
1 banana, sliced
1 tablespoon pure maple syrup
1/2 teaspoon cinnamon

In a medium-size saucepan combine the water and coconut milk. Bring to a boil and reduce heat to medium. Add the remaining ingredients and cook uncovered over medium heat for 15 to 20 minutes. Serve hot or cold with rice milk or soy milk.

SERVES 2.

CREAMY RISOTTO WITH CARDAMOM

2 1/2 cups water
2 1/2 cups unsweetened soy milk
1 tablespoon pure maple syrup
1/4 teaspoon cardamom powder
1/8 cup raisins
3 tablespoons ground unsalted almonds or pistachios

In a medium-size saucepan combine the water and soy milk. Bring to a boil and reduce heat to medium. Add the maple syrup, cardamom, and raisins and stir well. Continue to cook uncovered over medium heat for 10 to 15 minutes, stirring periodically. Sprinkle with the nuts and serve hot or cold.

SERVES 2.

CREAM OF BARLEY WITH OATS

3 cups water
2 cups Barley Plus (Erewhon)
1 cup rolled oats
1 banana, sliced
1 teaspoon pure vanilla extract

In a medium-size saucepan bring the water to a boil then reduce heat to medium. Add the barley cereal and whisk in to prevent clumping. Add the remaining ingredients, stir well, and continue to cook uncovered over medium heat for 10 to 15 minutes. Serve hot or cold with soy milk or rice milk.

SERVES 2.

MILLET WITH CINNAMON AND SPICE

3 cups water
1/2 cup millet
1/2 cup rolled oats
1/3 cup raw unsalted sunflower seeds
1/3 cup raisins
1 teaspoon pure vanilla extract
1/4 teaspoon cinnamon
1/2 cup toasted wheat germ

In a medium-size saucepan bring the water to a boil and reduce heat to medium. Add the remaining ingredients, except the wheat germ. Simmer uncovered over medium heat for 15 to 20 minutes until all of the water is absorbed. Serve hot or cold with soy milk or rice milk.

SERVES 2.

CREAM OF BUCKWHEAT WITH HONEY

4 1/2 cups water
1 1/2 cups Cream of Buckwheat cereal (Erewhon)
1/2 cup unsweetened flaked coconut
1 cup sliced banana
2 tablespoons light pure honey (tupelo or wildflower)
1/2 teaspoon pure vanilla extract
1/4 cup raw unsalted sunflower seeds
1 teaspoon cinnamon

In a medium-size saucepan bring the water to a boil then reduce heat to medium. Whisk in the buckwheat. Add the remaining ingredients and continue to cook uncovered for an additional 10 to 15 minutes until all of the water is absorbed. Serve hot or cold with soy milk or rice milk.

SERVES 2.

QUINOA WITH DATES AND PECANS

2 1/2 cups water
1 cup apple juice
1 1/2 cups quinoa
1/4 cup unsalted pecans
1/8 cup chopped pitted dates
1 tablespoon pure maple syrup
1 teaspoon pure vanilla extract
2 1/2 teaspoons unsweetened carob powder

In a medium-size saucepan combine the water and juice. Bring to a boil and reduce heat to medium. Add the remaining ingredients and stir well. Continue cooking uncovered over medium heat for 10 to 15 minutes or until all of the liquid is absorbed. Serve hot or cold with soy milk or rice milk.

SERVES 2.

QUINOA WITH PEACHES AND CREAM

2 1/2 cups water
1 1/4 cups rice milk (Rice Dream)
1 1/2 cups quinoa
1 teaspoon pure vanilla extract
3 tablespoons pure maple syrup
1/2 cup sliced peaches (fresh or frozen)
1/2 cup sliced bananas

In a medium-size saucepan bring the water and rice milk to a boil. Reduce heat to medium and add the quinoa. Continue to cook over medium heat until the liquid is absorbed, about 15 minutes. Stir in the remaining ingredients and serve with additional rice milk.

SERVES 2.

GOOD MORNING KASHA

1 cup raw kasha
2 cups water
1 cup rice milk (Rice Dream)
1/2 cup unsweetened flaked coconut
1/4 cup raisins
1/3 cup unsalted walnuts
3 tablespoons pure maple syrup
2 teaspoons pure vanilla extract
1/2 teaspoon cinnamon

Rinse the kasha and remove any small stones. In a medium-size saucepan bring the water and rice milk to a boil. Reduce heat to medium and add the remaining ingredients. Cook uncovered over medium heat for 15 minutes or until all of the liquid is absorbed. Serve hot or cold with rice milk or juice.

SERVES 2.

MILLET WITH CHERRIES

3 cups water
2/3 cups millet
3 tablespoons pure maple syrup
1 teaspoon pure almond extract
1/8 cup unsweetened coconut
1/3 cup chopped unsalted almonds
1/4 cup unsweetened pitted cherries (fresh or frozen)

Bring the water to a boil in a medium-size saucepan. Add the millet and cook uncovered over high heat for 15 minutes. Stir in the remaining ingredients and serve hot or cold with rice milk or soy milk.

SERVES 2.

PUMPKIN AND SPICE PANCAKES

2 eggs (use egg replacer)
1/2 cup unsweetened pumpkin puree
1 cup water
1 teaspoon pure vanilla extract
1 1/4 cups buckwheat flour
1/2 teaspoon baking soda
1/2 teaspoon baking powder
dash of cinnamon
3 tablespoons canola oil

In a large bowl whisk together the eggs or egg replacer, pumpkin puree, water, and vanilla. Add the dry ingredients and stir well. Heat a frying pan over high heat until a drop of oil placed in the pan sizzles. Pour one tablespoon of the canola oil into the frying pan and heat for one minute. Reduce the heat to medium and pour one-third of the batter into the frying pan. Cook uncovered over medium heat for 3 to 5 minutes or until bubbles form on top of the pancake. Flip the pancake over and cook it for an additional 2 minutes. Cut the pancake into nine pieces with a knife and continue cooking an additional minute. Serve hot with fruit canton (see pages 272–273) or pure maple syrup. Repeat procedure to make the remaining pancakes.

SERVES 2 TO 3.

BLUE CORN AND PECAN PANCAKES

2 eggs (use egg replacer)
1 cup rice milk (Rice Dream)
1 teaspoon pure almond extract

1 1/4 cups stone-ground whole wheat flour
1/2 cup blue cornmeal
3/4 teaspoon baking powder
1/2 teaspoon baking soda
dash of nutmeg
3 tablespoons canola oil

In a large bowl whisk together the eggs or egg replacer, rice milk, and almond extract. In a medium bowl sift together the dry ingredients and add to the egg mixture. Heat a frying pan over high heat until a drop of oil placed on the pan sizzles. Pour one tablespoon of canola oil into the frying pan and heat for one minute. Reduce heat to medium and pour one-third of the batter into the frying pan. Cook uncovered over medium heat for 3 to 5 minutes until bubbles form on top of the pancake. Flip the pancake over and cook for an additional 2 minutes. Cut the pancake into nine pieces with a knife and cook an additional minute. Serve hot with fruit canton (see pages 272–273) or pure maple syrup. Repeat this procedure to make the remaining pancakes.

SERVES 2 TO 3.

BARLEY GRITS WITH BANANAS AND COCONUT

3 cups water
1 cup barley grits
1 banana, sliced
1/3 cup unsalted Brazil nuts
1/3 cup unsweetened flaked coconut
1 teaspoon pure vanilla extract

In a medium-size saucepan bring the water to a boil. Whisk in the grits, then add the remaining ingredients and stir well. Reduce heat to medium and cook uncovered for 10 to 15 minutes or until all of the water is absorbed. Serve hot or cold with rice milk or juice.

SERVES 2.

BARLEY PANCAKES WITH PUMPKIN SEEDS

2 eggs (use egg replacer)
2 1/4 cups water
1 1/2 cups stone-ground barley & soy flour
1 1/4 teaspoons baking powder
1/2 teaspoon baking soda
1/2 cup unsalted pecans
1/2 cup unsalted pumpkin seeds
1 teaspoon pure almond extract
1/4 teaspoon nutmeg
1/4 cup unsweetened flaked coconut
4 to 6 tablespoons canola oil for frying

In a large mixing bowl combine the eggs or egg replacer with the water. Whisk in the flour, baking powder, and baking soda. Add the remaining ingredients except the oil and mix well. Heat a large frying pan until a drop of oil placed on the pan sizzles, then add 1 tablespoon of the oil and heat for 20 seconds. Pour one-quarter of the batter into the pan, reduce heat to medium, and cook for 2 to 3 minutes. Turn the pancake over and cook for 2 more minutes then cut into twelve pieces. Cook an additional 1 to 2 minutes. Serve hot with pure maple syrup or any other sweetener. Repeat this procedure for the remaining pancakes.

SERVES 2.

KASHA WITH PUMPKIN SEEDS AND PEARS

3 cups water
1 cup kasha
1/4 cup unsweetened flaked coconut
1/4 cup pumpkin seeds
1 cup diced pears
3 tablespoons pure light honey (tupelo or wildflower) or pure maple syrup

In a medium-size saucepan bring the water to a boil. Add the kasha, reduce heat to medium, and cook for 3 minutes. Add the remaining ingredients and continue to cook uncovered for an additional 5 to 10 minutes or until the water is absorbed. Serve hot or cold with soy milk or rice milk.

SERVES 2.

CREAM OF RICE WITH APPLES AND PEARS

4 1/2 cups water
1 1/2 cup Cream of Rice cereal (Erewhon)
1 cup sliced banana
2 tablespoons pure maple syrup
1 teaspoon pure vanilla extract
1/4 cup chopped unpeeled apples
1/4 cup chopped unpeeled pear

In a medium-size saucepan bring the water to a boil then reduce heat to medium. Whisk in the rice cereal. Add the remaining ingredients and continue to cook uncovered for an additional 10 to 15 minutes, until all of the water is absorbed. Serve hot or cold with soy milk or rice milk.

SERVES 2.

CREAM OF BARLEY WITH QUINOA

3 cups water
2 cups Barley Plus (Erewhon)
1 cup quinoa
1 banana, sliced
1 teaspoon pure almond extract
1/2 cup chopped dates

In a medium-size saucepan bring the water to a boil then reduce heat to medium. Whisk in the barley cereal. Add the remaining ingredients, stir well, and continue to cook uncovered over medium heat for 10 to 15 minutes. Serve hot or cold with soy milk or rice milk.

SERVES 2.

CAROB CHIP GRANOLA

1 cup rolled oats
1 1/4 cups unsweetened flaked coconut
1/2 cup unsalted walnuts
1/4 cup raisins
1/4 cup diced dried unsulfured apple slices
3/4 cup unsweetened carob chips
1/4 cup diced dried unsulfured apricots
1/4 cup sesame seeds

1/4 cup unsalted sunflower seeds
1/4 cup unsalted pumpkin seeds
3/4 tupelo honey (any light honey may be substituted)
1/2 teaspoon nutmeg

Preheat oven to 350 degrees. In a large mixing bowl combine the above ingredients and mix well. Place the mixture onto a greased cookie sheet and bake for 15 to 20 minutes or until light brown in color. Cool and store at room temperature in an airtight container for up to one week.

MAKES 5 CUPS.

VERY BERRY GRANOLA

2 cups rolled wheat flakes (rye flakes may be substituted)
1/2 cup sweet brown rice syrup
1/4 cup pure maple syrup
1/4 cup dried unsulfured cherries
1/2 cup dried unsulfured blueberries
1/2 cup finely chopped pitted dates
1 cup unsweetened flaked coconut
1/2 teaspoon pure almond extract
1/2 teaspoon cinnamon

Preheat oven to 350 degrees. Combine the above ingredients in a large mixing bowl and mix well. Place the mixture onto a greased cookie sheet and bake for 15 to 20 minutes or until light brown in color. Let the granola cool and store in an airtight container at room temperature for up to one week.

MAKES 4 1/4 CUPS.

NUTTY GRANOLA

2 cups rolled oats
1/4 cup pitted and chopped dates
1/4 cup dried blueberries (raisins may be substituted)
1/2 cup unsalted almonds
1/4 cup unsalted walnuts
1/4 cup unsalted pecans
1 teaspoon pure almond extract
1/4 cup sweet rice syrup
1/4 cup pure maple syrup

Preheat the oven to 350 degrees. Combine the above ingredients in a large mixing bowl and toss well. Spread the mixture onto a greased cookie sheet. Bake for 15 to 20 minutes or until light brown in color. Let the granola cool and store in an airtight container at room temperature for up to one week.

MAKES 3 1/4 CUPS.

Soups

NAVY BEAN AND SWEET POTATO SOUP

10 cups water
1 1/4 cups navy beans (uncooked)
2 teaspoons canola oil (or any flavorless oil)
1/4 cup chopped leeks
1/4 cup chopped sweet potatoes with skin
1/4 cup chopped parsnips
1/2 teaspoon sea salt
1/2 teaspoon black pepper

In a large saucepan bring the water to a boil. Add the remaining ingredients and cook over medium to high heat for 2 1/2 to 3 hours. When the beans are done the soup is done. Serve hot with whole grain bread.

SERVE 2 TO 4.

MINESTRONE SOUP

1/4 cups chopped yellow onion
1/4 cup chopped leeks
2 cups diced tomatoes (canned or fresh)
1/4 cup extra virgin olive oil
3 1/2 to 4 cups water
1 1/2 cups diced carrots
1 cup diced russet potatoes
2 cloves garlic, crushed
2 tablespoons chopped Italian parsley
1 1/2 tablespoons chopped basil
1 bay leaf
1/2 teaspoon sea salt
1/2 teaspoon black pepper
1 cup macaroni or noodles (De Bole's pasta)
1/2 cup chopped kale
1 cup white beans (cooked)
1/4 cup diced zucchini squash

In a large saucepan sauté the onions, leeks, and tomatoes in the olive oil for 5 minutes. Add the water and bring to a boil. Reduce heat to medium and add the carrots, potatoes, garlic, parsley, basil, bay leaf, salt, and pepper. Cook partially covered over medium heat for 15 to 20 minutes. Add the noodles, kale, beans, and zucchini and cook for an additional 15 to 20 minutes or until the noodles are done. Serve hot with whole grain bread.

SERVES 2 TO 4.

SPICY VEGETABLE SOUP STOCK

8 cups water
1 cup sliced carrots
1/2 cup sliced onions
1/2 cup sliced celery
2 cloves garlic, crushed
1 cup sliced leeks
1/2 cup diced tomatoes (canned or fresh)
1 teaspoon black peppercorns
4 to 5 whole cloves
2 bay leaves
2 tablespoons chopped parsley
1/2 teaspoon sea salt

In a large saucepan bring the water to a boil. Add the remaining ingredients and simmer partially covered for 1 hour and 20 minutes. Pour the mixture through a sieve over a large bowl. Reserve the liquid and discard the vegetables. This broth can be frozen or stored for three days refrigerated. Try adding ¼ cup fish, whole grain noodles, or vegetables for a simple soup.

MAKES 1 1/4 CUPS.

SPINACH DUMPLING SOUP

1 cup chopped spinach leaves
2 eggs (use egg replacer)
1/2 cup stone-ground whole wheat flour (oat flour may be substituted)
1/4 teaspoon sea salt
1 recipe Spicy Vegetable Soup Stock (see page 212)

In a blender or food processor combine everything except the soup stock. Process for 30 seconds or until a dough is formed. Flour your hands and roll the dough into twelve ¾-inch balls. In a medium-size saucepan bring the soup stock to a boil. Add the dumplings and cook for 4 to 5 minutes. Serve hot with salad.

SERVES 2.

HEARTY SPLIT PEA SOUP

2 cups Spicy Vegetable Soup Stock (see page 212)
6 cups water
1 cup green split peas
1 1/2 cups chopped tomatoes (canned or fresh)
1/4 cup chopped yellow onion
1/2 cup chopped celery
1 clove garlic, chopped
1/2 cup diced carrots
1/2 teaspoon sea salt
1/2 teaspoon black pepper

In a medium-size saucepan bring the soup stock and water to a boil. Reduce heat to medium and add the split peas. Continue to cook for 30 minutes. Add the remaining ingredients and cook an additional 20 to 30 minutes or until the split peas are soft. Serve hot with whole grain bread.

SERVES 2 TO 4.

CREAM OF MUSHROOM SOUP

2 1/2 cups sliced mushrooms
1/2 cup sliced celery
2 tablespoons canola oil
2 1/4 cups unsweetened soy milk or rice milk (Rice Dream)
1/4 cup chopped fresh dill
1/4 cup chopped fresh parsley
1/2 teaspoon sea salt
1/4 teaspoon black pepper
2 to 4 tablespoons millet (optional)

In a medium-size saucepan sauté the mushrooms and celery in the oil. Add the remaining ingredients and bring to a boil. Reduce the heat and simmer covered for 15 minutes. Serve hot with salad and whole grain bread.

SERVES 2.

Salads

LEAFY SALAD WITH ROASTED RED PEPPERS

4 cups Boston lettuce
1 1/2 cups sliced tomatoes
1/2 cup sliced roasted red peppers
1/2 cup sliced Bermuda onion
1/4 cup sliced basil leaves
1/2 cup Honey Mustard Dressing (*see page 241, 243*)

Combine the above ingredients in a large salad bowl and toss. Serve with almost any meal.

SERVES 2.

ARTICHOKE SALAD WITH MUSTARD DILL DRESSING

2 cups steamed, sliced beets
1 1/2 cups marinated artichoke hearts
1 1/4 cups garbanzo beans (cooked)
1/2 to 2 cups Mustard Dill Dressing (see page 239)

Combine the above ingredients in a large mixing bowl and toss gently. Serve chilled or at room temperature with fish or a sandwich.

SERVES 2.

FENNEL SALAD WITH LIME DRESSING

2 cups sliced fresh fennel (uncooked)
1 cup sliced avocado
1 cup mung bean sprouts
1/2 cup sliced Bermuda onion
1/2 cup Lime Dressing (see page 239)

Combine the fennel, avocado, sprouts, and onion in a large salad bowl and drizzle with the salad dressing. Serve with soup or a sandwich.

SERVES 2.

ARUGULA SALAD WITH RASPBERRY VINAIGRETTE

3 cups arugula leaves
2 cups Boston lettuce
1 cup halved cherry tomatoes
1/2 cup pignoli nuts
1/2 cup Raspberry Vinaigrette (see page 235)

Combine the above ingredients in a large salad bowl and toss well. Serve with soup or whole grain bread.

SERVES 2.

BRAISED LEEK SALAD

6 halved leeks, steamed for 5 minutes then allowed to cool to room temperature
1/2 cups Lemony Herb Dressing (see page 237)

Place the leeks onto a plate and drizzle with the dressing. Serve at room temperature with soup and whole grain bread.

SERVES 2.

TANGY CABBAGE SALAD WITH ORANGES AND GINGER

1 1/2 cups thinly sliced purple cabbage
1/2 cup seeded orange segments
1 cup thinly sliced green cabbage
1 cup very thinly sliced carrot strips
1/2 cup diced Bermuda onion
1/2 cup black walnuts
1/2 cup raisins
1/2 to 2/3 cups Orange Ginger Dressing *(see page 236)*

Combine the above ingredients in a large salad bowl and toss well. Serve chilled or at room temperature with almost any dish.

SERVES 2.

DANDELION SALAD

3 cups sliced dandelion greens
1 cup chopped apricots
1 cup sliced red bell pepper
1/2 cup Cherry Vinaigrette *(see page 234)*

Combine the above ingredients in a salad bowl and toss well. Serve chilled or at room temperature with soup and whole grain bread.

SERVES 2.

WATERCRESS SALAD

3 cups watercress
1 cup diced apples with skin
1 cup thinly sliced beets (peeled and steamed for 10 minutes)
1/2 to 2/3 cups Basil Vinaigrette (see page 242)

Combine the above ingredients in a large salad bowl and toss well. Serve chilled or at room temperature with soup or a sandwich.

SERVES 2.

SWISS CHARD SALAD WITH SWEET TARRAGON DRESSING

1 cup mache leaves
1/2 cup sliced basil leaves
2 cups sliced Swiss chard
1 cup sliced avocado
1 cup lentil sprouts (almost any type may be substituted)
1/2 to 2/3 cups Sweet Tarragon Dressing (see page 238)

Combine the above ingredients in a large salad bowl and mix well. Serve chilled or at room temperature with almost any meal.

SERVES 2.

BELGIAN ENDIVE SALAD

2 cups Belgian endive leaves
2 cups mache leaves
1 cup diced red bell pepper

1/4 cup walnut oil (optional)
1/2 cup black walnuts
1/2 to 2/3 cups Basil Vinaigrette (see page 242)

Combine the endive, mache, red pepper, and walnut oil, if using, in a large salad bowl. Sprinkle the walnuts on top of the salad and drizzle with the vinaigrette dressing. Serve with soup or a sandwich.

SERVES 2.

ARAME SALAD WITH PECANS

2 cups arame (soaked in boiling water then drained)
1 1/2 cups deseeded tangerine segments
1/2 cup unsalted pecans
2/3 cups Orange Ginger Dressing (see page 236)
2 tablespoons sweet rice vinegar

Combine the above ingredients in a large salad bowl and toss well. Serve chilled or at room temperature with soup and whole grain bread.

SERVES 2.

CHINESE GREEN BEAN SALAD

1 cup steamed wax beans
1 1/2 cups steamed Chinese long beans
1 cup steamed green beans
1/2 to 2/3 cup Tomato Vinaigrette (see page 241)
1/4 cup sesame seeds

Place the beans on a plate and drizzle with the salad dressing. Sprinkle with sesame seeds and serve at room temperature with any whole grain entrée.

SERVES 2.

ASSORTED ZUCCHINI SALAD

2 cups baby zucchini or diced large zucchini (steamed for 5 minutes)
1 1/2 cups tiny patty pan squash or diced yellow zucchini (steamed for 5 minutes)
1 cup sliced red bell pepper
1/2 to 2/3 cups Spicy Thai Dressing (see page 236)
1/4 cup black sesame seeds (white may be substituted)

Combine everything except the sesame seeds in a large salad bowl and toss well. Top with sesame seeds and serve at room temperature with soup and whole grain bread.

SERVES 2.

BRUSSELS SPROUT SALAD WITH CREAMY CHESTNUT SAUCE

3 cups brussels sprouts (halved then steamed for 5 minutes)
1/2 to 2/3 cups Creamy Chestnut Sauce (see page 246)
1 cup unsweetened chopped chestnuts (steamed for 10 to 15 minutes)

Place the brussels sprouts in a salad bowl and drizzle with the chestnut dressing. Sprinkle with the chestnuts and serve chilled or at room temperature with almost any meal.

SERVES 2.

WALDORF WATERCRESS SALAD

3 to 4 cups watercress
1 tablespoon lemon juice
1 cup chopped apples with skin
1/2 cup unsalted walnuts
1/4 cup Sweet Tarragon Dressing (see page 238)

Combine the above ingredients into a medium-size mixing bowl, toss well, and chill for one hour. Serve with almost any meal.

SERVES 2.

CURLY ENDIVE AND CRUNCHY SPROUT SALAD

1 cup chopped curly endive
1/2 cup whole arugula leaves
1 cup sliced Swiss chard
1 1/2 cups crunchy sprouts (any type may be substituted)
1 cup sliced red bell pepper
2 to 4 tablespoons Dijon Dressing (see page 235)

Combine the above ingredients in a large mixing bowl, toss well, and serve with almost any meal.

SERVES 2.

PAPAYA AND AVOCADO SALAD

1 cup sliced papaya
2 tablespoons papaya pits
1 cup sliced avocado
1/2 cup diced Bermuda onion
1 cup peeled and diced cucumber
1/4 cup Honey Mustard Dressing (see page 241, 243)

Combine the above ingredients in a large mixing bowl, toss well, and serve with almost any meal.

SERVES 2.

ESCAROLE WITH BRAZIL NUTS

2 cups sliced escarole
1 cup sliced red leaf lettuce
1 1/2 cups butternut squash (steamed for 10 minutes then diced)
1/2 cup chopped Brazil nuts
1/4 cup Creamy Garlic Dressing (page 238)

Combine the above ingredients in a medium-size mixing bowl, toss well, and serve with almost any meal.

SERVES 2.

PURPLE CABBAGE AND POPPY SEED SALAD

2 cups thinly sliced purple cabbage
2 cups finely chopped curly escarole
2/3 cup poppy seeds
1/4 cup Basil Vinaigrette (page 242)

Combine the above ingredients in a medium-size mixing bowl, toss well, and serve with almost any meal.

SERVES 2.

MACHE WITH GREEN GRAPES AND RADISH SPROUTS

1 cup Belgian endive leaves
2 cups mache leaves
1/2 cup halved, seedless green grapes
1/2 cup radish sprouts
1/2 cup Dijon Dressing (see page 235)

Combine the above ingredients in a medium-size mixing bowl, toss well, and serve with almost any meal.

SERVES 2.

ROMAINE WITH FRESH BASIL

1 1/2 cups sliced escarole
1 1/2 cups sliced romaine lettuce
1/2 cup thinly sliced basil leaves
1/2 cup peeled and thinly sliced daikon radish
1/4 cup Dijon Dressing (page 235)

Combine the above ingredients in a medium-size mixing bowl, toss well, and serve with almost any meal.

SERVES 2.

ASPARAGUS AND CARROTS DIJON

3 cups white and green asparagus (steamed for 5 minutes)
1 cup very thinly sliced carrot strips (steamed for 3 minutes)
1/4 cup Dijon Dressing (see page 235)

Combine the above ingredients in a medium-size mixing bowl, toss well, and serve with almost any meal.

SERVES 2.

ARUGULA WITH LEMON AND HERBS

3 cups arugula leaves
1 cup diced beets (peeled and steamed for 10 minutes)
2 tablespoons sesame seeds
1/4 cup Lemony Herb Dressing (see page 237)

Combine the above ingredients in a medium-size mixing bowl, toss well, and serve with almost any meal.

SERVES 2.

SORREL AND RADICCHIO DI VERNON SALAD

2 cups sorrel leaves
1 cup sliced radicchio leaves
1/4 cup pignoli nuts
1/4 cup Honey Mustard Dressing (see page 241, 243)

Combine the above ingredients in a large mixing bowl, toss well, and serve with almost any meal.

SERVES 2.

PURPLE CABBAGE AND PINEAPPLE SALAD

3 cups thinly sliced purple cabbage
1 cup cubed fresh pineapple
1/2 cup deseeded orange slices
1/4 cup unsalted pecans
1/4 cup Orange Ginger Dressing (see page 236)

Combine the above ingredients in a large salad bowl, toss well, and serve with soup and whole grain bread.

SERVES 2.

MIDDLE EASTERN SALAD

2 cups chopped tomatoes
1 1/2 cups chopped cucumber
1/4 cup chopped Bermuda onion
1 teaspoon chopped fresh mint
1/2 cup chopped Italian parsley
3/4 cup chopped green bell pepper
1/2 cup Tomato Vinaigrette (see page 241)

Combine the above ingredients in a large salad bowl, mix well, and serve with soup and whole grain bread.

SERVES 2.

RED LEAF AND BEET SALAD

1 1/2 cups chopped red leaf lettuce
1 1/2 cups sliced Boston lettuce
1 cup chopped cucumber
1 cup chopped beets (peeled and steamed for 10 minutes)
1/4 cup Mustard Dill Dressing (see page 239)

In a large salad bowl toss together everything except the salad dressing. Drizzle the dressing over the salad and serve with soup and whole grain bread.

SERVES 2.

SOUTHERN TOMATO SALAD

4 cups sliced tomatoes
1 cup sliced Bermuda onion
2 cups peeled and sliced cucumber
1/4 cup apple cider vinegar
3 cups Boston lettuce leaves

Combine the tomatoes, onion, cucumber, and vinegar in a large bowl and refrigerate for one-half hour. Serve chilled over a bed of Boston lettuce leaves with almost any meal.

SERVES 2.

TRICOLOR PEPPER SALAD

1 cup sliced red bell pepper
1 cup sliced green bell pepper
1 cup sliced yellow or orange bell pepper
3 cups sliced red leaf lettuce
1/4 cup Basil Vinaigrette (see page 242)

Combine the above ingredients in a large salad bowl. Toss well and serve with almost any meal.

SERVES 2.

ASSORTED BOK CHOY SALAD

1 cup sliced long bok choy
1 cup chopped short bok choy
1 cup diced Tientsin bok choy
1 cup mung bean sprouts
1/4 cup unsalted walnuts
1/4 cup poppy seeds
1/4 cup Spicy Thai Dressing (see page 236)

Combine the above ingredients in a large salad bowl, toss well, and serve with soup and whole grain bread.

SERVES 2.

FIVE-SPROUT SALAD

1/2 cup radish sprouts
1 cup crunchy lentil sprouts
2 cups alfalfa sprouts
1 cup sunflower sprouts
1/4 cup mung bean sprouts
1/4 cup Tomato Vinaigrette or Dijon Dressing (see page 241 or 235)

Combine the above ingredients in a large salad bowl, mix well, and serve with almost any meal.

SERVES 4.

CAESAR SALAD

4 cups sliced romaine lettuce
1 cup Croutons with French Herbs (see page 247)
1/4 cup pignoli nuts
1/4 cup Creamy Garlic Dressing (see page 238)

Combine the above ingredients in a large salad bowl, toss well, and serve with almost any meal.

SERVES 2.

DANDELION AND FENNEL SALAD

3 cups sliced dandelion leaves
1 1/2 cups diced fennel (steams and leafy portion)
1/4 cup diced unsalted almonds
1/4 cup Sweet Tarragon Dressing (see page 238)

Combine the above ingredients in a large salad bowl and toss well. Serve with an entrée or soup.

SERVES 2.

BOSTON AND FRESH PEACH SALAD

3 cups torn Boston lettuce leaves
1/4 cup unsalted walnuts
1 1/2 cups peeled and diced peaches
1/2 cup dice beets (peeled and steamed for 10 minutes)
1/4 cup Lemony Herb Dressing (see page 237)

Place the lettuce in a large salad bowl. Top with the nuts, peaches, and beets then drizzle on the salad dressing. Serve with soup or an entrée.

SERVES 2.

SWEET POTATO SALAD WITH DIJON DRESSING

1 1/2 cups cubed red potatoes (steamed for 20 minutes)
2 cups diced sweet potatoes (steamed for 20 minutes)
1/4 cup diced yellow onion
1/4 cup Dijon Dressing (see page 235)

Combine the above ingredients in a large salad bowl and toss well. Serve with almost any meal.

SERVES 2.

CARROT SALAD

3 1/2 cups shredded carrots
1 cup crunchy lentil sprouts
1/2 cup unsalted sunflower seeds
1/4 cup sesame seeds
1/4 cup raisins
1/4 cup Orange Ginger Dressing (see page 236)
2 cups Boston or mache lettuce leaves

Combine everything except the Boston or mache leaves in a large salad bowl and mix well. Serve over a bed of Boston or mache lettuce leaves to accompany almost any meal.

SERVES 2.

SUMMER FRUIT SALAD

1 cup sliced bananas
1 cup diced, peeled peaches
1 cup diced, peeled mango
1 cup blueberries
1/2 cup chopped fresh figs (optional)
2 tablespoons lemon juice
dash of cinnamon

Combine the above ingredients in a large salad bowl, toss well, and serve alone or as a side dish to any meal.

SERVES 2.

SALMON SALAD WITH BASIL VINAIGRETTE

2 8-ounce salmon steaks
1 recipe Five-Sprout Salad (see page 227)
1/4 cup Basil Vinaigrette (see page 242)

Preheat the broiler. Broil the salmon steaks for 15 minutes on the first side, then turn the steak over and broil for an additional 10 minutes. Allow the steaks to cool to room temperature, then slice them into six pieces. Place the fish segments onto two separate plates with the prepared salads and drizzle with dressing.

SERVES 2.

FILLET OF SOLE SALAD WITH DIJON DRESSING

2 8-ounce pieces fillet of sole
1 recipe Red Leaf and Beet Salad (see page 225)
1/4 cup Dijon Dressing (see page 235)

Preheat the broiler. Broil fillets for 10 minutes on one side then turn them over and broil for an additional 3 to 5 minutes. Let the fish cool to room temperature and place them on the two prepared salads. Drizzle with additional dressing and serve.

SERVES 2.

FARM-RAISED BROOK TROUT SALAD

2 8-ounce fillets brook trout (ask for farm raised)
1 recipe Red Leaf and Beet Salad (see page 225)
1/4 cup Mustard Dill Dressing (see page 239)

Preheat the broiler. Broil the fillets for 10 minutes on one side then turn them over and broil them for an additional 5 minutes on the other side. Let the fish pieces cool to room temperature, then place them on the prepared salads on two separate plates. Drizzle the fish with the salad dressing. Serve at room temperature for a tasty complete protein meal.

SERVES 2.

ITALIAN RICE SALAD

4 cups short-grain brown rice (cooked)
1/2 cup chopped yellow onion
1/2 cup chopped green bell pepper
1 cup chopped tomato
2 cloves garlic, finely chopped
1 tablespoon finely chopped parsley
1 tablespoon finely chopped basil
1/4 teaspoon black pepper
1/4 cup Basil Vinaigrette Dressing (see page 242)

In a large bowl combine the above ingredients, mix well, and serve with a tossed salad.

SERVES 4.

ASIAN RICE SALAD

4 cups white basmati rice (cooked)
2 cups cooked garbanzo beans
1/4 cup sliced scallions
1/2 cup chopped green bell pepper
1 cup chopped tomatoes
2 tablespoons chopped cilantro
1/2 teaspoon minced fresh gingerroot
1 clove garlic, minced
1/4 teaspoon minced red hot chili
1/4 cup Orange Ginger Dressing (see page 236)

Combine the above ingredients in a large bowl and mix well. Serve on a bed of salad greens.

SERVES 4.

ZESTY TOFU SALAD

1 1/2 cups diced firm tofu
2/3 cups diced celery
1/4 cup diced yellow onion
1 1/2 cups diced butternut squash (steamed for 15 minutes)
1 cup diced turnips (steamed for 15 minutes)
1 teaspoon chopped fresh basil
1/4 teaspoon black pepper
1/4 cup Lemony Herb Dressing (see page 237)

Combine the above ingredients in a large bowl and mix well. Serve over salad greens.

SERVES 2.

TEMPEH SALAD

2 tablespoons canola oil (for sautéing the tempeh)
1 cup cubed tempeh
2 cups broccoli florets (steamed for 2 minutes)
1 cup diced yellow squash (steamed for 3 minutes)
1 tablespoon diced scallions
1/2 teaspoon chopped fresh gingerroot
1 tablespoon chopped basil
2 tablespoons chopped cilantro
1 tablespoon unsweetened rice vinegar
1/4 cup Spicy Thai Dressing (see page 236)

In a large frying pan heat the oil until it is very hot. Add the tempeh and brown on all sides. Remove the browned tempeh and set aside on a paper towel to drain. In a large bowl combine the remaining ingredients with the tempeh and mix well. Serve at room temperature or chilled over salad greens.

SERVES 2.

TANGY ARAME SALAD

1 1/2 cups arame (soaked in boiling water then drained)
1/2 cup chopped red bell pepper
1/2 cup diced burdock (steamed for 10 minutes)
1/4 cup Spicy Thai Dressing (see page 236)

Combine the above ingredients in a large salad bowl and mix well. Serve with any meal.

SERVES 2.

Dressings, Sauces, and Gravies

CHERRY VINAIGRETTE

1 cup flavorless oil (safflower, sunflower, or soy)
1 1/2 cups pitted cherries (fresh or frozen)
1 1/2 cups chopped tomatoes
1/4 cup apple cider vinegar
1 tablespoon chopped basil leaves

Combine the above ingredients in a blender or food processor. Process for 1 to 2 minutes or until a homogeneous dressing is obtained. This dressing may be refrigerated for up to three days or frozen for up to three weeks.

MAKES 2 1/4 CUPS.

DIJON DRESSING

1 cup flavorless oil (safflower, sunflower, or soy)
2 tablespoons apple cider vinegar
1 tablespoon Dijon mustard
1 tablespoon fresh herbs (basil, parsley, and thyme)
dash of salt

In a blender or food processor combine the above ingredients and process until creamy, about 1 minute. Serve over almost any salad.

MAKES 1 1/4 CUPS.

RASPBERRY VINAIGRETTE

1 cup flavorless oil (safflower, sunflower, or soy)
1/3 cup fresh lime juice
1 1/2 cups raspberries (fresh or frozen)
3/4 cup water
2 1/2 teaspoons saffron threads

Combine the above ingredients in a blender or food processor. Process for 1 to 2 minutes or until a homogeneous dressing is obtained. This dressing may be refrigerated for up to three days or frozen for up to three weeks.

MAKES 3 CUPS.

SPICY THAI DRESSING

1 cup flavorless oil (safflower, sunflower, or soy)
1/4 cup fresh lime juice
1/2 cup sweet rice vinegar
1 teaspoon curry powder
4 cloves garlic
1 teaspoon chopped fresh gingerroot
2 teaspoons chopped cilantro
2 teaspoons chopped parsley
2 teaspoons chopped hot red chili

Combine the above ingredients in a blender or food processor. Process for 1 to 2 minutes or until a homogeneous dressing is obtained. This dressing may be refrigerated for up to three days or frozen for up to three weeks.

MAKES 1 3/4 CUPS.

ORANGE GINGER DRESSING

1 cup flavorless oil (safflower, sunflower, or soy)
1 cup fresh orange juice
1/4 cup fresh lemon juice
1 1/4 teaspoons chopped fresh gingerroot
1 1/4 teaspoons curry powder
1 tablespoon Dijon mustard

Combine the above ingredients in a blender or food processor. Process for 1 to 2 minutes or until a homogeneous dressing is obtained. This dressing may be refrigerated for up to three days or frozen for up to three weeks.

MAKES 2 1/4 CUPS.

COCONUT TERIYAKI SAUCE

1 cup flavorless oil (safflower, sunflower, or soy)
1 cup fresh orange juice
1/4 cup fresh lemon juice
1 1/4 teaspoons chopped fresh gingerroot
1 1/4 teaspoons curry powder
1 tablespoon prepared Dijon mustard
1/4 cup wheat-free tamari soy sauce
1 teaspoon kudzu (dissolved in 2 tablespoons water)
1 teaspoon chopped hot red chili
1/4 cup unsweetened flaked coconut

Combine the above ingredients in a blender or food processor. Process for 1 to 2 minutes or until a homogeneous dressing is obtained. This dressing may be refrigerated for up to three days or frozen for up to three weeks.

MAKES 2 1/4 CUPS.

LEMONY HERB DRESSING

1 cup flavorless oil (safflower, sunflower, or soy)
1/4 cup fresh lemon juice
1 1/2 tablespoons Dijon mustard
1 1/2 teaspoons chopped fresh marjoram (dry may be substituted)
1 1/2 teaspoons chopped fresh parsley
1 1/2 teaspoons chopped fresh dill

Combine the above ingredients in a blender or food processor. Process for 1 to 2 minutes or until a homogeneous dressing is obtained. This dressing may be refrigerated for up to three days or frozen for up to three weeks.

MAKES 1 1/4 CUPS.

SWEET TARRAGON DRESSING

¾ cup flavorless oil (safflower, sunflower, or soy)
3 tablespoons eggless mayonnaise
2 tablespoons apple cider vinegar
1 tablespoon fresh chopped tarragon (dry may be substituted)
3 tablespoons water
1/4 teaspoon black pepper

Combine the above ingredients in a blender or food processor. Process for 1 to 2 minutes or until a homogeneous dressing is obtained. This dressing may be refrigerated for up to three days or frozen for up to three weeks.

MAKES 1 1/4 CUPS.

CREAMY GARLIC DRESSING

1 cup extra virgin olive oil
2 1/2 tablespoons fresh lemon juice or apple cider vinegar
4 cloves garlic
2 teaspoons chopped fresh basil
2 teaspoons chopped fresh parsley
2 to 3 tablespoons eggless mayonnaise
1/4 teaspoon sea salt
dash of black pepper

Combine the above ingredients in a blender or food processor. Process for 1 to 2 minutes or until a homogeneous dressing is obtained. This dressing may be refrigerated for up to three days or frozen for up to three weeks.

MAKES 1 1/4 CUPS.

MUSTARD DILL DRESSING

1 cup flavorless oil (safflower, sunflower, or soy)
2 1/2 to 3 tablespoons apple cider vinegar
2 1/2 to 3 tablespoons eggless mayonnaise
3 3/4 teaspoons chopped fresh dill
dash of sea salt
dash of black pepper

Combine the above ingredients in a blender or food processor. Process for 1 to 2 minutes or until a homogeneous dressing is obtained. This dressing may be refrigerated for up to three days or frozen for up to three weeks.

MAKES 1 1/4 CUPS.

LIME DRESSING

3/4 cup flavorless oil (safflower, sunflower, or soy)
3 tablespoons fresh lime juice
1 1/2 teaspoons chopped cilantro
1 teaspoon saffron threads
dash of black pepper
dash of sea salt

Combine the above ingredients in a blender or food processor. Process for 1 to 2 minutes or until a homogeneous dressing is obtained. This dressing may be refrigerated for up to three days or frozen for up to three weeks.

MAKES 1 CUP.

SESAME TAHINI DRESSING

1/2 cup flavorless oil (sunflower, safflower, or soy)
2/3 cup pure sesame tahini
2 teaspoons wheat-free tamari soy sauce
3 to 4 tablespoons fresh lemon juice
2 cloves garlic
1/4 cup plus 1 tablespoon water

Combine the above ingredients in a blender or food processor and process until creamy, about 45 seconds. Serve over almost any entrée or salad.

MAKES 1 2/3 CUPS.

LIME TERIYAKI SAUCE

3/4 cup flavorless oil (safflower, sunflower, or soy)
1/4 cup fresh lime juice
1 1/2 teaspoons chopped cilantro
1 teaspoon saffron threads
1 1/2 tablespoons wheat-free tamari soy sauce
dash of black pepper
dash of sea salt

Combine the above ingredients in a blender or food processor. Process for 1 to 2 minutes or until a homogeneous dressing is obtained. This dressing may be refrigerated for up to three days or frozen for up to three weeks. Serve over any type of cooked fish.

MAKES 1 1/4 CUPS.

TOMATO VINAIGRETTE

1 cup flavorless oil (safflower, sunflower, or soy)
1 1/2 cups chopped tomatoes
3/4 teaspoon chopped hot red chili
2 teaspoons saffron threads
3 cloves garlic
1/4 cup apple cider vinegar
1/2 teaspoon chopped fresh basil
1/2 teaspoon sea salt
2 tablespoons eggless mayonnaise (optional)

Combine the above ingredients in a blender or food processor. Process for 1 to 2 minutes or until a homogeneous dressing is obtained. This dressing may be refrigerated for up to three days or frozen for up to three weeks.

MAKES 2 1/4 CUPS.

HONEY MUSTARD DRESSING

3/4 cup flavorless oil (safflower, sunflower, or soy)
1 tablespoon Dijon mustard
3 tablespoons pure light honey (tupelo or wildflower)
1 teaspoon wheat-free tamari soy sauce
1/2 teaspoon chopped fresh gingerroot

Combine the above ingredients in a blender or food processor. Process for 1 to 2 minutes or until a homogeneous dressing is obtained. This dressing may be refrigerated for up to three days or frozen for up to three weeks.

MAKES 1 CUP.

HONEY MUSTARD TERIYAKI SAUCE

3/4 cup flavorless oil (safflower, sunflower, or soy)
1 tablespoon Dijon mustard
3 tablespoons pure light honey (tupelo or wildflower)
1/2 teaspoon chopped fresh gingerroot
3 tablespoons wheat-free tamari soy sauce
1/2 teaspoon chopped red hot chili

Combine the above ingredients in a blender or food processor. Process for 1 to 2 minutes or until a homogeneous dressing is obtained. This dressing may be refrigerated for up to three days or frozen for up to three weeks. Serve over almost any type of fish.

MAKES 1 CUP.

BASIL VINAIGRETTE

1 cup flavorless oil (safflower, sunflower, or soy)
1 tablespoon Dijon mustard
1 tablespoon chopped fresh basil
1/4 cup fresh lemon juice
dash of salt
dash of pepper

Combine the above ingredients in a blender or food processor. Process for 1 to 2 minutes or until a homogeneous dressing is obtained. This dressing may be refrigerated for up to three days or frozen for up to three weeks.

MAKES 1 1/4 CUPS.

CRUDITÉ TOMATO SAUCE

2 cups crushed tomatoes
1 tablespoon extra virgin olive oil
1/2 teaspoon crushed garlic
1/2 teaspoon apple cider vinegar
1/4 teaspoon oregano

Combine the above ingredients in a medium-size saucepan and bring to a boil. Reduce heat to medium and continue to cook covered for 15 minutes. Serve hot or cold with almost anything.

MAKES 2 CUPS.

HONEY MUSTARD DRESSING

2 tablespoons balsamic vinegar
2 1/2 teaspoons chopped hot red chili
1/2 teaspoon dry mustard
2 tablespoons light pure honey (tupelo or wildflower)
1/2 cup canola oil

Combine the above ingredients in a blender or food processor and process for 2 to 3 minutes. Chill for 20 minutes and serve over salads or fish.

MAKES 3/4 CUP.

PARSNIP DEMIGLACE

2 1/2 cups sliced parsnip
8 whole cloves
1/2 teaspoon cinnamon
1 tablespoon saffron threads
2 cups water
1 1/2 cups apple juice
2 tablespoons pure maple syrup

Combine the above ingredients in a medium-size saucepan and cook over high heat for 1 hour and 20 minutes. Approximately 1 cup of liquid should be remaining. Remove the mixture from the heat and process it in a blender or food processor until creamy. Add ½ cup of water if necessary to obtain a creamy consistency. Serve hot or cold over fish, grains, or vegetables.

MAKES 1 CUP.

THAI DIPPING SAUCE

1 cup cilantro leaves
1/4 cup fresh lemon juice
1/3 cup unsweetened rice vinegar
3 tablespoons wheat-free tamari soy sauce
1/4 cup canola oil (any flavorless oil may be substituted)
3 cloves garlic
2 tablespoons chopped fresh gingerroot
3/4 teaspoon chopped hot red chili

Combine the above ingredients in a blender or food processor and process for 2 to 3 minutes. Chill or freeze then pour over fish or use as a salad dressing.

MAKES 1 CUP.

HEARTY ONION GRAVY

1 1/2 cups sliced onions
1/2 cup diced mushrooms
2 tablespoons canola oil
2 cups water
2 tablespoons agar-agar
1 1/2 tablespoons wheat-free tamari soy sauce

In a large saucepan sauté the onions and mushrooms in the oil until brown. Remove the onions to a dish and bring the water to a boil in the same pan. Add the agar-agar and simmer for 5 minutes. Add the tamari and reserved onions and continue to simmer for an additional 2 minutes. Remove from the heat and let cool to warm or room temperature. Serve over any entrée.

MAKES 2 CUPS.

CREAMY TOMATO GARLIC SAUCE

1/4 cup extra virgin olive oil
1/2 cup diced tomatoes
3 tablespoons tomato paste
1 tablespoon minced parsley
1 tablespoon minced basil
1/3 cup rice milk (Rice Dream)
2 cloves garlic
dash of sea salt
dash of black pepper

Combine the above ingredients in a blender or food processor and process until creamy, about 1 minute. Pour the mixture into a medium-size saucepan and bring to a simmer. Simmer for 5 minutes. Remove from the heat and serve over vegetables, grains, or pasta.

MAKES 1 1/2 CUPS.

CURRIED TOMATO SAUCE

1/4 cup extra virgin olive oil
1/2 cup diced tomatoes
3 tablespoons tomato paste
1 tablespoon minced parsley
1 tablespoon minced basil
1/3 cup rice milk (Rice Dream)
2 teaspoons curry powder
1/2 teaspoon cinnamon

Combine the above ingredients in a blender or food processor and process until creamy, about 1 minute. Pour the mixture into a medium-size saucepan and bring to a simmer. Simmer for 5 minutes. Remove from the heat and serve over vegetables, grains, or pasta.

MAKES 1 1/2 CUPS.

CREAMY CHESTNUT SAUCE

1/2 cup unsweetened cooked chestnuts
1/2 cup rice milk (Rice Dream)
2 to 4 tablespoons pure maple syrup
2 tablespoons unsalted pecans
dash of cinnamon

Combine the above ingredients in a blender or food processor and process for 2 minutes or until smooth. Serve over grains, soba noodles, or vegetables.

MAKES 1 CUP.

PEANUT SAUCE

1/2 cup amazake
1/2 cup unsalted peanut butter (almond butter may be substituted)
1/4 cup pure maple syrup

Combine the above ingredients in a food processor and process until smooth, about 2 minutes. Serve over soba noodles, vegetables, or veggieburgers.

MAKES 1 1/4 CUPS.

CROUTONS WITH FRENCH HERBS

1 cup whole grain bread pieces
1 tablespoon finely chopped parsley
1 teaspoon finely chopped basil
1/2 teaspoon finely chopped rosemary
2 to 4 tablespoons extra virgin olive oil

Preheat oven to 375 degrees. Combine the above ingredients in a bowl, toss, and bake on a cookie sheet for 15 to 20 minutes or until light brown in color.

MAKES 1 CUP.

Entrées

MOZZARELLA IN CARROZZA

1/4 cup virgin olive oil
8 4-inch strips of mozzarella-style soy cheese
1/2 cup oat flour
2 eggs (use egg replacer)
1/2 cup whole grain bread crumbs
1 recipe Crudité Tomato Sauce (see page 243)

In a large frying pan heat the oil for 2 to 3 minutes. Roll the mozzarella sticks first in the flour then in the egg mixture. Next coat them with flour again and end by dipping them in bread crumbs. Place them in the hot oil and cook over medium heat for 3 to 4 minutes on each side or until they are light brown in color. Remove them from the pan and place on a paper towel to drain. Serve hot with the Crudité Tomato Sauce.

SERVES 2.

SOBA NOODLES WITH TOASTED ONION SAUCE

1 cup sliced yellow onion
1 1/2 cups water
1 clove garlic, sliced
2 tablespoons virgin olive oil
1/2 teaspoon sea salt
dash of black pepper
1/2 cup unsweetened soy milk
1/4 teaspoon fresh oregano leaves (dry may be substituted)
4 1/2 cups cooked soba noodles

In a blender or food processor combine the onions and the water. Blend for 5 minutes or until smooth. In a small, heavy-bottomed saucepan toast the garlic over high heat for 2 to 3 minutes. Do not allow the garlic to brown or it will be bitter. Add the onion-water mixture, olive oil, salt, and pepper and simmer for 15 minutes. Stir in the soy milk and oregano and serve hot or at room temperature over the soba noodles.

SERVES 2.

FETTUCCINI WITH SWEET RED PEPPER SAUCE

1/4 cup extra virgin olive oil
1 cup diced sweet red bell pepper
3 cups chopped tomatoes
1/2 cup chopped yellow onion
2 tablespoons fresh chopped basil
dash of salt
4 cups cooked fettuccini

In a medium-size saucepan combine everything except the fettuccini and cook over medium-high heat for 5 to 10 minutes. Toss with fettuccini and serve hot with whole grain bread.

SERVES 3.

RICE THREADS WITH THAI PAI

1/4 cup canola oil (any flavorless oil may be substituted)
3 1/2 cups sliced purple cabbage
2 cups thinly sliced carrots
1 cup cauliflower florets
3 cups chopped bok choy
1 cup sliced red bell pepper
2 tablespoons wheat-free tamari soy sauce
1/4 cup sesame seeds
1 teaspoon finely chopped hot red chili
4 cups soaked rice threads (rice cellophane noodles)
2 tablespoons gomasio

Heat the oil in a large saucepan. Add everything except the rice threads and the gomasio. Stir-fry over high heat for 5 minutes; the vegetables should be crunchy when done. Remove from heat, toss with the rice threads, and sprinkle with the gomasio. Serve hot or at room temperature.

SERVES 3.

COUSCOUS WITH PARSNIP DEMIGLACE

1 1/4 cups diced parsnips with skin
1 cup sliced purple cabbage
1 cup sliced carrots
1 tablespoon flavorless oil (soy, safflower, or canola)
3 cups cooked couscous (molded into two teacups)
1 recipe Parsnip Demiglace (see page 244)
2 tablespoons toasted black sesame seeds

In a medium-size saucepan sauté the vegetables in the oil for 4 minutes, covered, over high heat. Remove from the heat. Place a plate over the teacup filled with couscous; holding it firmly, invert the plate and cup together, then gently lift off the cup. Do the same for the other teacup mold. Top with the vegetables then with sauce. Sprinkle with the seeds and serve.

SERVES 4.

RICE PASTA WITH SHIITAKE MUSHROOMS AND BUTTERNUT SQUASH

2 1/2 cups destemmed and sliced shiitake mushrooms
1 1/2 cups diced butternut squash (steamed for 10 minutes)
2 tablespoons toasted sesame oil
2 tablespoons wheat-free tamari soy sauce
3 1/2 cups cooked rice pasta (Pastariso)
2 tablespoons gomasio (optional)

In a medium-size saucepan sauté the mushrooms and squash with the oil and tamari for 5 minutes. Toss with the pasta and top with gomasio, if using. Serve hot with almost any salad.

SERVES 2.

CAPELLINI WITH GARLIC AND FRESH VEGETABLES

2 cups chopped yellow squash
1 cup diced zucchini
3 cups broccoli florets
4 1/2 cups sliced mushrooms
1/4 cup chopped garlic
1/4 cup finely chopped basil
1/2 teaspoon sea salt
1/4 cup extra virgin olive oil
4 cups cooked capellini

In a large saucepan sauté the vegetables, garlic, basil, and salt in the oil over high heat for 5 minutes. Remove from the heat and toss with the pasta. Serve hot with salad.

SERVES 4.

MATAR PANEER

1 cup extra firm tofu in 1/2 inch cubes
2 tablespoons canola oil
4 recipes Curried Tomato Sauce (see page 246)
1 cup frozen peas
1/4 teaspoon cinnamon

In a large frying pan brown the tofu in the oil over high heat. Stir in the sauce then the peas and cinnamon and continue to cook for an additional 5 minutes. Serve over rice or any grain.

SERVES 2.

BROCCOLI AND CAULIFLOWER GREENS WITH SESAME TAHINI

1 1/2 cups broccoli florets
1 cup cauliflower florets
1 cup chopped cauliflower greens
2 recipes Sesame Tahini Dressing (see page 240)
1/2 cup poppy seeds
3 cups cooked millet

Preheat the oven to 450 degrees. In a large baking dish toss together the vegetables. Spread them out evenly and top with the dressing, followed by the poppy seeds. Cover and bake for 20 to 25 minutes. Place over the millet and serve with salad.

SERVES 3.

CURRIED RED LENTIL STEW

1 tablespoon canola oil
4 cups water
1 cup dried red lentils
1/2 cup diced butternut squash
1/2 cup frozen peas
1 tablespoon chopped parsley (1 teaspoon dry may be substituted)
1 tablespoon chopped basil (1 1/2 teaspoons dry may be substituted)
1 teaspoon curry powder
1/2 teaspoon cinnamon
1/2 cup cubed unsweetened pineapple

In a large saucepan brown the onions in the oil. Add the water and bring to a boil. Add the lentils and the butternut squash. Cook uncovered for 15 minutes or until most of the water is absorbed. Add the remaining ingredients and cook for an additional 2 to 4 minutes. Serve hot over any grain or with salad.

SERVES 2.

GREEN CABBAGE STUFFED WITH FRUITS AND NUTS

1 cup cooked brown basmati rice
1/4 cup chopped apple
1/4 cup chopped carrot
1 tablespoon chopped yellow onion
1/4 cup chopped seeded orange
1/4 cup chopped unsweetened pineapple
2 tablespoons chopped pecans (optional)
2 tablespoon raisins
1 teaspoon cinnamon
1 recipe Orange Ginger Dressing (see page 236)
6 large green cabbage leaves (steamed for 5 minutes)
2 recipes Creamy Tomato Garlic Sauce (see page 245)

Preheat the oven to 450 degrees. In a large bowl combine everything except the tomato sauce and cabbage leaves. Mix these ingredients well. Place a cabbage leaf on a flat surface and put one tablespoon of stuffing in its center. Fold the portion of the leaf closest to you up over the filling. Next, fold in each side of the leaf. Last, fold down the top segment to enclose the filling. The leaves should be rolled tightly to ensure that they don't fall apart. Repeat this procedure with each remaining leaf. Place the stuffed leaves into a shallow baking dish and cover with tomato sauce. Cover and bake for 30 minutes. Serve hot with salad.

SERVES 2.

SWEET POTATO PUREE

3 cups chopped sweet potatoes (peeled then steamed for 20 minutes)
1 cup rice milk (Rice Dream)
1/4 teaspoon cinnamon

Combine the above ingredients in a blender or food processor and blend until creamy, about 2 minutes. Serve warm with almost anything.

MAKES 2 CUPS.

LENTIL-STUFFED PEPPERS

2 hollowed green bell peppers
2 hollowed red bell peppers
1 recipe Curried Red Lentil Stew (see page 253)
2 recipes Creamy Tomato Garlic Sauce (see page 245)

Preheat the oven to 375 degrees. Place the peppers in a small baking dish and fill with the stew. Top with the tomato sauce. Cover and bake for 30 minutes. Serve hot with salad.

SERVES 2.

INDONESIAN BEAN SAUTÉ

2/3 cup sliced yellow onion
2/3 cup chopped tomato (fresh or canned)
2 tablespoons canola oil (any flavorless oil may be substituted)
1/4 cup rice milk (Rice Dream)
1 1/2 to 2 teaspoons curry powder
1/2 teaspoon cinnamon
1/2 teaspoon chopped basil
2 cups cooked garbanzo beans
2/3 cups sliced red bell pepper
1/2 cup hijiki seaweed (soaked in hot water then drained; optional)

In a large saucepan sauté the onions and tomatoes in the oil. Add the rice milk then whisk in the spices. Add the garbanzo beans and bell pepper and simmer, covered, for 5 to 7 minutes. Remove from the heat and stir in the seaweed, if using. Serve hot over rice or with salad.

SERVES 2.

GUAMOCO

2 cups cooked short-grain brown rice
1 recipe Tangy Arame Salad (see page 234)
2 cups steamed carrots and assorted squash (steamed for 10 minutes; try acorn and butternut)
2 cups cooked beans (try black or kidney)
1 recipe Hearty Onion Gravy (see page 245)

Combine everything except the gravy on two separate plates and then drizzle on the gravy.

SERVES 2.

BRAISED STUFFED PURPLE CABBAGE

6 purple cabbage leaves (steamed for 5 minutes)
1 recipe Indonesian Bean Sauté (see page 256)
1 recipe Curried Tomato Sauce (see page 246)

Preheat oven to 450 degrees. Place a cabbage leaf onto a flat surface and put 2 to 3 tablespoons of the bean filling in its center. Fold the portion of the leaf closest to you up over the stuffing. Next, fold in each side of the leaf. Last, fold down the top segment to enclose the filling. Fill the remaining leaves in this way. The leaves should be rolled tight to ensure that they will not fall apart. Place the leaves into a baking dish and cover with the sauce. Cover and bake for 20 minutes. Serve hot with salad.

SERVES 2.

GARY'S BEAN THING

1 cup diced onions
3 tablespoons canola oil
2 cups pinto beans (cooked)
1 teaspoon chopped elephant garlic
1 cup chopped tomatoes (fresh or canned)
2 tablespoons curry powder
1/4 cup sesame tahini
2 tablespoons ketchup
2 cups chopped green bell peppers
1 cup cubed firm tofu or tofu dogs, sliced

In a medium-size saucepan sauté the onions in the oil until transluscent. Add everything except the tofu or tofu dogs and cook over high heat for 15 minutes. Add tofu or tofu dogs. Serve hot with rice and salad.

SERVES 2.

TUNA WITH LIME AND GINGER

2/3 cup chopped papaya, peeled and pitted
2 tablespoons fresh lime juice
1 teaspoon grated gingerroot
1 teaspoon chopped garlic
1/2 teaspoon minced hot red chili
1/4 cup canola oil
2 teaspoons balsamic vinegar
1/4 cup water
1/4 cup fresh lemon juice
1 teaspoon wheat-free tamari soy sauce
2 8-ounce tuna steaks

Combine everything except the tuna in a blender or food processor, and process for 3 minutes. Marinate the tuna steaks in the sauce for 20 minutes. Preheat the broiler. Broil the steaks on each side for 10 minutes, reserving the marinade in a bowl. Pour the marinade over the cooked steaks and serve with rice or salad.

SERVES 2.

FILLET OF SKATE WITH LIME TERIYAKI SAUCE

2 8-ounce fillets of skate
1 recipe Lime Teriyaki Sauce (see page 240)

Preheat the broiler. Broil the fillets for 15 minutes on one side, remove from the broiler, and top with sauce. Serve hot with salad and any whole grain.

SERVES 2.

FILLET OF SOLE WITH TOMATOES AND GARLIC

1/2 cup Italian parsley
1/3 cup garlic cloves
1/2 cup basil leaves
1/5 cup extra virgin olive oil
1/4 teaspoon sea salt
1/4 teaspoon black pepper
2 cups chopped tomatoes
2 8-ounce fillets of sole

Preheat the broiler. In a blender or food processor combine the parsley, cloves, basil, olive oil, salt, and pepper. Process for 5 minutes. In a medium-size saucepan, sauté the tomatoes in the above sauce over high heat for 5 minutes. Broil the fish for 10 to 15 minutes or until done. Pour the sauce over it and serve with rice and salad.

SERVE 2.

BRUSSELS SPROUTS WITH CHESTNUT SAUCE AND MILLET CROQUETTE

3 cups Gary's Croquette (see page 262)
3 cups brussels sprouts (halved and steamed for 4 minutes)
1/4 cup Creamy Chestnut Sauce (see page 246)
1/4 cup chopped unsalted pecans

Divide the croquettes evenly between two plates then top with the brussels sprouts. Next drizzle on the chestnut sauce and sprinkle with nuts.

SERVES 2.

SOBA NOODLES WITH PEANUT SAUCE

3 cups cooked soba noodles
2 cups diced butternut squash (steamed for 15 minutes)
2 tablespoons black sesame seeds
1/4 cup Peanut Sauce (see page 247)

In a large bowl combine the above ingredients and toss well. Separate the dish into two portions and serve chilled or at room temperature.

SERVES 2.

THANKSGIVING MUSHROOMS WITH BASMATI RICE AND HEARTY ONION GRAVY

4 1/2 cup chopped mushrooms, stems and caps
3/4 cup sliced celery
3/4 cup chopped yellow onion
1/3 cup extra virgin olive oil

3 cloves garlic
3/4 cup chopped parsley
3/4 teaspoon fresh thyme
3/4 teaspoon fresh sage
12 large mushroom caps
3 cups cooked white basmati rice
1 cup Hearty Onion Gravy (see page 245)

Preheat oven to 425 degrees. In a blender or food processor combine the chopped mushrooms, celery, onion, olive oil, garlic, and herbs. Process for 10 seconds. Place a mound of stuffing into each cap then place the caps onto a cookie sheet and cover with aluminum foil. Bake for 30 minutes. Separate the rice into two portions then top each rice-covered plate with six mushroom caps and drizzle with warm gravy.

SERVES 3.

TEMPEH HONG KONG

2 cups tempeh in 1/2-inch cubes
2 tablespoons canola oil
1 cup sliced Canton bok choy
1 cup sliced short bok choy
1 cup sliced red bell pepper
2 cups sliced purple cabbage
2 recipes Spicy Thai Dressing (see page 236)

In a large frying pan brown the tempeh on all sides in one tablespoon of the oil. Remove browned tempeh and set aside. Using the same pan stir-fry the vegetables in the remaining tablespoon of oil for 3 minutes. Add the tempeh and the sauce and toss well. Serve hot over rice.

SERVES 2.

STIR-FRIED TEMPEH WITH ORANGE GINGER SAUCE

1 cup tempeh in 1/2-inch cubes
2 tablespoons canola oil
1 cup sliced yellow squash
1 cup sliced red bell pepper
2 cups broccoli florets
1 teaspoon chopped cilantro
1/4 cup Orange Ginger Dressing (see page 236)

In a large frying pan brown the tempeh on all sides in one tablespoon of the oil. Remove the tempeh and set aside. Using the same pan, stir-fry the vegetables in the remaining tablespoon of oil for 3 minutes. Toss in tempeh and dressing. Mix well and serve.

SERVES 2.

GARY'S CROQUETTE

1 cup sunflower seeds
1/4 cup almond butter
2/3 cup raw carrot pieces
1/3 cup celery pieces
1/4 cup yellow onion
1 tablespoon chopped parsley
1 teaspoon chopped dill
1/4 teaspoon celery seed
1/4 teaspoon sea salt
1/4 teaspoon black pepper
1/3 cup cooked toasted kasha
1/3 cup cooked millet

1/2 cup rolled oats
3 tablespoons canola oil
1 cup alfalfa sprouts

In a blender or food processor combine the sunflower seeds, almond butter, carrots, celery, onion, parsley, dill, and spices. Process for 20 seconds and transfer to a large mixing bowl. Stir in the kasha and millet and sprouts. Shape the mixture into two to four burgers and bread both sides with the oats. Set aside. Heat the oil in a large frying pan. Fry the burgers over high heat for 5 minutes or until light brown in color. Serve with salad and almost any dressing. These can also be frozen for up to three weeks.

MAKES 2 TO 4 BURGERS.

VEGETABLE SPROUT BURGER

1 cup tempeh in 1/2-inch cubes
1 tablespoon canola oil
1/4 cup carrot pieces
2 tablespoons celery pieces
1/2 cup crunchy lentil sprouts
1/4 cup sunflower seeds
1/4 teaspoon sea salt
1 teaspoon chopped basil
1/4 cup Curried Tomato Sauce (see page 246)

Preheat oven to 325 degrees. Brown the tempeh on all sides in the oil. Combine the tempeh and the remaining ingredients in a blender or food processor and process for 1 minute. Shape into two to four burgers and bake on a greased cookie sheet for 20 to 25 minutes. Serve with salad and almost any dressing.

MAKES 2 TO 4 BURGERS.

Desserts

BASIC PIE CRUST

1 cup flour (1/2 whole wheat, 1/2 unbleached buckwheat flour)
1/2 teaspoon cinnamon
3 tablespoons safflower oil margarine
7 tablespoons cold water or soy milk

In a medium-size bowl, combine the flour and cinnamon. With a fork or pastry cutter, cut the margarine into the flour mixture until it becomes a mealy consistency. Add the cold water or soy milk by the tablespoon, tossing gently with a fork, until the dough holds together. Roll the dough into a ball. Flour a smooth surface and a rolling pin then roll the dough from the center out until it is ½ inch larger than the pie plate. Check by placing the plate on top of the rolled dough. Remove the crust to the pie plate by gently sliding a floured spatula underneath the crust toward its center. Do this around the entire area of the crust, then fold it over on itself and slide into the pie plate. For a prebaked pie shell, bake in a preheated 350-degree oven for 15 minutes or until light brown in color. For a double-crust pie, simply double the recipe.

MAKES ONE 9-INCH CRUST.

GARY'S SURPRISE COOKIES

1 1/2 cups unsalted almonds
1 1/2 cups unsalted pecans
1/4 cup safflower margarine

1 egg (use egg replacer)
1/4 cup pure light honey (tupelo or wildflower)
1 teaspoon pure vanilla extract
2 1/3 cups stone-ground whole wheat flour
1/2 teaspoon baking powder
1/2 teaspoon baking soda
1 cup chopped pitted dates
3/4 cup unsweetened carob chips (raisins may be substituted)

Preheat the oven to 350 degrees. Place the almonds and pecans on an ungreased cookie sheet and bake for about 10 minutes, stirring frequently. Remove the toasted nuts and allow to cool. Meanwhile, in a large bowl cream the margarine with the egg or egg replacer, honey, and vanilla. In a separate bowl sift together the flour with the baking powder and baking soda. Add the dry ingredients to the egg mixture and mix well with a sturdy spoon. Add the cooled nuts, dates, and carob chips to the batter and mix well. Press the dough into 2- to 3-inch cookies and bake on an ungreased cookie sheet for 10 to 15 minutes or until light brown in color. Remove from the oven and cool thoroughly. Store for up to one week in an airtight container.

MAKES 2 DOZEN.

GINGERBREAD COOKIES

1/2 cup pure date sugar
1/4 cup pure blackstrap molasses
1/3 cup pure maple syrup
1 egg
1/4 cup safflower margarine
4 cups stone-ground whole wheat flour
1/4 teaspoon ground cloves
1 1/2 teaspoons ground ginger
1 teaspoon cinnamon
1 1/4 teaspoons baking soda
dash of salt

In a large bowl cream the sugar, molasses, maple syrup, egg, and margarine. In a separate bowl sift together the dry ingredients. Add the sifted dry ingredients to the creamed mixture and mix well with a sturdy wooden spoon. Roll the dough into a ball, wrap in plastic wrap, and chill for 1 to 2 hours. Preheat the oven to 350 degrees. Turn the chilled dough onto a floured surface and roll to a thickness of 1/4 to 1/2 inch with a rolling pin. Use cookie cutters to press out special shapes. Bake on an ungreased cookie sheet for 8 to 12 minutes or until light brown in color.

MAKES 3 DOZEN.

PEANUT BUTTER COOKIES

1 cup unsalted peanut butter (almond butter may be substituted)
2 tablespoons egg replacer
1/4 cup pure maple syrup
1 teaspoon pure almond extract

1 teaspoon pure vanilla extract
1 1/2 cups stone-ground whole wheat flour
1 teaspoon baking soda
1 teaspoon baking powder
1/2 cup unsalted peanuts

Preheat oven to 350 degrees. In a blender or food processor combine the peanut butter, egg or egg replacer, maple syrup, almond and vanilla extract. Process for 2 minutes or until smooth. Transfer to a mixing bowl. In a separate bowl sift together the dry ingredients. Blend the sifted ingredients into the peanut butter mixture until a dough is formed. Stir in the peanuts. Wrap the dough in plastic wrap and refrigerate for one hour. Form the dough into twelve large cookies or twenty-four small ones and bake on a greased cookie sheet for 15 to 20 minutes or until light brown in color. Remove from the cookie sheet and let cool on a cookie rack for 5 to 10 minutes.

MAKES 2 DOZEN.

AMBROSIA CRUNCH

3 cups coarsely chopped unsalted pecans
1/4 cup chopped pitted dates
3/4 cups pure tupelo honey (any light honey may be substituted)
3/4 cup chopped unsweetened pineapple
1 1/2 cups diced unsweetened peaches
1 cup fresh pitted cherries (any variety)
1 cup sliced bananas
1/4 cup lemon juice
3/4 cup unsweetened deseeded tangerine segments
1 cup unsweetened flaked coconut

Preheat oven to 350 degrees. In a large mixing bowl combine the pecans, dates, and 3/4 cup of the honey and mix well. Place onto a greased cookie sheet and bake for 15 minutes or until the nuts are light brown in color. Remove from the oven and allow to cool to room temperature; set aside. Combine the remaining ingredients in a large mixing bowl. Spread the ambrosia in a decorative serving dish such as a shallow casserole. Top with the pecan-date topping and serve chilled or at room temperature.

SERVES 2 TO 4.

CRANBERRY APPLE CRUNCH PIE WITH CANDIED ORANGE PEEL AND ROSEMARY

peel from 1 orange (cut into 15 to 20 thin slices)
1/4 cup sweet rice syrup
3 cups peeled and sliced Macintosh or Granny Smith apples
1 cup fresh cranberries
1/4 cup pure date sugar
1/4 cup pure maple syrup
1/2 teaspoon allspice
1/2 teaspoon finely chopped fresh rosemary
1/4 teaspoon grated lemon peel
1 double prepared pie crust (see page 264)

Preheat oven to 375 degrees. In a small mixing bowl toss together the orange peel and rice syrup. Bake on a greased cookie sheet, for 10 minutes. Let the candied peel come to room temperature and set aside. In a large mixing bowl combine the apples, cranberries, date sugar, maple syrup, allspice, rosemary, and lemon peel. Mix these ingredients well and place them into the prepared pie crust. Place the second half of the prepared crust on top of the pie. Fold the edges underneath the bottom crust and press the two crusts together tightly. The crust should be sealed. Cut four 1-inch slits, equally separated, toward the center of the pie. Bake the pie on a cookie sheet to catch any spilling over of the filling for 45 minutes to 1 hour. Serve the pie warm or at room temperature garnished with candied orange peels and Rice Dream ice cream.

MAKES 1 PIE.

AUTUMN HARVEST PIE

Filling

1 cup peeled and sliced granny smith apples
2 cups peeled and sliced pears
3/4 cup assorted unsulfured dried fruits, finely chopped
1/2 cup pure date sugar
1/2 cup pure maple syrup
1/2 teaspoon allspice
1/2 teaspoon pure almond extract
1 prepared pie crust (see page 264)

Topping

4 tablespoons safflower margarine
1/4 cup pure maple syrup
1/4 cup pure date sugar
1/2 teaspoon pure almond extract
1 1/2 teaspoons cinnamon
2 1/2 cups oat flour
1 1/4 cups rolled oats
1 1/4 cups pecans

Preheat oven to 350 degrees. In a large bowl combine the filling ingredients and mix well. Pour this mixture into the prepared crust and bake for 15 minutes while you prepare the topping. In a blender or food processor combine the margarine, maple syrup, date sugar, extract, and cinnamon. Cream this mixture for 2 minutes. Transfer this mixture into a medium-size mixing bowl and stir in the remaining ingredients. Remove the pie from the oven and crumble on the topping. Continue to bake for an additional 30 to 40 minutes. Serve warm or hot with Rice Dream ice cream.

MAKES 1 PIE.

ALMOND COCONUT CREAM PIE

3 tablespoons agar-agar dissolved in 1/2 cup apple juice)
2 cups extra firm silken tofu
1 1/2 cups amazake
1/4 cup pure maple syrup
1 1/2 teaspoons pure almond extract
1 tablespoon kudzu (dissolved in 1/4 cup boiling water)
1/4 cup unsweetened flaked coconut
1 prebaked pie crust (see page 264)

In a small saucepan bring the agar-agar and apple juice to a boil, reduce the heat, and simmer for 10 minutes. In a blender or food processor combine the tofu, amazake, maple syrup, almond extract, kudzu, and coconut and process for 2 minutes or until smooth. Pour this mixture into the prebaked pie crust and refrigerate for 1 hour. Serve chilled with fresh fruit.

MAKES 1 PIE.

COCOA PUDDING

2 1/2 cups rice milk (Rice Dream)
5 tablespoons agar-agar
2 tablespoons egg replacer
1/4 cup extra firm silken tofu
3 tablespoons pure unsweetened cocoa powder (try Droste)
1/4 cup pure maple syrup
1 teaspoon pure vanilla extract
1 teaspoon pure almond extract
1/2 teaspoon cinnamon

In a small saucepan bring the rice milk and agar-agar to a boil. Reduce the heat and simmer for 10 minutes. In a blender or food processor combine the remaining ingredients and process for 2 minutes or until smooth. Pour into shallow glasses and refrigerate. Serve chilled with Peanut Butter Cookies (see page 266) as a tasty accompaniment

SERVES 2.

ALMOND CREAM PUDDING

1 1/2 cups amazake
2 cups extra firm silken tofu
1/4 cup pure maple syrup
1/4 cup egg replacer
2 teaspoons pure almond extract
1/2 teaspoon cinnamon

Combine all of the ingredients in a blender or food processor and process for 2 minutes or until smooth. Pour into shallow glasses and chill. Serve chilled with Almond Coconut Cream Pie (see page 270).

SERVES 2.

PEACH CANTON

4 cups apple juice
5 tablespoons agar-agar
3 cups chopped peaches (fresh or frozen)
1 tablespoon kudzu (dissolved in 1/2 cup boiling water)
1 teaspoon pure lemon extract

In a large saucepan bring the apple juice and agar-agar to a boil, reduce the heat, and simmer for 15 minutes. Remove from the heat and pour into a shallow baking dish or bowl. Stir in the remaining ingredients and let cool to room temperature. When the canton is at room temperature refrigerate for 1 hour or until a loose gelatin consistency is reached. Serve cool for a refreshing treat.

SERVE 2 TO 4.

VERY BERRY CANTON

4 cups apple juice
1/4 cup agar-agar
1 tablespoon kudzu (dissolved in 1/2 cup boiling water)
1 teaspoon pure lemon extract
1 cup sliced strawberries
1 cup blueberries
1 cup raspberries

In a large saucepan bring the apple juice and agar-agar to a boil. Reduce heat to medium and simmer for 15 minutes. Remove from the stove and pour the mixture into a shallow baking dish or bowl. Stir in the remaining ingredients and allow the mixture to cool to room temperature. When the canton has reached room temperature place it into the refrigerator for an additional 30 minutes. Serve chilled.

SERVES 2.

TROPICAL CANTON

4 cups apple juice
5 1/2 tablespoons agar-agar
1 tablespoon saffron threads (optional)
1 tablespoon kudzu (dissolved in 1/2 cup boiling water)
1 teaspoon pure almond extract
1 cup unsweetened pineapple cubes
1 cup sliced mango pieces
1 cup seedless tangerine segments (unsweetened)
1/4 cup unsweetened flaked coconut

In a large saucepan bring the apple juice to a boil. Reduce heat to medium and add the agar-agar flakes and saffron, if using, and simmer for 15 minutes. Remove from the stove and pour the mixture into a shallow baking dish or bowl. Stir in the remaining ingredients and allow the mixture to cool to room temperature. When the canton has reached room temperature place it into the refrigerator for an additional 30 minutes. Serve chilled.

SERVES 2.

ALMOND BUTTER FRUIT-FILLED DROPS

1 cup unsalted almond butter
1/2 cup unsalted almonds
2 tablespoons egg replacer
1/4 cup pure maple syrup
1 teaspoon pure almond extract
1 1/2 cups stone-ground whole wheat or oat flour
1 teaspoon baking soda
1 teaspoon baking powder
1/2 cup unsweetened fruit preserves (try strawberry, peach, cherry, or blueberry)

Preheat the oven to 350 degrees. In a blender or food processor combine the almond butter, almonds, egg or egg replacer, maple syrup, and almond extract. Process for 2 minutes or until smooth. In a separate bowl sift together the dry ingredients. Add the sifted ingredients to the almond butter mixture and blend for 30 seconds or until a dough forms. Wrap the dough in plastic wrap and refrigerate for 1 hour. Shape the dough into twenty-four small cookies. Place the cookies onto a greased cookie sheet. Using a teaspoon or your thumb make circular ¼-inch indentations in the center of each cookie. Fill in the indentations with 1 teaspoon of preserves. Bake for 15 to 20 minutes or until light brown in color. Remove from heat and let cool for 10 minutes. Transfer the cookies to a cooling rack and continue to cool until they are room temperature. Wrap airtight and refrigerate for up to one week.

MAKES 2 DOZEN.

The Twenty-one-Day Menu Plan

Day 1

Juice	Watercress Cucumber
Breakfast	Pumpkin and Spice Pancakes
Juice	Cucumber Blueberry
Lunch	Farm-Raised Brook Trout Salad
Snack	Peanut Butter Cookies
Dinner	Cappellini with Garlic and Fresh Vegetables

Day 2

Juice	Orange Apricot
Breakfast	Kasha with Pumpkin Seeds and Pears
Juice	Asparagus Carrot
Lunch	Minestrone Soup
	Leafy Salad with Roasted Red Peppers
Snack	Carob Chip Granola
Dinner	Chinese Green Bean Salad
	Matar Paneer with brown basmati rice

Day 3

Juice	Watermelon Beet
Breakfast	Creamy Risotto with Cardamom
Juice	Kale and Purple Cabbage
Lunch	Fennel Salad with Lime Dressing
	Guamoco, Tuna
Snack	Almond Cream Pudding
Dinner	Watercress Salad
	Couscous with Parsnip Demiglace

Day 4

Juice	Carrot Ginger
Breakfast	Very Berry Granola
Juice	Arugula Cucumber
Lunch	Tempeh Salad
Snack	Summer Fruit Salad
Dinner	Swiss Chard Salad with Sweet Tarragon Dressing
	Rice Threads with Thai Pai

Day 5

Juice	Cranberry Grape
Breakfast	Cream of Barley with Oats
Juice	Apple Strawberry
Lunch	Navy Bean and Sweet Potato Soup
	Belgian Endive Salad
Snack	Gingerbread Cookies
Dinner	Assorted Zucchini Salad
	Tuna with Lime and Ginger

DAY 6

Juice	Cranberry Orange
Breakfast	Cream of Buckwheat with Honey
Juice	Cucumber Parsley
Lunch	Italian Rice Salad
Snack	Ambrosia Crunch
Dinner	Stir-Fried Tempeh with Orange Ginger Sauce

DAY 7

Juice	Peach Kiwi
Breakfast	Millet with Cinnamon and Spice
Juice	Apple Cabbage
Lunch	Carrot Salad, Vegetable Sprout Burgers, Waldorf Watercress Salad
Snack	Peach Canton
Dinner	Brussels Sprout Salad with Creamy Chestnut Sauce
	Soba Noodles with Toasted Onion Sauce

DAY 8

Juice	Apple Cherry
Breakfast	Quinoa with Dates and Pecans
Juice	Bok Choy Garlic
Lunch	Romaine with Fresh Basil
	Gary's Croquette
Snack	Cocoa Pudding
Dinner	Purple Cabbage and Poppy Seed Salad
	Curried Red Lentil Stew

Day 9

Juice	Cranberry Ginger
Breakfast	Amaranth with Peaches and Bananas
Juice	Alfalfa Sprout and Beet
Lunch	Zesty Tofu Salad
Snack	Very Berry Canton
Dinner	Escarole with Brazil Nuts
	Broccoli and Cauliflower Greens with Sesame Tahini, Salmon

Day 10

Juice	Pineapple Cabbage
Breakfast	Carob Chip Granola
Juice	Kale and Carrot
Lunch	Spinach Dumpling Soup
	Southern Tomato Salad
Snack	Autumn Harvest Pie
Dinner	Dandelion Salad
	Fillet of Sole with Tomatoes and Garlic

Day 11

Juice	Apricot Lemon
Breakfast	Good Morning Kasha
Juice	Apple Kale
Lunch	Cream of Mushroom Soup
	Arugula with Lemon and Herbs
Snack	Almond Coconut Cream Pie Custard
Dinner	Asparagus and Carrots Dijon
	Sweet Potato Puree, Fillet of Sole

Day 12

Juice	Nectarine Sprout
Breakfast	Quinoa with Peaches and Cream
Juice	Swiss Chard and Zucchini
Lunch	Sweet Potato Salad with Dijon Dressing
Snack	Very Berry Granola
Dinner	Mache with Green Grapes and Radish Sprouts
	Brussels Sprouts with Chestnut Sauce and Millet Croquette

Day 13

Juice	Plum Grape
Breakfast	Barley Pancakes with Pumpkin Seeds
Juice	Cauliflower Lemon
Lunch	Salmon Salad with Basil Vinaigrette
Snack	Cranberry Apple Crunch Pie with Candied Orange Peel and Rosemary
Dinner	Five-Sprout Salad
	Soba Noodles with Peanut Sauce

Day 14

Juice	Banana Orange
Breakfast	Nutty Granola
Juice	Swiss Chard Carrot
Lunch	Papaya and Avocado Salad
	Mozzarella in Carrozza
Snack	Summer Fruit Salad
Dinner	Assorted Bok Choy Salad
	Indonesian Bean Sauté with brown rice

Day 15

Juice	Watercress Cucumber
Breakfast	Barley Grits with Bananas and Coconut
Juice	Raspberry Pear
Lunch	Belgian Endive Salad, Black Bean Soup
Snack	Cocoa Pudding
Dinner	Dandelion and Fennel Salad
	Tempeh Hong Kong

Day 16

Juice	Crenshaw Melon
Breakfast	Very Berry Granola
Juice	Swiss Chard Celery
Lunch	Sorrel and Radicchio Di Vernon Salad
	Vegetable Sprout Burger
Snack	Peach Canton
	Braised Leek Salad
Dinner	Gary's Croquette

Day 17

Juice	Nectarine Carrot
Breakfast	Blue Corn and Pecan Pancakes
Juice	Parsley Kale
Lunch	Fillet of Sole Salad with Dijon Dressing
Snack	Gary's Surprise Cookies
	Boston and Fresh Peach Salad
Dinner	Thanksgiving Mushrooms with Basmati and Hearty Onion Gravy

Day 18

Juice	Tropical Surprise
Breakfast	Kasha with Pumpkin Seeds and Pears
Juice	Special Mixed Vegetable Surprise
Lunch	Hearty Split Pea Soup
	Arugula Salad with Raspberry Vinaigrette
Snack	Tropical Canton
Dinner	Middle Eastern Salad
	Green Cabbage Stuffed with Fruits and Nuts

Day 19

Juice	Casaba Watermelon
Breakfast	Cream of Rice with Apples and Pears
Juice	Cucumber Sprout
Lunch	Tangy Arame Salad
Snack	Very Berry Canton
Dinner	Fennel Salad with Lime Dressing
	Guamoco
	Brown Rice with Sauce

Day 20

Juice	Carrot Apple
Breakfast	Cream of Barley with Quinoa
Juice	Cucumber Parsley
Lunch	Swiss Chard Salad with Sweet Tarragon Dressing
Snack	Tempeh Salad
Dinner	Assorted Zucchini Salad
	Broccoli and Cauliflower Greens with Sesame Tahini, Brown Rice

Day 21

Juice	Apple Cherry
Breakfast	Millet
Juice	Watercress Cucumber
Lunch	Cream of Mushroom Soup
	Escarole with Brazil Nuts
Snack	Almond Butter Fruit-Filled Drops
Dinner	Belgian Endive Salad
	Fillet of Skate with Lime Teriyaki Sauce

Vegetarian's Vocabulary

Agar-agar A clear, flavorless variety of seaweed sold in flakes or in bars that is used like gelatin.

Almond butter Raw or roasted almonds ground until the consistency is creamy, like that of peanut butter. Usually available at health food stores.

Almond extract The oil that is obtained through mechanical means from the almond, then combined with alcohol.

Amaranth A high-protein grain native to Central and South America that has more fiber than wheat and rice. The grain was grown for nearly eight thousand years until it virtually disappeared for reasons unknown, in the early 1500s. Renewed interest in this tasty grain has revived its cultivation.

Amazake A beverage consisting of either a blend of almonds and water or a dilution of cultured rice. It is available at health food stores under a variety of brand names in a variety of flavors, such as chocolate, almond, vanilla, and carob.

Arame A black seaweed that is mild in flavor and aroma. Arame is usually in the form of thin strands and is added, reconstituted, to soups, grains, or stews, or served cold as a salad.

Arugula A dark green, somewhat peppery, leafy lettuce.

Barley A grain often lower in fiber than other grains, but one of the easiest to digest. Its tough outer hull makes barley almost impossible to cook and is removed in a process called "pearling."

Basmati rice A variety of rice grown in India that has a distinctive nutty flavor and comes in both brown and white varieties.

Blackstrap molasses The end product extracted from cane or beet juice. Contains 35 percent sucrose and is a source of iron, calcium, and B vitamins.

Bok choy An Asian variety of cabbage that has broad white stalks with dark green leaves projecting from them. Has a mild sweet flavor and can be eaten raw or enjoyed in soups and stir fries. Comes in several varieties.

Buckwheat flour A finely ground flour made from the buckwheat grain. Buckwheat is a type of grass. Its nutritional value and taste put it in the class of whole grains.

Bulgur A cracked-wheat grain made from parboiled crushed wheat.

Cardamom An East Indian plant whose seeds are used to produce a ground powder for a distinct Asian flavor.

Carob powder/Carob chips Carob is the seedpod of the Mediterranean evergreen tree. It can be ground into a powder or made into chips that taste like and can be used like cocoa and chocolate chips.

Celery seed A spice that comes from the celery plant.

Chickpeas/Garbanzo beans A bean grown in the Mediterranean and used in such Middle Eastern dishes as hummus.

Cilantro Also known as coriander or Chinese parsley. Used in Asian and Spanish cooking. Cilantro is the leafy portion of the plant.

Cocoa powder A powder made from cacao seeds after they have been roasted, ground, and freed of most of their fatty oil.

Coconut flakes Coconut that has been dried and flaked.

Coriander A spice made from the ground seeds of the cilantro plant. Used in Asian dishes.

Couscous Tiny pearls of semolina pasta, conscous is derived from a variety of wheat known as durum.

Cream of brown rice Fine-grain cereal made from whole grain rice that must be cooked before eating. It can be purchased in health food stores.

Daikon A variety of large, white Oriental radish.

Date sugar Dehydrated ground dates.

Dijon mustard A mustard produced in the Dijon province of France.

Egg replacer A nondairy, wheat-free powder used as an egg substitute, primarily for baking. This product can be purchased in most healthfood stores.

Gomasio A traditional Japanese seasoning composed of lightly toasted and ground sesame seeds and sea salt.

Kasha Also known as buckwheat, kasha is available in both whole and unhulled forms and is found either roasted or cut.

Kudzu, also kuzu A starch used to thicken sauces and puddings. Available from Oriental markets or healthfood stores.

Lemon extract Lemon oil and alcohol are combined to create an extract.

Mache Also known as corn salad, a spinachlike salad green very popular in Europe.

Millet A variety of grain high in protein and well tolerated by people allergic to other grains.

Null-Trim Protein Powder A complete protein in powder form that provides eight essential amino acids and is made from allergy-free vegetable ingredients.

Oat flour A flour milled from the whole oats.

Pignoli nuts Great-tasting nut that is low in protein and high in calories. Used occasionally as a vegetable or dessert garnish.

Quinoa A high-protein grain with a unique texture.

Radicchio A bitter red lettucelike vegetable frequently used in salads.

Red lentils Among the tastiest of beans. They're a good source of protein, vitamin A, thiamin, riboflavin, niacin, iron, calcium, phosphorus, and potassium.

Rice dream An unsweetened nondairy milk product made from brown rice.

Rice noodles Noodles made from rice flour.

Rice syrup A sweetener made from cooked rice. Available in Oriental markets or health food stores.

Rice vinegar Vinegar obtained from rice.

Safflower oil/Sunflower oil For general cooking purposes, both are mild-flavored salad oils. A good source of polyunsaturated fats and vitamin E.

Saffron threads The dried stigmas of the flower *Crocus sativus* used to color foods and as a cooking spice.

Sea salt From the sea or ocean, sea salt contains trace vitamins and minerals.

Sesame oil, hot Has a pleasant nutty flavor. Makes a good salad oil. Hot red pepper is added to create the hot spicy flavor.

Sesame oil, toasted Made from toasted sesame seeds ground into oil.

Sesame seeds The seeds from the sesame plant. A excellent source of protein, unsaturated fatty acids, calcium, magnesium, niacin, and vitamins A and E.

Shiitake mushrooms One of the variety of mushrooms used in soups, salads, and main dishes. These can be purchased in most grocery stores.

Silken tofu A creamy variety of soybean curd.

Soba noodles A noodle product made with 40 to 100 percent buckwheat flour.

Soybean oil Soybean oil is somewhat stronger in flavor than other oils and makes a good choice for frying foods.

Soy cheese A cheese made from soy beans.

Soy milk A nondairy "milk." Made from soybean mash.

Sprouts Any seed that has been sprouted. Sprouts are the best source of unsaturated fatty acids. They provide protein, minerals, and vitamins A, B, and E.

Sunflower seeds A rich source of protein, unsaturated fatty acids, phosphorus, calcium, iron, fluorine, iodine, potassium, magnesium, zinc, some of the B vitamins, and vitamins D and E.

Tahini Sesame seeds that have been ground into a paste.

Tamari Naturally fermented soy sauce, 9 to 18 percent complete protein and easily digestible. It contains B vitamins, riboflavin, and niacin and is the best nonmeat source of vitamin B12. Also available in wheat-free form.

Tempeh A fermented soybean product.

Wheat germ This is the central base of the wheat kernel. It is the richest source of vitamin E and is a good source of B vitamins.

PART THREE

Resource Guide

▲

▲

▲

Basic Immune-Building Nutrients and Herbs

THE FOUNDATION NUTRIENTS

While a multitude of nutrients contribute to a healthy and balanced immune system, a smaller list of vitamins and minerals should be considered of higher priority and importance. There are so many nutrients on the shelves in health food and similar stores that the consumer is often overwhelmed. To make matters more complicated, new and highly advertised substances with great claims appear all the time.

In the same way that you build a house with a strong foundation as the first step, you should maintain immune health by keeping the most basic nutrients in adequate supply. After building this foundation, you might consider some products to fulfill a second level of nutritional need. The ideal situation would be to find an environmental or nutritionally oriented physician who has experience in the use of appropriate laboratory testing and, probably even more important, the interpretation of those test results. After you have obtained a metabolic profile of the pattern of deficient nutrients, the second phase is to develop a food and supplement program to address those deficiencies. In the early stages, supplementary vitamin and mineral concentrates may be required to rescue the body from its deficit. As the deficit decreases, foods may play a greater role in the maintenance of immune balance.

The foundation, or level one, nutrients include: vitamin A, zinc, vitamin C, bioflavonoids, gamma linoleic acid (GLA), essential fatty acids (EFA), vitamin E, selenium, and B complex.

Vitamin A

Vitamin A, which is particularly important for immune functioning, comes in different forms. The emulsified vitamin A, which often comes from fish liver oil, works especially well because it is easily absorbed by the digestive apparatus.

Vitamin A also comes from nonanimal sources, such as lemon grass, which can work equally well. Many manufacturers produce this product, and it is relatively easy to find.

A third source of vitamin A is beta carotene, which the liver must convert to true vitamin A. Before taking beta carotene, it is a good idea to have your liver function analyzed. Although some persons have a known weakness of liver function, easily diagnosed by the presence of elevated enzymes such as SGOT, SGPT, or GGTP, there are also situations in which the liver is functioning less than optimally yet there is no simple laboratory test that will confirm that fact. The mechanism may not be known yet, but the clinical fact nevertheless exists that these persons do not convert beta carotene efficiently to vitamin A in the body. Women who have even a remote chance of becoming pregnant should ingest beta carotene rather than vitamin A, since there have been no reported fetal problems with the former, whereas there have been complications with true vitamin A. Beta carotene may be taken in doses from 10,000 up to 20,000 IU per day with safety, since the body will convert and use only as much vitamin A as it requires. Doses of vitamin A of 10,000 IU per day are in wide use and seem very compatible with body function. In my experience, many patients with allergy tend to have an immune-system imbalance that requires even higher doses of true vitamin A or beta carotene.

ZINC

Men over the age of forty commonly have zinc deficiencies. This may be due in part to the prostate gland, which often becomes irritated as men age. The gland uses up a certain amount of zinc in its basic day-to-day functioning, especially when the prostate is irritated or enlarged. The reproductive apparatus also utilizes zinc in the production of semen, such that zinc is lost to the body with each ejaculation. The problem is that any zinc used by the prostate gland cannot be used by the immune system because there is only so much zinc to go around.

Zinc is an essential mineral. The United States Recommended Daily Allowance (RDA) for adults is 15 mg per day. An average practical dose is 25 mg daily; however, if persons are zinc deficient, the dose required may be 40 or 50 mg. Zinc may be found in whole grains, seeds, and nuts.

The zinc found in these foods was removed from the soil and incorporated into living plant tissue, which makes it absorbable and usable by the body's metabolism. If taken in a supplement, the elemental zinc must be combined with a transporter that will enable it to be absorbed and then utilized. Some of the transporters commonly used are amino acid chelate, gluconate, or picolinate. Recent clinical work suggests that the picolinate form is a very effective vehicle for zinc, and my clinical experience has borne this out. When labeling a mineral supplement, the manufacturer must describe the form of zinc—namely, the transporter component of the mixture. The dose may be described with two numbers: the milligrams, or weight, of the entire zinc complex, but more important, the amount of elemental zinc present within the complex. The body only benefits from the actual elemental zinc, so this is the important quantity to note when you're seeking a specific dosage.

Vitamin C

Vitamin C is the most commonly supplemented nutrient and is by far the most popular vitamin of them all. People who take relatively low doses of vitamin C in supplement form daily are obtaining a very minimal benefit. Even very sophisticated and appropriately dosed multivitamin formulas tend to have in the range of 1,000 to 2,000 mg of vitamin C, which is a very moderate dose. While these doses will benefit people with a deficiency state, they would be inadequate for bringing those people's health up to an optimum level.

Although most attention to vitamin C focuses on its ability to assist weakened immune-system function and help with sore throats, colds, or similar situations in which one's resistance has failed, vitamin C also has a major role in the treatment of allergic symptoms. When in the midst of an immune-system breakdown, as with a severe viral infection or, at the other end of the spectrum, with a hyperactive immune system producing an asthmatic attack, very high doses of vitamin C should be considered. In either situation, an individual may attempt to determine dose by testing him- or herself for bowel tolerance. *Bowel tolerance* is the term used to describe the ability of the bowel to absorb the vitamin C ingested. When one has needs for higher doses of this vitamin, the bowel will absorb as much as is required. However, the portion of the vitamin C dose above the amount needed will not be absorbed and, rather, will pass rapidly through the digestive system, resulting in diarrhea. Therefore, to find the right dosage progressively increase the vitamin C dose until bowel tolerance is reached, and then reduce the ingested dose until the loose bowel movements cease. When ingesting high doses of vitamin C, one should use powdered vitamin C. This form should be buffered or rendered less acid; otherwise, the acid itself might irritate the stomach. The vitamin C should be taken in at least three separate portions per day.

Although most newcomers to the vitamin C arena recoil when they learn of some of the doses, when the immune system is off the beam doses of 3 to 5 grams three times daily are usually very well tolerated. Each half teaspoon of powder is about 2½ grams, so the physical amount one needs to ingest is small.

Beyond the high oral doses, many practitioners in the nutritional and environmental medicine community treat patients with high doses of vitamin C via intravenous drip. Many patients have reported great benefit and reduction of symptoms following a twice-weekly program of an intravenous vitamin C formula administered over a four-week period. A recipe that seems to have great benefit in repairing the overactive immune system of the allergic patient contains vitamin C (10 to 20 grams per infusion), magnesium, calcium, B complex, and B_{12}. For asthmatic patients, a similar formula with higher levels of magnesium is very effective in many patients. Certain illnesses are more responsive to certain nutrients. For example, most allergy sufferers seem to benefit from calcium, while asthma patients usually need extra magnesium.

Bioflavonoids

Bioflavonoids are immune-enhancing nutrients that are often found in foods containing vitamin C. In an orange, for example, bioflavonoids are part of the white inner peel that clings to the orange sections. Since bioflavonoids are found in nature along with vitamin C, it is not surprising that they work hand in hand with vitamin C in biochemical processes throughout the body. Dr. Feldman recommends a formula containing an equal dose of vitamin C and bioflavonoid complex for any patient with immune-system imbalance. One such formula contains 500 mg of vitamin C and 675 mg of bioflavonoid components, including lemon bioflavonoids and rutin (flavonol). A moderate daily dose of bioflavonoid complex would be 2,000 mg.

In addition to this general bioflavonoid–vitamin C complex, good results have been observed using additional guercetin, a noncitrus bioflavonoid. Quercetin would be used in a much lower dose, such as 100 to 200 mg per day.

Another excellent bioflavonoid that has a role in all allergic or underactive immune-system patients is picnogenol.

GLA

GLA, or gamma linoleic acid, plays a primary role in restoring immune function. It is available in three sources: evening primrose oil, borage oil, and black currant seed oil capsules. Generally, a black currant seed oil capsule contains 85 mg of GLA; approximately 500 mg per day is an effective dose.

Vitamin E

Although vitamin E participates in many body processes, including ovarian function and skin rejuvenation, it also has a role as a building block of immune function. My clinical experience has been that women are more likely to become deficient in this nutrient. When there are female problems such as irregular menstrual cycle, premenstrual syndrome (PMS), adult acne, or infertility, there is a much higher probability of vitamin E depletion. These female malfunctions thus may indirectly weaken the female immune system's integrity, since the body's supply and store of vitamin E have been diverted in the body's attempt to correct the female problems mentioned. Vitamin E supplements are available in a natural form derived from soybean oil; this source yields a natural unesterified d-alpha tocopherol with accompanying mixed tocopherols, namely d-beta, d-delta, and d-gamma. This form of vitamin E seems to work well as an immune-system nutritional source. In persons with difficulty absorbing the oil-based natural vitamin E, there is a water-soluble form that is very digestible. In addition to the natural source, many synthetic variants are in wide use; these have good biological activity, but my experience leads me to favor the natural form. Women with allergy, and especially with any of the female problems mentioned, will usually require at least 200 to 400 IU of vitamin E daily. Men with immune problems require vitamin E in adequate supply but very often will require only 400 IU per day. In some patients with both vitamin E and selenium deficiency, taking these two nutrients at the same time seems to correct the deficiency of each more rapidly than when taken individually.

Selenium

Selenium, a true trace mineral or element, is one of the basic, or level one, components of immune-system function. It is in short supply in the soil in many of the farming areas of America, so that food sources of selenium are limited. Selenium in tablet form is rarely available; a natural form is Oceanic Selenium, which is powdered. Many other chemically produced forms that are digestible are L-Selenomethionine, amino-acid-complex selenium, and a liquid form, aqua selenious acid. A routine dose would be 100 mcg per day, but those with immune-system problems very often require 200 mcg or more. This element may also be injected intramuscularly in those patients with inefficient absorption or those in the early stages of a nutrient program in which it is desirable to accelerate immune repair by providing the body with more usuable selenium.

Vitamin B Complex

Although the B vitamins are intermediary metabolites in the body's energy systems, such as carbohydrate metabolism and brain and nervous system functions, they also participate in immune-system activities. Because this family of vitamins is water soluble, they are not stored and must be renewed from food or other nutrient sources daily. A practical program may be designed around a supplement containing all the B-complex nutrients in one formulation. A B-complex formula may also contain many other vitamins and minerals and still work effectively. In some patients vitamin B_6 and vitamin B_{12} seem to play an important role in immune-system rebalancing. An effective dose of vitamin B_6 may begin at 50 mg daily but go higher. Vitamin B_{12} is available as a sublingual, which is administered under the tongue; this route bypasses the digestion and presents the B_{12} to the circulating blood. When higher doses seem to be required, the B vitamins may be injected by intramuscular route or dripped intravenously.

NONSPECIFIC STIMULANT HERBS

Herbs that have nonspecific stimulating effects bolster the entire immune system. Rather than promote the immune system to act against one particular type of organism, as a vaccine would do, they make the immune system more active against all kinds of invading organisms. These herbs also work by building up the overall endurance and stamina of the body.

ECHINACEA

Echinacea, also known as purple coneflower, is an American botanical that has long been known for its powerful immune-stimulating properties. This was the foremost medicinal plant used by many American Indian tribes. And when the Europeans who colonized this country became familiar with it, echinacea rapidly became their most popular medicine too. By the turn of the century, echinacea was the number one selling herbal tincture and it remains so to this day because of its effectiveness in building immune resistance.

Echinacea stimulates every aspect of the immune system. It has been shown to increase the number of developing immune cells in the bone marrow and in the lymphatic system. As a result, these cells can be released into the circulation at a much faster rate and become more active in attacking bacteria, viruses, and aberrant cells that could be the start of cancerous conditions.

Modern research on echinacea comes primarily from Europe, and especially Germany, where hundreds of studies have been conducted. Echinacea has been grown and used in Europe since the 1930s and it is one of their most popular herbal compounds. The most recent European research suggests that echinacea and most other immune stimulants have effects that last from four to five days. European clinics prefer to use these stimulants on a schedule; they will give you the herbs for three or four days and then stop it for the same time period to let your immune system rest before it receives another boost. This on/off procedure allows it to be taken to an even higher level of activity.

Echinacea, which can easily be found in your local health food store, is most popular as a liquid extract, but also comes in capsules and tablets. You can judge its quality to some extent by its taste. If it has a peculiar tingling effect and a numbing effect on the tongue and it increases salivation, the compound generally contains more echinacea.

It is difficult to recommend specific doses of echinacea since the active ingredients may differ from preparation to preparation. There are also different species of echinacea that may be combined in different proportions. Moreover, the components of a capsule or a tablet may be quite different from the components of the alcohol tincture or other liquid forms.

Astragalus

Astragalus is one of the best-researched immune-system stimulants now available. It has been shown to reduce tumor cell growth and to reverse cancerous conditions. In one study done at the University of Texas, astragalus completely restored the immune function of cells taken from cancer patients, which is a very difficult task to accomplish.

Astragalus is found in America as well as in China. In China it has been used since ancient times to strengthen the body. The historical Chinese philosophy of what we call disease focused instead upon the energy flows within the body and ascendance to these energies—which they called ill humors or destructive energies—that attacked the organism and caused imbalance. Astragalus was thought to shield against these hazards.

In some ways, astragalus works with much like echinacea. Both herbs increase the number and activity of immune cells in circulation; however, astragalus concentrates more on building the immune system. And in the Orient, people take it on a longer-term basis than they do echinacea. They also use astragalus as an ingredient in soups because it is energizing and nourishing. Astragalus has been proven to reduce the frequency and duration of colds and flus by boosting the immune system rather than by killing viruses. Today the HIV-infected community is taking a close look at both echinacea and astragalus because of their immune-stimulating effects.

Licorice Root

Although licorice root is not known predominantly for its immune-stimulating effects, some preliminary evidence shows that it fosters anti-HIV activity. The element within the licorice that promotes this activity is the one that makes it sweet.

You can buy licorice root in liquid extract form, in capsules and tablets, or as a whole herb.

Panax and Siberian Ginseng

Both panax (meaning "all healing") ginseng and Siberian ginseng (eleutherococcus) have powerful immune-stimulating effects. Both ginsengs are known to build stamina, energy, and endurance by stabilizing the body. For this reason, they are popular with athletes and with people who suffer from conditions that zap them of their strength and energy, like chronic fatigue syndrome.

The latest research on Siberian ginseng is especially impressive because of a new tool that's now being used to measure the herb's activity in the immune system. This tool actually allows you to see how the cells circulating in each area of the immune system increase in activity and number.

Garlic

Garlic not only stimulates the immune system but also serves as an antibacterial, antiviral, and antifungal element. Garlic is a mild natural antibiotic that increases the activity of natural killer cells so that they can better fight off viruses and tumor cells. It also works actively to fight off infections. Other members of the allium genus, such as onions, have anticancer properties as well. They also assist in the circulatory system and help to protect the liver.

It's beneficial to take garlic every day as a preventive measure and to enhance your well-being. You can take garlic tablets and use a lot of garlic in your cooking. Much research has been done on garlic in the last five to ten years to make garlic products more potent and concentrated while eliminating their effects on the breath.

SPECIFIC ANTIVIRAL STIMULANT HERBS

The following herbs have more specific antiviral effects on the immune system. In general, they are less well understood than the nonspecific stimulant herbs mentioned above.

Philanthus

Philanthus, also called life plant, is used in Oriental medicine. It has been shown to act against hepatitis B and is now being researched for its antiretroviral and anti-HIV activity. Philanthus is a new herb in this country and as such may be difficult to find, but evidence of its effectiveness is promising.

Usnea and Lomacium

Usnea and lomacium, both new to the marketplace, are known for their specific antiviral activity. They seem to help fight off influenza and chronic fatigue syndrome. In addition, they appear to promote antifungal activity against candida.

St.-John's-Wort

St.-John's-wort, a common weed found in California, is now being studied by AIDS researchers because it seems to help prevent infections of T cells by making it harder for the AIDS virus to get into cells. In addition, the National Cancer Institute is looking at hypericum, a chemical found in the weed, because researchers believe it to be the active component of the plant.*

Ephedra

Ephedra, or mahuang, is a powerful short-term energy herb. The plant has a long and interesting history. As the oldest known medicinal plant, ephedra was first cultivated more than five thousand years ago. In ancient China, it was used specifically for the treatment of respiratory disease.

Ephedra contains two ingredients that are commonly used in our more chemical pharmacopeia today. One of these, ephedrin, is used for the treatment of asthma. And the second is known as pseudoephedrine.

Ephedra serves as a decongestant and a stimulant that's similar to caffeine but less detrimental. Its stimulating effect is short term; when you take ephedra or an extract of it, you feel its effect within fifteen to thirty minutes and it lasts for as long as the boost you get from a cup of coffee or tea. Ephedra is safer to use than caffeine because its composition more closely resembles the adrenaline produced by your body. In fact, ephedrin is the closest chemical found in the plant kingdom to adrenaline.

It should be emphasized that ephedra is meant to be used only for a short period of time. There is a saying in

*Unfortunately, a clinical trial of hypericum conducted in San Francisco was altered when the project's natural source of hypericum was replaced by a semisynthetic form of the chemical. Thus, the effects of hypericum taken in its natural context could not be observed.

Scientists often assume that they know which chemical in a plant is most important. However, they may overlook some essential ingredients or not realize the importance of looking at whole plant extracts instead of taking plants apart. For example, some studies now show that plants relatively low in hypericum exhibit significant antiretroviral activity, which means that scientists may have misidentified the active ingredient in the plant. Or it may mean that the combination of ingredients enhances the plant's overall effectiveness.

China that long-term ephedra use is like beating a tired horse, and long-term ginseng use is like feeding a tired horse. The ginseng builds physical and mental energy and endurance more slowly over the long term.

Ganoderma (Reishi Mushroom)

The mushroom fungi used in Oriental medicine have powerful immune-stimulating effects. The type of mushroom gaining the most ground in this country is ganoderma. The mushroom's Japanese name, reishi, is commonly used in America as well. The Chinese call it ling zhe.

Through its immune-stimulating activity, ganoderma reduces the cholesterol, triglycerides, and total serum lipids, which are the fats in the bloodstream. It also has potent anticancer properties that are creating great excitement.

The Chinese produce some very interesting products from ling zhe. They sell it in liquid extracts in glass vials or ampules and in a concentrated form as well, often adding honey to it for taste. Some excellent American products are also made from reishi mushrooms.

Shiitake and Agaricus Mushrooms

Shiitake mushrooms have a particular polysaccharide complex sugar that appears to have some powerful antitumor and antimutagenic qualities. For this reason, the mushrooms are now being researched in Japan at a feverish pace.

The Japanese are taking a close look at the genus Agaricus, which includes the ordinary mushroom found in the grocery store. It is not yet known whether this mushroom's activity even approaches that of the better-known medicinal mushrooms, but it does appear to have health-promoting properties such as combating the effects of free radicals.

Poria Cocos

Poria cocos, better known as poria, is another fungus used in Asia for its beneficial effects on the blood. The fungus reduces fat levels in the blood and lessens the deposition of fats within organs, thereby preventing fatty degeneration within the liver and other organs. It also helps to increase stamina and endurance.

Iknowki Mushroom

Iknowki mushrooms are the long, thin, white mushrooms now showing up in salad bars in America. The area in Japan where iknowki mushrooms are grown has the lowest incidence of cancer in that country.

CLEANSING HERBS

Herbs that detoxify the body appear to increase the activity of the liver and the secretion of bile, which helps to eliminate some of the poisons from the liver and blood.

Many of these herbs are diuretics (like dandelion leaves) and laxatives (like senna, cascara sagrada, and Chinese rhubarb), and therefore are meant for short-term use only. Laxative herbs should just be used for a brief period of time to eliminate toxins from the body. Long-term use will make you dependent on them because your intestines will become accustomed to working with a stimulant and then have a hard time working without one. By discontinuing the herbs you allow your digestive system to return to normal.

The same is true of diuretics because long-term use can lead to dehydration. When you begin any cleansing program that involves the use of diuretics, drink plenty of liquids to maintain your nutrient levels, and take vitamin supplements if necessary. Some cleansing herbs are listed below:

Burdock Root

Burdock root is one of the best-known cleansing herbs, according to folklore. It works as a liver and bile stimulant and also acts to increase digestion.

Burdock is a very popular vegetable in the Orient. In fact, the Japanese consume it more than carrots and it can be found in any sushi bar. In America, you can find burdock root in extracts, capsules, or bulk form in natural food stores.

Dandelion Root and Leaves

Dandelion root helps to stimulate the liver, the gall bladder, and the bile secretion. Dandelion leaves prove useful in a detoxification program because they act as a diuretic. One advantage dandelion leaves have over chemical diuretics is that chemical ones deplete potassium from your body. Dandelion leaves, on the other hand, contain high levels of potassium. In a sense, eating these leaves is like taking a diuretic with a potassium supplement. One report showed dry dandelion leaves to have a potassium content of 4½ percent, which is a substantial amount.

Red Clover

Many cleansing programs include red clover, partly because of its high nutritional content and its anti–free radical effect. Red clover protects liver cells and cells in other organs from oxidation damage. This damage may be caused by any number of things, including rancid fats that can throw off free radicals and attack the DNA of the cells, thereby causing mutations that could conceivably lead to cancer. And since free radicals contribute to the aging process, red clover and other herbs like ginkgo and garlic can have a rejuvenating effect and enhance longevity.

REGENERATIVE HERBS FROM ANCIENT TIMES

Some other ancient healing herbs are being rediscovered today for their immune-enhancing effects and other beneficial properties. They include the following:

Gurmar

Gurmar, known scientifically as gymnea, was used in Ayurvedic medicine in India more than six hundred years ago for the treatment of what they called honey urine. This was their name for the modern-day diabetes. It's astonishing to think that a culture knew six centuries ago that diabetes was a condition characterized by increased sugar or sweetness in the urine, especially when you consider that Western scientists discovered this in the eighteenth century.

Today, scientific studies of extracts of this plant confirm that its properties are beneficial to diabetes patients. In fact, it has been found effective not only in the reduction of blood sugar, which is an antidiabetic agent's primary function, but also in the repair of damage to the kidneys, liver, and pancreas as well.

Recent studies in India have also shown that extracts of this plant actually increase beta cells, which are the insulin-producing cells in the pancreas. This finding is virtually medical heresy because modern Western medicine believes that pancreas damage can never be repaired. The study, which was reported in *The Journal of Ethnopharmacology*, a well-respected peer-review journal, found an actual improvement in the insulin output of the diabetic pancreas. And in follow-up testing of insulin-dependent and insulin-independent diabetics, the amount of medication needed was reduced in both cases. In many instances, subjects did not need anything but this plant compound, which rather than damaging the liver and kidneys actually improved them. But despite the importance of these findings, the Western medical community has refused to recognize these amazing Indian studies, and attempts have not yet been made to duplicate the experiment here.

Milk Thistle

Another herb whose use dates back to ancient history is milk thistle. This botanical has long been known to protect and regenerate the liver. In the past, the seeds of the plant were eaten or crushed and brewed into a tea as a remedy for liver ailments. Now a high-tech, standardized extract of the plant is being used not just as a folk medicine but also as a respected modern plant medicine sold throughout the pharmacies of Europe.

One milk thistle compound, called silverin, is an injectible drug used as a life-saving treatment to stop the progress of fatal or potentially fatal mushroom poisoning. It is the only thing in the world known to counteract poisoning from the deadly amanita mushroom.

Environmentally Oriented Health-Care Practitioners

Health-Care Practitioners

Lorraine Abbey, M.D.
Warren Place West
Route 130
East Windsor, NJ 08512
(609) 443-6393
Acupuncture

John Ackerman, M.D.
2417 Castillo Street
Santa Barbara, CA 93105
(805) 682-1011

John Adams, M.D.
711 East End Boulevard South
Marshall, TX 75670
(214) 938-4363
Family Practice

Neil Adams, M.D.
123 North Tower
Centralia, WA 98531
(206) 736-1171
Otolaryngology, Rhinology

Hartwig Adler, M.D.
4208 Vendome Place
New Orleans, LA 70125
(504) 865-1767
Otolaryngology

Majid Ali, M.D.
95 E. Main St.
Denville, NJ 07834
(201) 586-4111
Pathology, Self-Regulation

Jeffry Anderson, M.D.
45 San Clemente Road 100b
Corte Madera, CA 94925
(415) 927-7140
Clinical Immunology, Internal Medicine

Barbara Ardoin, M.D.
123 Ridgeway Drive
Lafayette, LA 70505
(318) 981-8204
Preventative Medicine

Robert Armer, M.D.
8803 North Meridian Street
Indianapolis, IN 46260
(317) 846-7341
Pediatrics

Terry Armheim
7 Marcy Drive
New York, NY 11766
(516) 473-4314
Nutrition Counselor

Dr. Robert Atkins
400 East 56th Street
New York, NY 10022
(212) 758-2110
Holistic Medicine

Howard Aylward, M.D.
4512 Carriage Hill Drive
Santa Barbara, CA 93110
(805) 967-5955
Otolaryngology

Richard Bahr, M.D.
2353 West Stroop Road
Dayton, OH 45439
(513) 299-8788
Family Practice

Sidney Baker, M.D.
60 Washington Avenue
Hamden, CT 06518
(203) 287-1800
Pediatrics

Wyrth Post Baker, M.D.
4701 Willard Avenue
Chevy Chase, MD 20815
(301) 656-8940
Internal Medicine

E. G. Barnet, M.D.
550 West Thomas Road 233D
Phoenix, AZ 85013
(602) 264-7957
Clinical Immunology

John Baron, D.O.
4807 Rockside
Suite 100
Cleveland, OH 44145
(216) 642-0082
Preventative Medicine

Ervin Barr, D.O.
2350 West Oakland Park Boulevard
Ft. Lauderdale, FL 33311
(305) 731-8080
Family Practice

Gerald Bart, M.D.
10004 Kennerley Road #310
St. Louis, MO 63128
(314) 842-5082
Otolaryngology

Bruce Battleson, M.D.
18124 Culver City Drive #G
Irvine, CA 92715
(714) 786-3433
Allergist, Nutritionist

John Beaty, M.D.
40 East Putnam Avenue
Cos Cob, CT 06807
(203) 869-6302
Allergy

Iris Bell, M.D.
Department of Psychiatry
University of Arizona
Tucson, AZ 85724
(602) 626-6254
Psychiatry

Thomas Benson, M.D.
1200 North East Street
Olney, IL 62450
(618) 395-5222
Pediatrics

Adam Ber, M.D.
20635 North Cave Creek Road
Phoenix, AZ 85024
(602) 279-3795
Homeopathic Physician

Thomas Bernawsky, M.D.
4 Ivy Knoll
Westport, CT 06880
(203) 454-5963
General Medicine, Nutrition, Preventative Medicine, Allergist

Robert Bettis
224 East 47th Street
New York, NY 10017
(212) 556-1025
Nutrition Counselor

Murray Black, D.O.
609 South 48th Avenue
Yakima, WA 98908
(509) 966-1780
Family Practice

Miklos Boczko, M.D.
12 Greenridge Avenue
White Plains, NY 10605
(914) 949-8817
Neurology

Marvin Boris, M.D.
75 Froelich Farm Boulevard
Woodbury, NY 11797
(516) 921-9000
Pediatrics

Robert Boxer, M.D.
64 Old Orchard Road
Skokie, IL 60077
(708) 677-0260
Allergist

John Boyles, M.D.
7076 Corporate Way
Centerville, OH 45459
(513) 434-0555
Otolaryngology

Cecil Bradley, M.D.
27206 Calaroga Avenue #205
Hayward, CA 94545
(415) 783-9900
Addiction Medicine

Muriel Bramwell
2435 Chester Street
Eureka, CA 95501
(707) 443-2306
Nutritionist

William Brauer, M.D.
2545 Chicago Avenue
Minneapolis, MN 55404
(612) 871-2611
Psychiatrist

Nachman Brautbar, M.D.
201 South Alvarado #202
Los Angeles, CA 90057
(213) 662-8866
Internal Medicine, Nephrology

Harold Brenner, M.D.
8622 Liberty Plaza Mall
Randallstown, MD 2113
(301) 922-1133
Pediatric and Adolescent Medicine

Jennifer Brett
6 Hollyhock Road
Wilton, CT 06897
(203) 834-9788
Naturopathic Physician

Brian Briggs, M.D.
718 SW 6th Street
Minot, ND 58701
(701) 838-6011
Family Practice, General Practice, Nutritional Therapy

Martin Brody, M.D., D.D.S.
7100 West 20th Avenue
Hialeah, FL 33016
(305) 822-9035
Otolaryngology

Richard Brody, M.D.
37 Burr Farms Road
Westport, CT 06518
(203) 227-5311
Psychologist, Nutritionist

Clifton Brooks, M.D.
2114 Martingdale
Norman, OK 73072
(405) 329-8437
Preventative and Environmental Medicine, Pediatrics

Andrew Brown, M.D.
515 South Third Street
Gadsen, AL 35901
(205) 547-4971
Otolaryngology

David Brown, M.D.
830 Fidelity Building
Dayton, OH 45402
(513) 223-3691
Ear, Nose, and Throat Allergist

Don Bryan, M.D.
P.O. Box 1857
Alabaster, AL 35007
(205) 663-5840
Otolaryngology

William Bryce, M.D.
1254 Irvine Boulevard #160
Tuslin, CA 92580
(714) 544-3900
Colonic and Chelation Therapist

Thurman Bullock, M.D.
104 East 7th Avenue
Chadbourn, NC 28431
(919) 654-3143
Family Practice

David Buscher, M.D.
1370-116th Avenue NE #102
Bellevue, WA 98004
(206) 453-0388
Family Practice, Preventative Medicine

Harold Buttram, M.D.
R.D. #3 Clymer
Quakertown, PA 18951
(215) 536-1890
Nutrition, Internal Family Practice

Christopher Calapai, M.D.
1900 Hempstead Turnpike #502
East Meadow, NY 11554
(516) 794-0404
Allergy Testing and Treatment, Arthritis, and Osteopathic Medicine

Herbert Camp, M.D.
4011 Orchard Drive 3004
Midland, MI 48641
(517) 631-1254
Otolaryngology

Stanley Cannon, M.D.
9085 Southwest 87th Avenue
Miami, FL 33176
(305) 279-3020
Otolaryngology

Lawrence Caprio, M.D.
830 Post Road East
Westport, CT 06880
(203) 226-4167
Naturopathic Medicine

Francis Carroll, M.D.
104 East 7th Avenue
Chadbourn, NC 28431
(919) 654-3143
Internal Medicine

Dr. H. Richard Casdorph
1703 Termino Avenue
Suite 201
Long Beach, CA 90804
(310) 597-8716
Internal Medicine, Cardiologist

Hyla Cass, M.D.
20522 Roca Chica Drive
Malibu, CA 90265
(310) 456-5432

Rocco Cassone, M.D.
1175 Cook Road #230
Orangeburg, SC 29116
(803) 536-5511
Otolaryngology

William Cates, M.D.
2885 West Dublin Granville Road
Columbus, OH 43235
(614) 261-0151
Psychiatry, Homeopathy

Robert Cathcart, M.D.
127 Second Street
Los Altos, CA 94322
(415) 949-2822
Orthomolecular Physician, Allergist, Environmental Medicine

Hana Chaim, D.O.
595 West Granada Boulevard
Ormond Beach, FL 32174
(904) 672-9000
Family Practice

I-Tsu Chao, M.D.
1641 East 18th Street
Brooklyn, NY 11229
(718) 998-3331
Immunologist, Allergist

Dr. Emmanuel Cheraskin
Park Tower 904–906
2717 Highland Ave. South
Birmingham, AL 35205
(205) 934-4750
Clinical Research

Tom Chesnick
289 Lake Shore Drive
Parsippany, NJ 07054
(201) 386-5773
Nutrition Counselor

Chin Chung, M.D.
210 East 2nd Street
Erie, PA 16507
(814) 455-4429
Pediatric Cardiology

Mary Cody, Ph.D.
Box 355A Meadowbrook Road
Boontown Township, NJ 07005
(201) 335-9841
Nutritionist

Harold Cohen, M.D.
Six Wind Northwest
Albuquerque, NM 87120
(505) 898-7115
Medical Doctor; Psychiatrist

Jack Cohen, M.D.
184 Upper Mountain Avenue
Montclair, NJ 07042
(201) 239-6688
Internal Medicine

Linda Cohen
25 Central Park South #17H
New York, NY 10023
(212) 957-9002
Nutrition Counselor

Thomas Collins, M.D.
4737 Sonoma Highway
Santa Rosa, CA 95409
(707) 538-3554
Chiropractor

Vicki Conrad, M.D.
1616 South Boulevard
Edmond, OK 73013
(405) 341-5691
GP, Environmental, Nutritional Medicine

George Constanti, M.D.
115 Medical Drive #201
Victori, TX 77904
(512) 576-4182
Neuropsychiatrist

Albert Corrado, M.D.
750 Swift Avenue
Suite #22
Richland, WA 99352
(509) 946-4631
Dermatology, Internal Medicine

Serafina Corsella, M.D.
200 West 57th Street
12th Floor
New York, NY 10019
(212) 517-0222
Chelation, Homeopathy for Children, Chronic Fatigue, Candidiasis, Stress Management

Carrie Cossaboon, Ph.D.
342 Meadowbrook Road
North Wales, PA 19454
(215) 699-4600
Radiational Physics

Dr. Alan Cott
160 East 38th Street
New York, NY 10016
(212)679-6694

Dr. Elmer M. Cranton
Ripshin Road
P.O. Box 44
Trout Dale, VA 24378
(703) 677-3631
Family Practioner

William Crook, M.D., P.C.
681 Skyline Drive
Jackson, TN 38301
(901) 423-5400
Pediatrician, Environmental Medicine

Linwood Custalow, M.D.
1832 Todds Lane
Hampton, VA 23666
(804) 826-0232
Head and Neck Surgery, Otolaryngic Allergy, Otolaryngology

Peter D'Adamo
54 Lafayette Place
Greenwich, CT 06830
(203) 661-7375
Naturopathic Physician

David Darbro, M.D.
2124 East Hanna Avenue
Indianapolis, IN 46227
(317) 783-5433
Preventative Medicine

Martin Dayton, D.O., M.D.
18600 Collins Avenue
North Miami Beach, FL 33160
(305) 931-8484
Osteopathic, Holistic, Homeopathic, Acupuncture

Sharon De Kadt
94 Center Road
Woodbridge, CT 06525
(203) 785-1154
Naturopathic Physician

Sandra Denton, M.D.
5080 List Drive
Colorado Springs, CO 80919
(719) 548-1600
Diabetes, Family Practice, Mercury Toxicity

Cornelius Derrick, M.D.S.
1821 King Road
Trenton, MI 48183
(313) 675-0678
Otolaryngology, Dermatology

John Dogden, M.D.
5185 Comanche Drive #A
La Mesa, CA 92116
(619) 464-8924
Psychiatry

Nedra Downing, D.O.
7650 Dixie Highway
Clarkston, MI 48016
(313) 625-6660
Hypertension, Osteoporosis

Crawford Duhon, M.D.
4841 Eldorado Springs Drive
Boulder, CO 80303
(303) 499-9386
Allergy, Environmental Medicine

Paul Dunn, M.D.
715 Lake Street
Oak Park, IL 60301
(312) 383-3800
Psychiatry

Carl Ebnother, M.D.
20430 Town Center Lane
Suite 5G
Cupertino, CA 95014
(415) 969-0708
Holistic Medicine

Dr. Jeanne Eckerley
5851 Duluth Street
Suite 110
Minneapolis, MN 55422
(612) 593-9458
Chelation Therapy, Environmental Medicine

Robert Elghammer, M.D.
723 North Logan Avenue
Danville, IL 61832
(217) 446-3259
Pediatrics

Leander Ellis, M.D.
2746 Belmont
Philadelphia, PA 19131
(215) 477-6444
Phobias, Lupus, Anxiety

Stephen Elsasser, D.O.
206 South Engelwood
Metamora, IL 61548
(309) 367-2321
Osteopath, Family Practice

Kenneth Emonds, Ph.D.
65 Newburyport Turnpike
Newbury, MA 01950
(617) 465-5009
Nutritional Biochemistry

Carol Englander, M.D.
1340 Centre Street
Newton Center, MA 02159
(617) 965-7770
Holistic Physician

Walter Evans, Ph.D.
102 Midway Drive
Clinton, MS 39056
(601) 924-5605
Nutrition Counselor

Hobart Feldman, M.D.
16800 Northwest Second Avenue
#301
North Miami Beach, FL 33169
(305) 652-1062
Allergy and Immunology Specialist

Dr. Martin Feldman
132 East 76th Street
New York, NY 10021
(212) 744-4413
(718) 376-5032
Neurologist

David Filkoff, M.D.
760 Framington Avenue
West Hartford, CT 06105
(203) 523-8462
Holistic Medicine

Howard Fine
468 Main Street N.
Westport, CT 06880
(203) 221-0216
Homeopathic Physician

Jerold Finnie, M.D.
1185 New Litchfield Street
Torrington, CT 06790
(203) 489-8977
Nutrition, Otolaryngology

James Fish, M.D.
3030 North Hancock Avenue
Colorado Springs, CO 80907
(719) 471-2273
Dermatology, Urology, Hypnoanalysis, Allergy

J. W. Fitzsimmons, M.D.
591 Hidden Valley Road
Grants Pass, OR 97527
(503) 474-2166
Environmental Medicine

Molly Fleming
600 George Street
New Haven, CT 06511
(203) 772-3000
Naturopath

Dr. Richard Frey
1170 Broadway
New York, NY 10019
(212) 545-1140
Chiropractor, Nutrition Counselor

Milton Fried, M.D.
4426 Tilly Mill Road
Atlanta, GA 30360
(404) 451-4857
Environmental Medicine

Suzanne Fromherz, B.S., R.N.
327 West Meadow
Fayetteville, AR 72701
(501) 442-7959
Homeopathy

John Furlong, M.D.
902 Main Street #2D
Willimantic, CT
(203) 456-3349
Naturopath

Fred Furr, M.D.
9217 Park West Boulevard Building East
Suite 1
Knoxville, TN 37923
(615) 693-1502
Family Practice

Estelle Futterman
200 Central Park West
New York, NY
(212) 765-8056
Nutrition Counselor

Charles Gabelman, M.D.
24953 Paseo De Valencia
#16C
Laguna Hills, CA 92653
(714) 859-9851
Allergist, Fatigue and Thyroid Specialist

Leo Galland, M.D.
133 E. 73rd St.
New York, NY 10021
(212) 861-9000
Evaluation and Treatment of Disease Involving Food and Environmental Sensitivity, Asthma, Chronic Fatigue, Arthritis

John Gambee, M.D.
66 Club Road
Eugene, OR 97401
(503) 686-2536
Preventative Medicine

Tierry Garcia, M.D.
1500 Albany Street
Beech Grove, IN 46107
(317) 783-8830
Otolaryngology

Zane Gard, M.D.
P.O. Box 231309
San Diego, CA 92123
(619) 571-0300
Immunotoxicology Consultant, Family Practice

James Gensenig
600 George Street
New Haven, CT 06511
(203) 772-3000
Naturopath

Kendall Gerdes, M.D.
1617 Vine Street
Denver, CO 80206
(303) 377-8837
Internal Medicine

Jacqueline Germaine, M.D.
67 Bernie O'Rourke Drive
Middletown, CT 06457
(203) 347-8600
Naturopathic Physician

Debra Gibson
15 East Main Street
New Milford, CT 06776
(203) 350-8959
Naturopath, Holistic Medicine, Allergist

Peter Gilbert, M.D.
415 South Second
Geneva, IL 60134
(708) 232-7761
Family Practice

Robert Gillcash, M.D.
P.O. Box 37
North Franklin, CT 06524
(203) 642-4145
Otolaryngology

Donald Goehring, M.D.
503 Union Bank Building
Butler, PA 16001
(412) 287-4241
Otolaryngology

Sheldon Goldberg, M.D.
2 Medical Center Drive #110
Springfield, MA 01107
(413) 732-7426
Otolaryngology

William Goldwag, M.D.
7499 Corritos Avenue
Stanton, CA 90680
(714) 827-5180
Preventative Medicine

Nicholas Gonsalez, M.D.
737 Park Avenue
New York, NY 10021
(212) 535-3993
Treatment of Cancer Including AIDS and Other Degenerative Disorders

Thomas Goodwin, M.D.
6111 Harrison Street #343
Merrillville, IN 46410
(219) 980-6117
Family Practice

Dr. Ross Gordon
405 Kains Street
Albany, CA 94706
(510) 526-3232
Nutritionist, Preventative Medicine

John Green, M.D.
P.O. Box
Aurora, OR 97002
(503) 678-2233
Environmental Physician

Leyland Green, M.D.
P.O. Box 508
Lansdale, PA 16001
(412) 287-4241
Otolaryngology

Howard Greenspan, M.D.
Mountainview Medical
Nyack, NY 10960
(914) 368-4700
Nutritional and Preventative Medicine

Howard Hagglund, M.D.
2227 West Lindsey #1401
Norman, OK 73069
(405) 329-4458
Family Practice

William Halcomb, D.O.
4830 East Main Street #27
Mesa, AZ 85205
(602) 832-3014
Preventative Medicine, General Practice

Vicker Halloran, M.D.
5629 FM 1967 West #225
Houston, TX 77069
(713) 440-0800
Pediatrics

Bruce Halstead, M.D.
22607 Barton Road
Grand Terrace, CA 92324
(714) 783-2773
Preventative Medicine, Chelation

Charles Hamel, M.D.
4412 Matlock Road #300
Arlington, TX 77069
(713) 440-0800
Otolaryngology

Stanley Hansen, M.D.
440 Fair Drive #J
Costa Mesa, CA 92626
(714) 557-5500
Psychiatry, Internal Medicine

Mechtold Van Hardenbroek, M.D.
205 Country Club Park
Grand Junction, CO 81503
(303) 241-8554
Family Practice, Nutrition

Dennis Harper, D.O.
1675 North Freedom Boulevard
200 W #11E
Provo, UT 84604
(801) 373-8500
Bariatrics, Family Practice

Robert Hazelwood, M.D.
711 West 38th Street C-4
Austin, TX 78705
(512) 458-9286
Psychiatry

Harold Hedges, M.D.
424 North University
Little Rock, AR 72205
(501) 664-4810
Family Practice

Edwin Helleniak, M.D.
811 Madison Avenue
Dunellen, NJ 08812
(908) 752-2216
Psychiatric and Nutritional Practice

Neil Henderson, M.D.
30 South East Seventh Street
Boca Raton, FL 33432
(407) 368-2915
Allergist

Pearlyn Goodman Herrick
21 Trails End Road
Weston, CT 06883
(203) 227-5534
Naturopathic Physician

Ralph Herro, M.D.
5115 North Central Avenue
Phoenix, AZ 85012
(602) 266-2374
Family Practice, Internal Medicine

Aaron Herschfus, M.D.
62 South Main Street
P.O. Box 336
Sharon, MA 02067
(617) 784-2082
Internal Medicine

Norene Hess, M.D.
700 Oak
Winnetka, IL 60093
(708) 446-1923
Environmental Medicine

James Hill, M.D.
780 Eagle Creek Court
Zionsville, IN 46007
(317) 846-7341
Allergist

Charle Hinshaw, M.D.
1133 East Second
Wichita, KS 67214
(316) 262-0951
Pathology, Nuclear Medicine

Dr. Abram Hoffer
Suite 3A
2727 Quadra Street
Victoria, British Columbia
Canada V8T 4E5
(604) 386-8756
Orthomolecular Psychiatrist

Ronald Hoffman, M.D.
40 East 30th Street
New York, NY 10014
(212) 779-1744
Arthritis and Allergy

Harris Hosen, M.D.
2001 Holcomb Boulevard
#1301
Houston, TX 77030
(713) 799-2148
Allergist

Richard Hrdlicka, M.D.
123 South Street
Geneva, IL 60134
(708) 232-1900
Family Practice, Nutrition

Reed Hyde, M.D.
2225 East Flamingo Road
#301
Las Vegas, NV 89119
(702) 731-3117
Environmental Allergist

Herbert Insel, M.D.
894 Madison Avenue
New York, NY 10021
(212) 772-7782
Specialist in Cardiology and Internal Medicine

Joe Izen, M.D.
3912 Brookhaven
Pasadena, TX 77504
(713) 941-2444
Otolaryngology

Mary James
94 Center Road
Woodbridge, CT 06525
(203) 397-8890
Naturopath

Scott Jamison, M.D.
369 South Franklin #300
Juneau, AK 99801
(907) 586-6810
Naturopathic Physician

Michael Janson, M.D.
2557 Massachusetts Avenue
Cambridge, MA 02140
(617) 661-6225
Nutrition, Holistic Medicine

Deidre J'Occoner, M.D.
19 East Main Street
Mystic, CT
(203) 572-9566,
(203) 572-9566
Naturopath

Alfred Johnson, D.O.
8345 Walnut Hill Lane #205
Dallas, TX 75231
(214) 368-4312
Internal Medicine

George Juetersonke, D.O.
3090 North Academy Boulevard #10
Colorado Springs, CO 80917
(719) 596-9040
Family Practice

James Julian, M.D.
1654 Cahuenga Boulevard
Hollywood, CA 90025
(213) 467-5555
Chelation

Eleazar Kadile, M.D.
1901 South Webster
Green Bay, WI 54301
(414) 468-9442
Psychiatry, Hypnosis

Leonard Kaplan, M.D.
NW Professional Plaza
Columbus, OH 43220
(614) 431-9393
Weight Loss and Hypnosis

John Keebler, M.D.
6701 Airport Boulevard B123
Mobile, AL 36608
(205) 633-2323
Otolaryngology, Head and Neck Maxillofacial Cosmetic Surgery

Joseph Keenan, M.D.
75 Springfield
Westfield, MA 01085
(413) 568-2304
Otolaryngology

Roy Kerry, M.D.
17 6th Avenue
Greenville, PA 16125
(412) 588-2600
Head and Neck Surgery, Allergy Environmental Medicine, Facial Plastic Surgery

Gerald Keyte, D.O.
388 Inkster
Inkster, MI 48141
(313) 278-3050
GP

Howard Kimball, M.D.
c/o Garst Clinic
Mt. View, AR 72560
(501) 269-4301
Family Practice

Jeffrey Klase, N.D.
625 East Main Street
Bramford, CT 06405
(203) 481-5219
Naturopath

Wayne Konetzki, M.D.
403 North Grand Avenue
Waukesha, WI 53186

(414) 547-3055
Allergist

Kenneth Krischer, M.D., Ph.D.
910 South West 40th Avenue
Plantation, FL 33317
(305) 584-6655
Nutrition

Jacqueline Krohn, M.D.
Los Alamos Medical Center
#136
Los Alamos, NM 87544
(505) 662-9620
Pediatrics

George Kroker, M.D.
615 South 10th
P.O. Box 2408
La Crosse, WI 54602
(608) 782-2027
Allergist

Richard Kunin, M.D.
2698 Pacific Avenue
San Francisco, CA 94115
(415) 346-2500
Psychiatric, Nutritional, Orthomolecular Medicine

Howard Lang, D.O.
1404 Brown Trail
Bedford, TX 76022
(817) 268-1171
Allergist, Family Practice

Randall Langston, M.D.
1005 Mar Walt Drive
Ft. Walton Beach, FL 32548
(904) 863-8287
Otolaryngology

Richard Layton, M.D.
901 Dulaney Valley Road #602
Towson, MD 21204
(301) 337-2707
Pediatrics

Thomas Le Cava, M.D.
1084 Main Street
Holden, MA 01520
(508) 829-5321
Pediatrics

Ralph Lee, M.D.
110 Lewis Drive #B
Maritta, GA 30068
(404) 423-0064
Family Practice, Preventative Medicine

Richard Leigh, M.D.
2314 Library Lane
Grand Forks, ND 58201
(701) 775-5527
Nutritional Medicine

Michael Lesser, M.D.
2340 Parker Street
Berkeley, CA 94704
(510) 845-0700
Nutritionist

Warren Levin, M.D.
444 Park Avenue South
New York, NY 10016
(212) 696-1900
Chelation, Clinical Ecology, Parasitiology, Candida

Allan Lieberman, M.D.
7510 Northforest Drive
North Charleston, SC 29420
(803) 572-1600
Clinical Toxicology

Cathie Ann Lippman, M.D.
8383 Wilshire Boulevard #360
Beverly Hills, CA 90211
(213) 653-0486
Environmental Medicine, Psychiatry

Enrico Liva, M.D.
87 Bernie O'Rourke Drive
Middletown, CT 06457
(203) 347-8600
Naturopathic Methods to Treat Heart Disease

Paul Lynn, M.D.
345 West Portal Avenue
San Francisco, CA 94127
(415) 566-1000
Preventative Medicine

Laura Maeates
185 Cedar Lane
Teaneck, NJ 07666
(201) 836-0888
Nutrition Counselor

Allan Magaziner, M.D.
1907 Greentree Road
Cherry Hill, NJ 08003
(609) 424-8222
Family Practice, Nutrition, Osteopathy, Preventative Medicine

Hamid Mahmud, M.D.
1610 North Broadway
Salem, IL 63881
(618) 548-4613
Pediatrics, Family Practice

Marshall Mandell, M.D.
3 Brush Street
Norwalk, CT 06850
(203) 838-4706
Somatic, Cerebral, and Visceral Allergy, Ecologic Mental Illness, Neuro Allergy

Russel Manuel, M.D.
4200 Lake Otis Parkway #304
Anchorage, AK 99508
(907) 562-7070
Family Practice, Acupuncture

Vincent Mark, M.D.
P.O. Box 760
Aptos, CA 95001
(408) 688-8514
Environmental Medicine

George Marsh, M.D.
P.O. Drawer H
Grand Saline, TX 75140
(214) 962-4247
Family Practice

Robert Marshall, M.D.
700 Oak
Winnetka, IL 60093
(708) 446-1923
Internal Medicine

Lisa Carberry Masini, M.D.
164 East Elm Street #F
Greenwich, CT 06830
(203) 661-6164
Naturopath

Conrad Maulfair, D.O.
RR#2, Box 71
Main Street
Mertztown, PA 19539
(215) 682-2104
Osteopathy; Family Practice

Lynne Mauss
23 Brewster Street
Huntington Station, NY 11746
(516) 673-4588
Nutrition Counselor

Adelia McCord
30072 Running Deer Lane
Laguna Niguel, CA 92677
(714) 495-1454
Environmental Facilitator, Allergy Technician, Environmental Medicine, Hypothermic Detoxification

Edward McDonagh
2800 A Kendallwood
Glaston Parkway
Kansas City, MO 64119
(816) 453-5940
Chelation Therapy

Dr. John McDougall
Saint Helena Health Center
P.O. Box 25
Deer Park, CA 94576
(800) 358-9195
(800) 862-7575
Internist, Preventative Medicine

Charles McGee, M.D.
1717 Lincoln Way #108
Coeur D'alene, ID 83814
(208) 664-1478
Preventative Medicine

Anita Millen, M.D.
1010 Cranshaw Boulevard #170
Torrance, CA 90501
(213) 320-1132
Naturopath

John Miller, M.D.
5901 Airport Boulevard B123
Mobile, AL 36608
(205) 342-8540
Otolaryngology, Head and Neck Maxillofacial Cosmetic Surgery

Billy Mills, D.O.
4725 Gus Thomasson
Mesquite, TX 75150
(214) 279-6767
Family Practice

Anne Mitchell
600 George Street
New Haven, CT 06511
(203) 772-3000
Naturopath

George Mitchell, M.D.
2639 Connecticut Avenue North
Washington, D.C. 20018
(202) 265-4111
Nutrition

Paul Mittman, M.D.
Laura Ra Mittman, M.D.
19 East Main Street
Mystic, CT
(203) 572-9566
Naturopath

Michele Moore, M.D.
115 Key Road
Keene, NH 03431
(603) 357-2180
Family Practice, Acupuncture

Peter Moreo
71-50 Loubet Street
Forest Hills, NY 11375
(718) 268-8258
Nutrition Counselor

Heather Morgan, M.D.
138 South Main Street
Centerville, OH 45459
(513) 439-1797
Holistic, Preventative Medicine

Joseph Morgan, M.D.
1750 Thompson Road
Coos Bay, OR 97420
(503) 269-0333
Pediatrics

Herbert Moselle, M.D.
201 N.W. 82nd Avenue #103
Plantation, FL 33324
(305) 472-1212
Ear, Nose, and Throat Specialist

Abraham Moskowitz
1101 Whalley Avenue
New Haven, CT 06515
(203) 572-9388
Naturopath

Charles Moss, M.D.
8950 Villa La Jolla Drive 2162
La Jolla, CA 92037
(619) 457-1314
Acupuncture, Environmental Medicine

Sara C. Murnane N.M., A.N.P.
Box 15071 FCB
Homer, AK 99603
(907) 235-7268
Certified Nurse Midwife, Adv. Nurse Practitioner

Donald Nelson, M.D.
544 White Pond #B
Akron, OH 44320
(216) 836-3016
Allergist

Joseph Nemecek, M.D.
344 Sherwood Court
La Grange, IL 60525
(708) 354-1600

Robert Noble, M.D.
6757 Arapaho Road #757
Dallas, TX 75248
(214) 458-9944
Family Practice, Allergist

John O'Brian, M.D.
3217 Lake Avenue
Fort Wayne, IN 46805
(219) 422-9471
Family Practice

Eugene Oliveto, M.D.
8031 West Center
Omaha, NB 68124
(402) 392-0233
Psychiatrist, Chelation Therapy

Gary Oberg, M.D.
31 North Virginia Street
Crystal Lake, IL 60014
(815) 455-1990
Allergist, Adults

Harold Ofgang, M.D.
57 North Street #323
Danbury, CT 06811
(203) 798-0533
Naturopath

Henry Palacios, M.D.
1481 Chain Bridge Road #3101
McLean, VA 22101
(703) 356-2244
Dermatology

Harry Panjwani, M.D.
141 Dayton Street
Box 398
Ridgewood, NJ 07451
(201) 447-2033
Neurologist, Psychiatry, Preventative Medicine, Nutritionist

Gherald Parker, D.O.
6208 Montgomery Boulevard NE #D
Albuquerque, NM 87109
(505) 884-3506
Dietician

Carin Pavlinchak, M.D.
289 South Marshall Street
West Hartford, CT 06105
(203) 523-8462
Naturopath

Sunil Perera, M.D.
404 Sunrise Avenue
Roseville, CA 95661
(916) 782-7758
Allergist

Louis Petrucco, M.D.
6001 Outer Drive
Detroit, MI 48235
(313) 864-7400
Family Practice, Internal Medicine

Guy Pfeiffer, M.D.
R.R. 4
#200 Professional Plaza
Mattoon, IL 61938
(708) 231-3649
Otolaryngology

Charles Platt, M.D.
522 South West Street
Versailles, OH 45380
(513) 526-3271
Family Practice

Richard Podell, M.D.
29 South Street
New Providence, NJ 07947
(908) 464-3800
Internal Medicine

Harold Posner, M.D.
111 Bala Avenue
Bala Cynwynd, PA 19004
(215) 667-2927
Internal Medicine, Nutritionist

Bhaskar Power, M.D.
P.O. Box 1132
Roanoke Rapids, NC 27870
(919) 535-1411
Otolaryngology

Gus Prosch, M.D.
759 Valley Stream
Birmingham, AL 35226
(205) 823-6180
Preventative Medicine

Johnathon Raistrick
7 Taft Point #60
Waterbury, CT
(203) 262-6755
Naturopath

Theoron Randolph, M.D.
161 South Lincoln Way #305
North Aurora, IL 60542
(708) 884-9898
Internal Medicine

Dr. Doris Rapp
1421 Colvin Road
Buffalo, NY 14233
(716) 875-5578
Allergist and Environmental Medicine

Bernard Raxlen, M.D.
22 Lafayette Pl.
Greenwich, CT 06830
(203) 629-0703
Biological Psychiatry, Nutritional Medicine, Clinical Ecology

William Rea, M.D.
8345 Walnut Hill Lane #205
Dallas, TX 75231
(214) 368-4132
Environmental Medicine

John Rechsteiner, M.D.
1116 South Limestone
Springfield, OH 45505
(513) 325-0223
Candida-Related Complex

Dennis Remington, M.D.
1675 North Freedom Boulevard
200 West #11E
Provo, UT 84604
(801) 373-8500
Bariatrics, Family Practice

Charles Ressenger, M.D.
853 South Norwalk
P.O. Box 374
Norwalk, OH 44857
(419) 668-9615
Family Practice

Emanuel Revici, M.D.
164 East 91st Street
New York, NY 10028
(212) 876-9667
Control Disorders of the Body Defense System

Richard Ribner, M.D.
25 Central Park West
New York, NY 10023
(212) 246-7010
Arteriosclerosis

Kathleen Riley
80 Dodgingtown
Bethel, CT 06801
(203) 790-6889
Naturopath

Hugh Riordan, M.D.
3100 North Hillside
Wichita, KS 67219
(316) 682-9241
Holistic Medicine

Robin Ritterman
600 George Street
New Haven, CT 06511
(203) 772-3000
Naturopath

Albert Robbins, D.O., M.S.P.H.
400 South Dixie Highway
Building 2 #210
Boca Raton, FL 33432
(407) 395-3282
Environmental Medicine, Allergist

Russel Roby, M.D.
3410 Far West Side #110
Austin, TX 78731
(512) 338-4336
Allergist

Sally Rockwell
4703 Stone Way North
Seattle, WA 98103
(206) 547-1814
Nutrition Counselor

Harvey Ross, M.D.
7060 Hollywood Boulevard
Los Angeles, CA 90028
(213) 466-8330
Psychiatrist

Robert Rowen, M.D.
615 East 82nd Street #300
Anchorage, AK 99518
(907) 344-775
Family Practice

Daniel Royal, D.O.
3720 Howard Hughes Parkway
Las Vegas, NV 89109
(702) 732-1400
Family Practice

Andrew Rubman
800 Main Street South
Southbury, CT 06488
(203) 262-6755
Naturopath

Jose Sanchez, M.D.
2615 Sunset Boulevard
Steubenville, OH 43952
(614) 264-1692
Ear, Nose, and Throat Specialist

William Sayer, M.D.
145 North California Avenue
Palo Alto, CA 94301
(415) 321-3361
Internal Medicine

Michael Schachter, M.D.
Two Executive Boulevard
Suffern, NY 10901
(914) 368-4700
Cancer, Cardio, Homeopathy

Tony Scarpa
16 McKeon Avenue
Valley Stream, NY 11580
(516) 561-8273
Nutrition Counselor

Paul Schlickler
662 Selfmaster Parkway
Union, NJ 07083
(201) 851-0244
Nutrition Counselor

Gene Schmutzer, D.O.
2425 North Alveron Way
Tucson, AZ 85712
(602) 795-0292
Environmental Allergies

James Schuler, M.D.
Box 297, Haight & Highland
Smith River, CA 95567
(707) 487-3405
Dermatology, Family Practice

Richard Schwimmer, M.D.
2635 Nostrad Avenue
Brooklyn, NY 11210
(718) 252-3622
Pediatrician

Joan Scott B.S.N., M.P.H.
2038 22nd Court South
Birmingham, AL 35223
(205) 871-1288
Bach of Science Nursing, Masters of Public Health

Shirley Scott, M.D.
P.O. Box 2670
Santa Fe, NM 87504
(505) 986-9960

Jack Seeley, M.D., M.P.H.
10796 West Overland
Boise, ID 83814
(208) 664-1478
Family Practice

Drescarlito Sevilla, M.D.
5437 Mahoning Avenue
Youngstown, OH 44514
(216) 792-1956
Ear, Nose, and Throat Specialist

George Shambaugh, M.D.
40 South Clay Street
Hinsdale, IL 60521
(708) 887-1130
Otolaryngology

William Shay, D.O.
407 East Philadelphia Avenue
Boyertown, PA 19512
(215) 367-5505
Family Practice

Young Shin, M.D.
3850 Holcomb Bridge Road #438
Atlanta/Norcros, GA 30092
(404) 242-0000
Allergist, Nutrition Counselor

Welma Shrader, M.D.
Opelo Plaza
Suite 12 2470
Kamuela, HI 96743
(808) 885-6860
Allergist, Environmental Medicine

Jacob Siegel
8300 Waterbury
Suite #305
Houston, TX 75956
(713) 973-8832
Allergist

Louis Silverman, M.D.
1000 South Columbia Road
Grand Forks, ND 58206
(701) 780-6000
Pediatrics

Robert Sinaiko, M.D.
450 Sutter Street 1124
San Francisco, CA 94108
(415) 788-2008
Clinical Immunology, Internal Medicine

Robert Sklovsky, N.D., Pharm.
6910 South East Lake Road
Milwaukie, OR 97267
(503) 654-3938
Naturopath

Priscila Slagle, M.D.
12301 Wilshire #300
Los Angeles, CA 90025
(213) 826-0175
Nutrition

Gerald Smith, M.D.
5320 Education Drive
Cheyenne, WY 82009
(307) 632-5589
Otolaryngology

Donald Soll, M.D.
708 North Center Street
Reno, NV 89501
(702) 786-7101
General Practitioner

Neil Solomon, M.D., O.H.D.
901 Dulaney Valley Road #602
Towson, MD 21204
(301) 337-2707
Internal Medicine

D. E. Sprague, M.D., M.C.
Medical Dept. USS Kittyhawk CV63
Navy Shipyard, San Diego, CA

Allan Spreen, M.D.
5627 Atlantic Blvd. Suite #2
Jacksonville, FL 32207
(904) 725-8725
Nutritionist

Nina Starr
15 West 72nd Street #2G
New York, NY 10023
(212) 496-5015
Nutrition Counselor

Philip Stavish, M.D.
136 Broadway, Newport-Mesa
Costa Mesa, CA 92627
(714) 722-0175
Nutritionist, Family Practice

Bruce Stayton, M.D.
1212 West Truman Road
Independence, MO 64050
(816) 836-5010
Family Practice

Rheeta Stecker, M.D.
3205 Albert Pike
Hot Springs, AR 71913
(501) 767-1144
Family Practice

Del Stiglr, M.D.
2005 Franklin Street #409
Denver, CO 80205
(303) 831-7335
Pediatrics

Thomas Stone, M.D.
1811 Hicks Road
Rolling Meadows, IL 60008
(312) 934-1100
Psychiatry

Tipu Sultan, M.D.
11585 West Florissant Road
Florissant, MO 63033
(314) 921-5600
Pediatrics

Marvin Sweitzer, M.D.
71 East Avenue #F
Norwalk, CT 06851
(203) 838-9355
Naturopath

Yiwen Y. Tang, M.D.
380 Brinkby
Reno, NV 89509
(702) 826-9500
Homeopathy

Rafael Tarnopolsky, M.D.
3200 Grand Avenue
Des Moines, IA 50312
(515) 271-1400
Otolaryngology

John Taylor, D.O.
6208 Montgomery Boulevard NE #D
Albuquerque, NM 87109
(505) 884-3506
Dietician

Phillip Taylor, M.D.
325 South Moorpark Road
Thousand Oaks, CA 91361
(818) 889-8249
Allergist, Nutritionist

Theodore Tepas, M.D.
1012 Lake Shore Boulevard
Evanston, IL 60202
(708) 328-5826
Psychiatry

John Trowbridge, M.D.
9816 Memorial Boulevard
Suite 205
Humble, TX 77338
(713) 540-2329
Nutritional Medicine, Laser Therapy, Chelation

Judy Trupin
143 Avenue B #12A
New York, NY 10009
(212) 533-9585
Nutrition Counselor

Jeffrey Tulin-Silver, M.D.
6330 Orchard Lake Road #110
West Bloomfield, MI 48322
(313) 932-0010
Internal Medicine

Robert Vance, D.O.
801 South Rancho
Suite F2
Las Vegas, NV 89106
(702) 385-7771
General Practice

Gary Vickar, M.D.
1245 Braham Road
Florissant, MO 63031
(314) 837-4900
Psychiatrist

Carol Wade
Route 4, Box 126E
Boonton Township, NJ 07005
(201) 627-5901
Nutrition Counselor

Francis Waickman, M.D.
544 White Pond Drive
Suite #B
Akron, OH 44320
(216) 867-3767
Immunology

R. O. Waiton, M.D., D.O.
221 Almendra Avenue
Los Gatos, CA 95030
(408) 354-2300
Preventative and Rehabilitative Physician

John Wakefield, M.D.
970 West El Camino Real #1
Sunnyvale, CA 94087
(408) 732-3037
Psychiatry

James Walker, M.D.
2000A Southbridge Parkway, Suite 300
Birmingham, AL 35209
(205) 871-4274
Radiologist

Jerry Walker, D.O.
5681 South Beech Daly Road
Dearborn Heights, MI 48125
(313) 292-5620
Family Practice, Allergist

Richard Wanderman, M.D.
5545 Murray Suite #330
Memphis, TN 38119
(901) 683-2777
Family Practice, Adolescent Medicine, Pediatrics

Wendy Wasdahl
17 White Street #3A
New York, NY 10013
(212) 966-6479
Nutrition Counselor

Deleno Webb, M.D.
401 11th Street #701
Huntington, WV 25701
(304) 525-9355
Psychiatrist

Harold Weiss, M.D.
8002 19th Avenue
Brooklyn, NY 11214
(718) 236-2202
Candida, Arthritis, Depression

Ronald Wempen, M.D.
3620 South Bristol Street #306
Santa Ana, CA 92704
(714) 546-4325
Homeopathy, Nutrition

Norman Wenger, M.D.
P.O. Box 502
Carbondale, PA 18407
(717) 222-9595
Family Practice

Melvyn Werbach, M.D.
4751 Viviana Drive
Tarzana, CA 90505
(818) 996-6110
Psychiatrist

Dr. Julian Whitaker
440 McArthur Blvd.
Newport Beach, CA 92660
(714) 851-1550
General Practitioner

Harold Whitcomb, M.D.
100 East Main Street #201
Aspen, CO 81611
(303) 925-5440
Internal Medicine

Jeffrey White, M.D.
3715 Azeele
Tampa, FL 33609
(813) 876-6117
Environmental Medicine, Ophthalmology

James Whittington, M.D.
1021 Seventh Avenue
Fort Worth, TX 76104
(817) 332-4585
Eye, Ear, Nose Allergist

Randall Wilkinson, M.D.
302 South 12th Avenue
Yakima, WA 98902
(509) 453-5506
Family Practice

Moke Williams, M.D.
50 N.E. 26th Avenue #302
Pompano Beach, FL 33062
(305) 782-8855
Nutrition Counselor

Hope Wing, N.D.
520 East 34th Street #305
Anchorage, AK 99503
(907) 561-2330 ·
Naturopathic Doctor

V. G. Clark Wismer, D.O.
1441 Kapiolani #1113
Honolulu, HI 96814
(808) 941-0522
Osteopathic Physician

Joseph Wojcik, M.D.
525 Bronxville Road
Yonkers, NY 10708
(914) 793-6161
Pediatrician, Allergist

David Wong, M.D.
3250 West Lomite Boulevard #209
Torrance, CA 90505
(310) 326-8625
Family Practice, Nutritionist

Jack Woodard, M.D.
1304 Whispering Pines Road
Albany, GA 31707
(912) 436-9535
Holistic Medicine

Otis Woodward, M.D.
1304 Whispering Pines Road
Albany, GA 31707
(912) 436-9535
Holistic Medicine, Psychiatrist

Aubrey Worrell, M.D.
3900 Hickory Street
Pine Bluff, AR 71603
(501) 535-8200
Allergy, Immunology, Environmental Medicine, Pediatrics

Harlan Wright, D.O.
4903 82 Street #50
Lubbock, TX 79424
(806) 794-9632
Nutrition Therapy, Osteopathic Manipulative Therapist

Jonathon Wright, M.D.
24030 132nd Avenue SE
Kent, WA 98042
(206) 631-8920
Diabetes

Linda Wright, M.D.
421 21st Avenue #7
Longmont, CO 80501
(303) 678-5891
Internal Medicine, Nutrition

Ray Wunderlich, M.D.
666 Sixth Street South
St. Petersberg, FL 33701
(813) 822-3612
Preventative and Nutritional Medicine

Conrad Wurtz, Ph.D.
18 Center Street
Brunswick, ME 04011
(207) 782-1035
Psychologist

Jose Yaryura-Tobias, M.D.
935 Northern Boulevard
Great Neck, NY 11021
(516) 487-7116
Psychiatrist

Robert Yee, M.D.
3317 Chanate Road #2-D
Santa Rosa, CA 95404
(707) 544-6891
Gynecology, Orthomolecular Medicine, Chronic Fatigue

George Zabrecky
158 Danbury Road
Ridgefield, CT 06877
(203) 431-6165
Life Extension, Chiropractic Techniques to Work with Cancer Patients

Eugene Zamperion
54 Lafayette Place
Greenwich, CT 06830
(203) 661-7375
Naturopath

Erhardt Zinke, M.D.
2131 Winter Warm Road
Fallbrook, CA 92028
(619) 728-4901
Family Practitioner

Holistic Dentists

Antony Ammirata, D.D.S.
Route 206 and Gordon Avenue
Lawrenceville, NJ
(609) 896-0050

Edward Arana, D.D.S., S.D.A.
107 Quien Sabe
Carmel Valley, CA 93924
(408) 659-5385
Biological Dentistry

Donald Barber
6010 Main Street
Williamsville, NY 14221
(716) 632-7310

Terry Bellman, D.D.S.
595 Madison Avenue
New York, NY 10022
(212) 838-0840

Israel Brenner, D.M.D.
14 West Neck Road
Huntington, NY 11743
(516) 271-1770

Norman Bressack, D.D.S.
1692 Newbridge Road
North Bellemore, NY 11710
(516) 221-7447

Ira Cohen, D.D.S.
Route 22
Goldens Bridge, NY 10526
(914)232-5004

Jay Doreck, D.D.S.
70 Glen Cove Road
Roslyn Heights, NY 11577
(516) 621-2430

Andrew Galante, D.M.D.
53 Mountain Boulevard
Warren, NJ 07059
(908) 561-3939

James Getchonis, D.D.S.
10 Henry Street
Norwich, NY 13815
(607) 336-2273

Steven Goldberg, D.D.S.
1600 Avenue M
Brooklyn, NY 11230
(212) 505-5055

Neil Gross, D.D.S.
30 East 60th Street
New York, NY 10022
(212) 888-9022

Marcella Halpert, D.D.S.
111 East 19th Street
New York, NY 10010
(212) 475-7912

William Hambree, D.M.D.
1510 Willow Branch Avenue
Jacksonville, FL 32205
(904) 387-3535

Vaughn Harada, D.D.S.
1752 Ocean Park Boulevard
Santa Monica, CA 90405
(213) 450-7120

Howard Hinden, D.D.S.
P.O. Box 628
Suffern, NY 10901
(914) 357-1595

Hal Huggins, D.D.S.
5080 Lift Dr.
Colorado Springs, CO 80919
(719) 548-1600

Joshua Kanner, D.D.S.
763 Clove Road
Stanton, NY 10310
(718) 442-5319

Melvin Landeu, D.D.S.
355 Chestnut Street
Union, NJ 07083
(908) 686-0409

Victor Penzer, D.M.D.
187 Grant Avenue
Newton, MA 02159
(617) 332-1234

William Pollak, D.D.S.
2130 Millburn Avenue
Maplewood, NJ 07040
(201) 763-3231

Claude Springer, D.D.S.
256-80 Horace Harding Expressway
Little Neck, NY 11362
(718) 428-7780

Roberta Tehans, D.D.S.
153 North Auten Avenue
Somerville, NJ 08876
(908) 722-6373

Holistic Veterinarians

Jeffrey Broderick
229 Wall Street
Huntington, NY 11743
(516) 427-7321
Ortho for Medicine for Pets, Herbs, Nutritional Medicine

Martin Goldstein
Box 262-B, Route 123
Vista, NY 10590
(914) 533-6066
Prevention, Nutrition, Cancer, Arthritis, Skin Conditions, and Other Chronic Ailments

Evan Kanouse
Brook Farm Veterinarian Center
B234
Patterson, NY 12563
(914) 878-4833
Acupuncture and Nutrition

Dr. Neil Wolff
530 East Putnam Avenue
Greenwich, CT 06830
(203) 869-7755
Acupuncture, Homeopathy, Herbs

Detox Support Groups

Lucy Alvarez
P.O. Box 4041
South Hackensack, NJ 07606

Mike Cassiola
45 Hollow Tree Ridge Rd.
Darien, CT 06820
(203) 656-2744

Franco Pantoni
1641 3rd. Ave., Apt. 9F
New York, NY 10128
(212) 722-7939

Delores Perri, M.S., R.V.
P.O. Box 53
Brooklyn, NY 11218
(718) 851-0707

Bernice Tanenbaum
18 Lighthouse Rd.
Great Neck, NY 11024
(516) 482-4652

Professional Organizations

Academy of Orthomolecular Psychiatry
P.O. Box 372
Manhassett, NY 11030

American Academy of Medical Preventics
6151 West Century Boulevard
Suite 114
Los Angeles, CA 90045
(213) 645-5350

American College of Advancement in Medicine
23121 Verdugo Drive
Suite 204
Laguna Hills, CA 92653

American Herb Association
P.O. Box 353
Rescue, CA 94672

American Holistic Medical Association
6932 Little River Turnpike
Annandale, VA 22003

American Holistic Nurses Association
P.O. Box 116
Telluride, CO 81435

Association for Cardiovascular Therapy
P.O. Box 706
Bloomfield, CT 06002
(203) 724-0082

Association for Heart Patients
P.O. Box 54305
Atlanta, GA 30308
(404) 523-0826

Cancer Control Society
2043 North Berendo
Los Angeles, CA 90027
(213) 663-7801

Fryer Research Center
30 East 40th Street
New York, NY 10016
(212) 808-4940

Huxley Institute for Biosocial Research
900 North Federal Highway
Suite 330
Boca Raton, FL 33432
(305) 393-6167
(800) 847-3802

International Academy of Preventive Medicine
34 Corporate Woods
Suite 469
Overland Park, KS 66210

International Association of Cancer Victims and Friends, Inc.
7740 West Manchester Avenue
Suite 110
Playa del Rey, CA 90291
(213) 822-5032

Long Island Schizophrenia Association
1691 Northern Boulevard
Manhasset, NY 11030
(516) 627-7530

Natural Health Association
600 George Street
New Haven, CT 06511
(203) 772-3000

Princeton Bio Center
Skillman, NJ 08558
(609) 924-8607
GP, Allergy, Arthritis

Society for Clinical Ecology
2005 Franklin Street
Suite 490
Denver, CO 80205

Studies and Articles on Environmental Medicine

For many years mainstream medicine rejected the legitimacy of environmental medicine or its predecessor, clinical ecology, because they claimed there was no scientific validation. However, individuals practicing environmental medicine who also have a background in science, such as Dr. William Rea, Dr. Theoron Randolph, Dr. William Crook, Dr. Marshall Mandell, Dr. Doris Rapp, and others, have extensively reviewed the scientific literature and have more than documented their articles and books to show there is a sound, voluminous body of evidence to support both the theoretical and actual applications in environmental medicine.

Rather than reinventing the wheel, I have reviewed all of their materials over the last three years and have included here the best sources that any serious researcher, scholar, or skeptical physician would require in order to get past any biases and begin to utilize environmental medicine as a healing tool.

ARTHRITIS

Brown, G. 1934. Allergic phases of arthritis. *Journal of Laboratory and Clinical Medicine:* 247–249.

Creip, L. 1946. Allergy of joints. *Journal of Bone and Joint Surgery:* 276–278.

Darlington, L., and J. Mansfield. 1983. Food allergy and rheumatoid disease. *Annals of Rheumatoid Diseases* 42:218.

Epstein, S. 1969. Hypersensitivity to sodium nitrate: A major causative factor in a case of aplindromic rheumatism. *Annals of Allergy* 27:343–349.

Feldman, S. 1989. Rheumatoid arthritis: Patient follow-up after hospitalization in a comprehensive environmental control unit. *Clinical Ecology* 6:94.

Kremer, J., J. Biguauoette, and A. Michalek. 1985. Effects of manipulation of dietary fatty acids on clinical manifestation of rheumatoid arthritis. *Lancet:* 184–187.

Kremer, J., W. Juviz, and A. Michalek. 1987. Fish oil fatty acid supplementation in active rheumatoid arthritis. *Annals of Internal Medicine,* 106:497–502.

Kroker, G., 1984. Fasting and rheumatoid arthritis: A multicenter study. *Clinical Ecology* 2:137–144.

Malone, D., and D. Metcalfe. 1988. Mast cells and arthritis. *Annals of Allergy* 61:27–30.

Marshall, R., R. Stroud, and G. Kroker. 1984. Food challenge effects on fasted rheumatoid arthritis patients: A multicenter study. *Clinical Ecology* 2:181–190.

Panush, R., R. Carter, P. Katz, B. Kowsari, S. Longley, and S. Finnie. 1983. Diet therapy for rheumatoid arthritis. *Arthritis and Rheumatism* 26:462–470.

Panush, R., R. Stroud, and E. Webster. 1990. Food-induced (allergic) arthritis: Inflammatory arthritis exacerbated by milk. *Arthritis and Rheumatism* 29:220–226.

Randolph, T. 1970. Ecologically oriented rheumatoid arthritis. In *Clinical Ecology*, edited by L. Dickey. Springfield, Ill.: Charles C. Thomas.

Ratner, D., E. Eshel, and K. Vigder. 1985. Juvenile rheumatoid arthritis and milk allergy. *Royal Society of Medicine Journal* 78:410–413.

Service, W. 1937. Hydroarthrosis of allergic origin. *American Journal of Surgery* 37:121–123.

Skoldstam, L., L. Larson, and F. Lindstrom. 1979. Effects of fasting and lactovegetarian diet on rheumatoid arthritis. *Scandinavian Journal of Rheumatology*, 8:249–255.

Talbot, F. 1917. Role of food idiosyncrasies in practice. *New York Journal of Medicine* 17:419–425.

Taub, L., et al. 1936. Allergic synovitis due to ingestion of English walnuts. *JAMA* 166:2144.

Turnbull, J. 1924. The relation of anaphylactic disturbances to arthritis. *JAMA* 82:1757–1759.

Turnbull, J. 1944. Changes in sensitivity to allergenic foods in arthritis. *Journal of Digestive Diseases* 15:182–190.

Vaughan, W. 1943. Palindromic rheumatism among allergic persons. *Journal of Allergy* 14:256–263.

Walker, V. 1956. Iritis of allergic origin. *South African Medical Journal* 30:132–134.

Zeller, M. 1949. Rheumatoid arthritis: Food allergy as a factor. *Annals of Allergy* 7:200–239.

Zussman, B. 1966. Food hypersensitivity simulating rheumatoid arthritis. *Southern Medical Journal* 59:935–939.

ASTHMA

Amirav, I. 1989. Letter. *Journal of Allergy and Clinical Ecology* 83(6):1138–1139.

Barker, A. 1989. Strategies in managing asthma. *Western Journal of Medicine* 150:303–308.

Barnes, P. 1989. New concepts in the pathogenesis of bronchial hyperresponsiveness and asthma. *Journal of Allergy and Clinical Immunology* 83:1013–1026.

Baughman, R., and R. Loudon. 1989. Stridor: Differentiation from asthma or upper airway noise. *American Review of Respiratory Disease* 139:1407–1409.

Benton, G., R. Thomas, B. Nickerson, J. McQuitty, and J. Okikawa. 1989. Experience with a metered-dose inhaler with a spacer in the pediatric emergency department. *American Journal of Disability in Children* 143:678–681.

Burrows, B., F. Martinez, M. Halonen, R. Barbee, and M. Cline. 1989. Association of asthma with serum IgE levels and skin-test reactivity to allergens. *New England Journal of Medicine* 320:271–277.

Chabra, S., and S. Gaur. 1989. Effect of long-term treatment with sodium cromoglycate on nonspecific bronchial hyperresponsiveness in asthma. *Chest* 95(6):1235–1238.

Croft, R. 1989. Two-year-old asthmatics can learn to operate a tube spacer by copying their mothers. *Archives of Dis. Child.* 64:742–743.

DeJongste, J., and E. Duiverman. 1989. Nebulised budesonide in severe childhood asthma (letter). *Lancet* 1:1388.

Dixon, C., R. Fuller, P. Barnes, and P. Ind. 1989. Anticholinergic blockade of beta-blocker-induced bronchoconstriction. *American Review of Respiratory Disease* 139:1390–1394.

Ekstrom, T., and L. Tibbling. 1987. Gastro-oesophageal reflux and triggering of bronchial asthma: A negative report. *European Journal of Respiratory Diseases* 71:177–180.

Fritz, G., and J. Overholser. 1989. Patterns of response to childhood asthma. *Psychosomatic Medicine* 51:347–355.

Gerrard, J., et al. 1989. A double-blind study on the value of low-dose immunotherapy in the treatment of asthma and allergic rhinitis. *Clinical Ecology* 6:43–46.

Gerstman, B., L. Bosco, D. Tomita, T. Gross, and M. Shaw. 1989. Prevalence and treatment of asthma in the Michigan Medicaid patient population younger than forty-five years: 1980–1986. *Journal of Allergy and Clinical Immunology* 83:1032–1039.

Gibson, P., J. Dolovich, J. Denburg, E. Ramsdale, and F. Hargreave. 1989. Chronic cough: Eosinophilic bronchitis without asthma. *Lancet* 1:1346–1348.

Kaslow, J., and H. Novey. 1989. Methotrexate use for asthma: A critical appraisal. *Annals of Allergy* 62:541–545.

Leung, A., and H. Hedge. 1989. Exercise-induced angioedema and asthma. *American Journal of Sports Medicine* 17(3):442–443.

Moffitt, J. 1989. Behavioral and cognitive effects of theophylline. *Pediatric Nurse* 15(3):277.

Olm, M., P. Munne, and M. Jimenez. 1989. Severe reactive airways disease induced by propafenone (letter). *Chest* 95(6):1366–1377.

Plaut, G. 1989. Exercise training, fitness, and asthma. *Lancet* 1:1147.

Pretolani, M., P. Ferrer-Lopez, and B. Vargaftig. 1989. From anti-asthma drugs to PAF-acether antagonism and back: Present status. *Biochemical Pharmacology* 38(9):1373–1384.

Rachelefsky, G., S. Siegel, R. Katz, S. Spector, and A. Rohr. 1989. Letter. *Journal of Allergy and Clinical Ecology* 83(6):1139.

Rogers, S. 1987–1988. Provocation/neutralization of cough and wheezing in a horse. *Clinical Ecology* 5:185–187.

Small, P. 1989. Anti-inflammatory therapy in asthma (editorial). *Annals of Allergy* 62:481–482.

Snider, G. 1989. Chronic obstructive pulmonary disease: Risk factors, pathophysiology, and pathogenesis. *Annual Review of Medicine* 40:411–429.

Stein, R., G. Canny, D. Bohn, J. Reisman, and H. Levison. 1989. Severe acute asthma in a pediatric intensive care unit: Six years' experience. *Pediatrics* 83:1023–1028.

Stenius, A., A. Aro, A. Hakulinen, I. Ahola, E. Seppala, and H. Vapaatalo 1989. Evening primrose oil and fish oil are ineffective as supplementary treatment of bronchial asthma. *Annals of Allergy* 62:534–537.

Tang, R., and K. Wu. 1989. Total serum IgE, allergy skin-testing, and the radioallergosorbent test for the diagnosis of allergy in asthmatic children. *Annals of Allergy* 62:432–435.

Thoracic Society of America. 1987. Standardization of spirometry: 1987 update. *American Review of Respiratory Disease.* 136:1285–1298.

Walling, A. 1990. Why is asthma mortality rising? (editorial). *American Family Physician* 42(2):358–359.

Zora, J., C. Lutz, and D. Tinkelman. 1989. Assessment of compliance in children using inhaled beta adrenergic agonists. *Annals of Allergy* 62:406–409.

AUTISM

Stubbs, E., S. Budden, R. Jacson, L. Terdal, and E. Rityo. 1986. Effects of fenfluramine on eight outpatients with the syndrome of autism. *Developmental Medicine and Child Neurology* 28:229–235.

CANDIDA

Axelrod, M. A. 1968. Suppression of delayed hypersensitivity by antigen and antibody. *Immunology* 15:159–171.

Bennett, J. 1990. Searching for the yeast connection. *New England Journal of Medicine* 323:1766–1767.

Crook, W. G. 1983. The coming revolution in medicine. *Tennessee Medical Association. Journal.* 76:145–149.

Crook, W. G. The yeast connection, 3d ed. Reprinted in *The Relationship of Food Sensitivities (and Other Dietary Factors) to Hyperactivity, Attention Deficits, and Other Nervous System Symptoms: A Compendium,* (edited by W. G. Crook).

Dismukes, W., S. Wade, J. Lee, B. Dockery, and J. Hain. 1990. A randomized, double-blind trial of nystatin therapy for the candidiasis hypersensitivity syndrome. *New England Journal of Medicine* 323:-1717–1723.

Fischer, A., J.-J. Ballet, and C. Griscelli. 1978. Specific inhibition of in vitro candida-induced lymphocyte proliferation by polysaccharide antigens present in the serum of patients with chronic mucocutaneous candidiasis. *Journal of Clinical Investigation* 62:1005–1013.

Gewurz, H., and T. F. Lint. 1977. Alternative modes and pathways of complement activation, in *Biological Amplification Systems in Immunology,* edited by N. K. Day and R. A. Good. New York: Plenum.

Hobbs, J. R., D. Brigden, F. Davidson, et al. 1977. Immunological aspects of candidal vaginitis. *Royal Society of Medicine. Proceedings* 70:11–14.

Iwata, K., and Y. Yamamoto. 1977. Glycoprotein toxins produced by *Candida albicans.* Proceedings of the Fourth International Conference on the Mycoses, PAHO, Scientific Publication 356. Reprinted in *The Relationship of Food Sensitivities (and Other Dietary Factors) to Hyperactivity, Attention Deficits, and Other Nervous System Symptoms: A Compendium,* edited by W. G. Crook.

Johnston, R. B., and R. M. Stroud. 1977. Complement and host defense against infection. *Journal of Pediatrics* 90:169–179.

Kirkpatrick, C. H. 1976. Mitogen- and antigen-induced lymphocyte responses in patients with infectious diseases. In *Mitogens in Immunobiology,* edited by J. J. Oppenheim and D. L. Rosenstreich. New York: Academic Press.

Kirkpatrick, C. H., R. R. Rich, and M. D. Bennett. 1971. Chronic mucocutaneous candidiasis: Model-building in cellular immunity. *Annals of Internal Medicine* 74:955–978.

Kirkpatrick, C. H., R. R. Rich, and T. K. Smith. 1972. Effect of transfer factor on lymphocyte function in anergic patients. *Journal of Clinical Investigation* 51:2948–2958.

Kirkpatrick, C. H., and P. G. Sohle. 1981. Chronic mucocutaneous candidiasis. In Part 1 of *Immunology of Human Infection,* edited by A. J. Nahmias and R. J. O'Reilly. New York: Plenum.

Miles, M. 1977. *Recurrent vaginal candidiasis: Importance of an intestinal reservoir. JAMA* 238:1836–1837.

Nelson, R. D., M. J. Herron, R. J. McCormack, et al. 1984. Two mechanisms of inhibition of human lymphocyte proliferation by soluble yeast mannan polysaccharide. *Infection and Immunology* 43:1041–1046.

Paterson, P. Y., R. Semo, G. Blumenschein, et al. 1971 Mucocutaneous candidiasis, anergy, and a plasma inhibitor of cellular immunity: Reversal after amphotericin B therapy. *Clinical and Experimental Immunology* 9:595–602.

Rogers, T. J., and E. Balish. 1980. Immunity to *Candida albicans. Microb. Rev.* 44:660–682.

Schinfeld J. 1987. PMS and candidiasis: Study explores possible link. *Female Patient* 12:66.

Schulkind, M. I., W. H. Adler, W. E. Altmeier, et al. 1972. Transfer factor in the treatment of a case of chronic mucocutaneous candidiasis. *Cellular Immunology* 3:606–615.

Stobo, J. D., 1977. Immunosuppression in man: Suppression by macrophages can be mediated by interactions with regulatory T cells. *Journal of Immunology* 119:918–924.

Stobo, J. D., S. Paul, R. E. Van Scoy, et al. 1976. Suppressor thymus-derived lymphocytes in fungal infections. *Journal of Clinical Immunology* 57:319–328.

Theofilopoulos, A. N., and F. J. Dixon. 1979. The biology and detection of immune complexes. *Advances in Immunology* 28:89–220.

Truss, C. O. 1978. Tissue injury induced by *Candida albicans:* Mental and neurological manifestations. *Journal of Orthomolecular Psychiatry* 7:17–37.

Truss, C. O. 1980. Restoration of immunologic competence to *Candida albicans. Journal of Orthomolecular Psychiatry* 9:287–301.

Twomey, J. J., C. C. Waddell, S. Krantz, et al. 1975. Chronic mucocutaneous candidiasis with macrophage dysfunction, a plasma inhibitor, and co-existent aplastic anemia. *Journal of Laboratory and Clinical Medicine* 85:968–977.

Valdimarsson, H., J. Higgs, R. Wells, et al. 1973. Immune abnormalities associated with chronic mucocutaneous candidiasis. *Cellular Immunology* 6:348–361.

Waldman, R. H., J. M. Cruz, and D. S. Rone. 1972. Intravaginal immunization of humans with *Candida albicans. Journal of Immunology* 109: 662–664.

Wilton, J. M. A., and T. Lehner. 1980. Immunology of candidiasis. In *Immunodermatology,* edited by B. Safai and R. A. Good. New York: Plenum.

Witkin, S. S. 1985. Defective immune responses in patients with recurrent candidiasis. *Infections in Medicine.* May/June: 129–32. Reprinted in *The Relationship of Food Sensitivities (and Other Dietary Factors) to Hyperactivity, Attention Deficits, and Other Nervous System Symptoms: A Compendium,* edited by W. G. Crook.

Witkin, S. S., I. R. Yu, and W. J. Ledger. 1983. Inhibition of *Candida albicans*–induced lymphocyte proliferation by lymphocytes and sera from women with recurrent vaginitis. *American Journal of Obstetrics and Gynecology* 147:809–811.

Zwerling, N., K. Owens, and N. Ruth. 1984. Think yeast: The expanding spectrum of candidiasis. *South Carolina Medical Association Journal* 80:454–456.

CHEMICAL SENSITIVITY

Ashford, N. A., and C. S. Miller. 1989. *Chemical Sensitivity: A Report to the New Jersey State Department of Health.*

Bryce-Smith, D. 1986. Environmental chemical influences of behavior, personality, and mentation. *International Journal for Biosocial Research* 8(2):115–150.

Finn, R. 1987–1988. Organic solvent sensitivity. *Clinical Ecology* 5:155–158.

Hoffman, R., P. Stehr-Green, K. Webb, G. Evans, A. Knutsen, W. Schramm, J. Staake, and B. Bigson. 1986. Health effects of long-term exposure to 2, 3, 7, 8-tetrachlorodibenzo-p-dioxin. *JAMA* 225:2031.

Johnson, R., D. Manske, D. New, and D. Podrebarac. 1981. Pesticide, heavy metals, and other chemical residue in infant and toddler total diet samples: August 1975–July 1976. *Pesticide Monitoring Journal* 15:39–50.

Johnson, R., D. Manske, and D. Podrebarac. 1981. Pesticide, heavy metal, and other chemical residues in adult total diet samples: August 1975–July 1976. *Pesticide Monitoring Journal* 15:54–69.

Laseter, J., and B. Dowty. 1976. The transplancental migration and accumulation in blood of volatile organic constituent. *Pediatric Research.* 10:696–701.

Lashford, S. 1988. *The Residue Report.* Northamptonshire, England: Thorsons Publishers.

Lewtas, J. 1989. Toxicology of complex mixtures of indoor air pollutants. *Annual Review of Pharmacology and Toxicology.* 29:415–439.

Lieberman, A., P. Hardman, P. Preston. 1981. *Academic, Behavioral, and Perceptual Reactions in Dyslexic Children When Exposed to Environmental Factors: Malathion and Petrochemical Ethanol.* Tallahassee, Fla.: Dyslexia Research Institute.

Pan, Y., W. Rea, A. Johnson, and E. Fenyes. 1989. Formaldehyde sensitivity. *Clinical Ecology* 6:79–84.

Rapp, D. 1978. Double-blind case report of chronic headache due to foods and air pollution. *Annals of Allergy* 40:289.

Rapp, D., J. McGovern, and F. Waickman. 1982. Video documentation of food and chemical sensitivities. *Annals of Allergy* 48:258.

Rea, W., A. Johnson, R. Smiley, B. Maynard, and O. Dawkins-Brown. 1989. Magnesium deficiency in patients with chemical sensitivity. *Clinical Ecology* 4:17–20.

Rea, W., Y. Pan, and A. Johnson. 1987–1988. Clearing of toxic volatile hydrocarbons from humans: A study. *Clinical Ecology* 5:166–170.

Rea, W., Y. Pan, A. Johnson, and E. Fenyves. 1987–1988. T and B lymphocytes in chemically sensitive patients with toxic volatile organic hydrocarbons in their blood. *Clinical Ecology* 5:171–175.

Rogers, S. 1989. Diagnosing the tight-building syndrome or diagnosing chemical hypersensitivity. *Environmental International* 15:75–79.

Root, D., et al. 1987. Excretion of a lipophilic toxicant through the sebaceous gland: A case report. *Journal of Toxicology* 6(1):13–17.

Ross, G. 1990. Confirmation of chemical sensitivity by double-blind inhalant challenge. Paper presented at the International Conference on

Food and Environmental Factors in Human Disease, July 3–6, Buxton, Derbyshire, England.

Stewart-Pinkham, S. 1989. Attention deficit disorder: A toxic response to ambient cadmium air pollution. *International Journal of Biosocial and Medical Research* 11(2):134–143.

U.S. Congress. House. Committee on Science and Technology. 1986. *Neurotoxins at Home and the Workplace.* Washington, D.C.: U.S. Government Printing Office.

Zebede, M., M. White, and J. Bellanti. 1988. Immunal suppressive effects following exposure to polychlorinated hydrocarbons: A future challenge for the allergist. *Annals of Allergy* 60:181.

CHILDHOOD ALLERGIES

Crook, W. G. 1961. Systemic manifestations due to allergy (allergic toxemia, or TFS). *Pediatrics* 27:790.

Crook, W. G. 1963. *The Allergic Child.* New York: Hoeber, Harper & Row.

Deamer, W. C. 1960. Allergy in childhood. *Advances in Pediatrics* 11:147.

Deamer, W. C. Pediatric allergy: Some impressions gained over a thirty-seven-year period. 1971. *Pediatrics* 486: 930–938. Reprinted in *The Relationship of Food Sensitivities (and Other Dietary Factors) to Hyperactivity, Attention Deficits, and Other Nervous System Symptoms: A Compendium,* edited by W. G. Crook.

Fontana, V. 1969. *Practical Management of the Allergic Child.* New York: Appleton-Century-Crofts.

Glasser, J. 1956. *Allergy in Childhood.* Springfield, Ill.: Charles C. Thomas.

Grow, M. H., and N. B. Herman. 1930. Intracutaneous tests in normal individuals: Analysis of 150 subjects. *Journal of Allergy* 7:108.

Herxheimer, H., P. Melnroy, K. H. Sutton, H. L. Utidjian, and H. M. D. Utidjian. The evaluation of skin tests in respiratory allergy. *Acta Allergologica* 7:380.

Holmes, T., H. Goodell, S. Wolf, and H. Wolff. 1950. *The Nose.* Springfield, Ill.: Charles C. Thomas.

Kaufman, W. 1952. The overall picture of rheumatism and arthritis. *Annals of Allergy* 10:49.

Miller, H. 1951. A study of the incidence of clinical and immunological (reaginic) allergy in a group of medical students. *Journal of Allergy* 22:475.

Rackemann, F. M., and F. A. Simon. 1935. Technic in intracutaneous tests and results of routine tests in normal persons. *Journal of* Allergy 6:184.

Randolph, T. G. 1947. Allergy as a causative factor of fatigue, irritability, and behavior problems of children. *Journal of Pediatrics* 31:560.

Randolph, T. G. 1959. Musculoskeletal allergy in children. *Int. Arch. Allergy* 14:84.

Roth, A. 1962. Detection of food allergy. *Postgraduate Medicine* 32:432.

Rowe, A. H. 1950. Allergic toxemia and fatigue. *Annals of Allergy* 8:72.

Samter, M. 1965. *Immunological Diseases.* Boston: Little, Brown.

Sherman, W. B. 1968. *Hypersensitivity.* Philadelphia: W. B. Saunders.

Speer, F. 1954. The allergic tension-fatigue syndrome. *Pediatric Clinics of North America* 1:1029.

Szentivanyi, A. 1968. The beta adrenergic theory of the atopic abnormality in bronchial asthma. *Journal of Allergy* 42:203.

Tuft, L., and H. Mueller. 1970. *Allergy in Children.* Philadelphia: W. B. Saunders.

Whitcomb, N. 1971. Incidence of positive skin tests among medical students. *Annals of Allergy* 29:67.

COLITIS

Lake, A. P. Whitington, and S. Hamilton. 1982. Dietary protein-induced colitis in breast-fed infants. *Journal of Pediatrics* 101:906–910.

Taylor, K., and S. Truelove. 1961. Circulating antibodies to milk protein in ulcerative colitis. *British Medical Journal* 2:924–929.

DELINQUENCY

Clark, T. W. 1950. The relationship of allergy to character problems in children: A Survey. *Annals of Allergy* 8:175.

Satterfield, J., C. Hope, and A. Schell. 1982. Prospective study of delinquency in 110 adolescent boys with attention deficit disorder and 88 normal adolescent boys. *American Journal of Psychiatry* 139:795–798.

Schauss, A. 1985. Research links nutrition to behavior disorders. *School Safety* 3:20–28.

Schauss, A. 1986. Nutrition, student achievement, and behavior: Insights from new research. *Intermediate Teacher* (Canada) 20.

Schoenthaler, S. 1982. The effect of sugar on the treatment and control of antisocial behavior: A double-blind study of an incarcerated juvenile population. *International Journal for Biosocial Research* 3:1.

Schoenthaler, S. 1983. Diet and delinquency: A multi-state replication. *International Journal for Biosocial Research* 5:70–117.

DEPRESSION

Randolph, T. 1950. Allergic factors in the etiology of certain mental symptoms. *Journal of Laboratory and Clinical Medicine* 36:977.

Randolph, T. 1951. An experimentally induced acute psychotic episode following the intubation of an allergic food. Presented at the Seventh Annual Congress College of Allergists, February, Chicago, Ill.

Randolph, T. 1955. Depression caused by home exposures to gas combustion products of gas, oil, and coal. *Journal of Laboratory and Clinical Medicine* 46:942.

Randolph, T. 1959. Ecologic mental illness: Psychiatry exteriorized. *Journal of Laboratory and Clinical Medicine* 54:936.

ECZEMA

Atherton, D. 1983. Breast feeding and atopic eczema. *British Medical Journal* 2:775–776.

Atherton, D. 1988. Role of diet in treating atopic eczema: Elimination diets can be beneficial. *British Medical Journal* 297:1458–1460.

Devlin, J., R. Stanton, and T. David. 1989. Calcium intake and cow's-milk-free diets. *Archives of Diseases in Childhood* 64:1183–1193.

Hathaway, M., and J. Warner. 1983. Compliance problems in the dietary management of eczema. *Archives of Diseases in Childhood* 58:-463.

Sampson, H. 1986. Immediate hypersensitivity reactions to foods: Blinded food challenges in children with atopic dermatitis. *Annals of Allergy* 57:209–212.

ENVIRONMENTAL ILLNESS

Beasley, J. D., and J. Swift. 1989. *The Kellogg Report: The Impact of Nutrition, Environment, and Lifestyle on the Health of Americans.* Annandale-on-Hudson, N.Y.: Institute of Health Policy and Practice, Bard College Center.

Brodsky, C. 1983. "Allergic to everything": A medical subculture. *Psychosomatics* 24(8):731–742.

Crook, W. G. 1989. Controversial techniques in allergy (letters). *Pediatrics* 83.

Hodgson, M., et al. 1989. Clinical diagnosis and management of building-related illness and the sick-building syndrome. *Occupational Medicine* 4(4):593–606.

Kniker, W. T. 1985. Deciding the future for the practice of allergy and immunology. *Annals of Allergy* 55:106–113.

LaVia, M., and D. LaVia. 1979. Phenol derivatives and immunodepressive in mice. *Drug and Chemical Toxicology* 2(1 and 2):167–177.

Moore, P. 1990. Clinical ecology: Medicine for the chemical-sensitive. *Coming Clean at Home—Garbage—The Practical Journal for the Environment,* pp. 30–35.

Rapp, D. 1986. Environmental medicine: An expanded approach to allergy. *Buffalo Physician,* pp. 15–24.

Terr, A. 1986. Environmental illness: A clinical review of fifty cases. *Archives of Internal Medicine* 146:145–149.

EPILEPSY

Bowen, R. 1933. *Balyeat-Bowen Hay Fever and Asthma Clinic. Proceedings.* 1:5.

Bridge, E. M. 1949. *Epilepsy and Convulsive Disorders in Children.* New York: McGraw-Hill.

Churchill, J. A., and G. D. Gammon. 1949. The effect of anti-histaminic drugs on convulsive disorders. *JAMA* 141:18.

Clarke, T. W. 1948. Neuro-allergy in childhood, *New York State Journal of Medicine* 48:393.

Cooke, R. A. 1947. *Allergy in Theory and Practice.* Philadelphia: W. B. Saunders.

Davison, H. 1952. Allergy of the nervous system. *Quart. Rev. Allergy* 6:157.

Dees, S. C., and H. Lowenbach. 1951. Allergic epilepsy. *Annals of Allergy* 9:446.

Feinberg, S. M. 1944. Allergy in Practice. Chicago: Year Book.

Forman, J. 1934. Atopy as a cause of epilepsy. *Arch. Neurol. & Psychiat.* 32:517.

Levin, S. J. 1929. Some allied manifestations of allergy in children. *Michigan State M. Soc.* 28:857.

Pleasants, H., Jr. 1935. Epilepsy of allergic origin. *Medical World* 53:-776.

Rowe, A. H. 1927. Allergy in etiology of disease, *Journal of Laboratory and Clinical Medicine* 13:31.

Spangler, A. H. 1927. Allergy and epilepsy: analysis of one hundred cases. *Journal of Laboratory and Clinical Medicine* 13:41.

Spratling, W. P. 1904. *Epilepsy and Its Treatment.* Philadelphia: W. B. Saunders.

Vaughn, W. T. 1948. *Practice of Allergy,* 2d ed. revised by J. H. Black. St. Louis: Mosby.

FOOD ALLERGIES

Bahna, S. 1978. Contol of milk allergy: A challenge for physicians, mothers, and industry. *Annals of Allergy* 41:1–12.

Blackley, C. 1873. *Experimental Research on the Cause and Treatment of* Catarrhus aestivus *(Hayfever or Hay Asthma)*. London: Baillere, Tindall and Cox.

Breneman, J. C. 1959. Allergic cystitis: The cause of nocturnal enuresis. *GP* 20:84.

Bullock, J. D., W. C. Deamer, O. L. Frick, J. R. Crisp III, S. P. Galant, and W. H. Ziering. 1970. Recurrent abdominal pain (letters). *Pediatrics* 46:969.

Clark, T. W. 1940. The relationship of allergy to childhood neuroses. *Child Psychiat.* 1:177.

Crayton, J. 1986. Immunologically mediated behavioral reactions to foods. *Food Technology* 40(1):153–157.

Crook, W. G. 1963. The allergic tension-fatigue syndrome. In *The Allergic Child,* edited by F. Speer. New York: Hoeber, Harper & Row.

Crook, W. G. 1970. Recurrent abdominal pain (letters) *Pediatrics* 46:-969.

Crook, W. G. 1972. School phobia? Or allergic tension-fatigue? (letters). *Pediatrics* 50:340.

Crook, W. G. 1973. Musculoskeletal allergy, genitourinary allergy. In *Allergy and Immunology in Children,* edited by F. Speer. Springfield, Ill.: Charles C. Thomas.

Crook, W. G. 1975a. *Can Your Child Read? Is He Hyperactive?* Jackson, Tenn.: Pedicenter Press.

Crook, W. G. 1975b. Food allergy: The great masquerader. *Pediatric Clinics of North America* 22.

Crook, W. G., ed. 1973. *Your Allergic Child.* New York: Medcom Press.

Crook, W. G., W. W. Harrison, S. E. Crawford, and B. S. Emerson. 1961. Systemic manifestations due to allergy. Report of fifty patients and a review of the literature on the subject (allergic toxemia and the allergic tension-fatigue syndrome). *Pediatrics* 27:790.

Deamer, W. C. 1973a. Recurrent abdominal pain: recurrent controversy (letters). *Pediatrics* 51:307.

Deamer, W. C., O. L. Frick, et al. 1970. Allergic tension-fatigue syndrome. Scientific Exhibition of the American Academy of Pediatrics, October, San Francisco.

Duke, W. W. 1923. Food Allergy as a cause of illness. *JAMA* 81:886.

Eich, W., E. Thim, and J. Crowder. 1979. Effect of the Feingold Kaiser Permanente diet in minimal brain dysfunction. *Journal of the Medical Association of the State of Alabama* 49:16–20.

Ellis, E. 1972. Quoted by W. G. Crook in Allergy . . . the great masquerader. *Pedia. Basics* (Gerber Products, Fremont, Mich.).

Farr, R. S. 1972. Presentation at the Annual Meeting of the American College of Allergists, March 5, Dallas, Texas.

Fries, J., and I. Glaser. 1950. Studies on the antigenicity of bananas, raw and dehydrogenated. *Journal of Allergy* 21:169.

Gerrard, J., and M. Shenassa. 1983. Food allergy: Two common types seen in breast- and formula-fed babies. *Annals of Allergy* 50:375.

Gerrard, J. W. 1966. Familial recurrent rhinorrhea and bronchitis due to cow's milk. *JAMA* 198:605.

Gerrard, J. W. 1973. *Understanding Allergies*. Springfield, Ill.: Charles C. Thomas.

Gerrard, J. W., and M. Esperance. 1969. Nocturnal enuresis: Studies in bladder function in normals and enuretics. *Canadian Medical Association* 101:269.

Gerrard, J. W., D. C. Heiner, E. J. Ives, and L. W. Hardy. 1963. Milk allergy: Recognition, natural history, and management. *Clinical Pediatrics* 2:634.

Gerrard, J. W., et al. 1971. Letters. *Pediatrics* 48:994.

Glaser, J. 1954. Migraine in pediatric practice. *Am. J. Dis. Child.*, 88:92.

Goldman, S., W. Sellars, S. Halpern, D. Anderson, T. Furlow, C. Johnson, et al. 1963. Milk allergy II: Skin testing of allergic and normal children with purified milk proteins. *Journal of Pediatrics* 32:572–79.

Harrison, A. 1971. Letters. *Pediatrics* 48:166.

Heiner, D. C., J. W. Sears, and W. T. Kniker. 1962. Multiple precipitins due to cow's milk in chronic respiratory diseases, including poor growth, gastrointestinal symptoms, evidence of allergy, iron deficiency anemia, and pulmonary hemosiderosis. A syndrome. *Am. J. Dis. Child.* 103:634.

Hoobler, B. R. 1916. Some early symptoms suggesting protein sensitization in infancy. *Am. J. Dis. Child.* 12:129.

Hughes, E., R. Weinstein, P. Gott, R. Bingelo, and K. Whitaker. 1982. Food sensitivity in attention deficit disorder with hyperactivity: A procedure for differential diagnosis. *Annals of Allergy* 49:276–280.

Jewett, D., et al. 1990. A double-blind study of symptom provocation to determine food sensitivity. *JAMA* 323:429–433.

Kahn, I. S. 1927. Pollen toxemia. *JAMA* 88:241.

Kaufman, W. 1955. The comprehensive management of patients suffering from food-induced allergies. *Int. Arch. Allerg.* 6:361.

Kemp, J. P. 1970. Recurrent abdominal pain (letters). *Pediatrics* 46:972.

Lothe, L., T. Lindberg, and I. Jakobsson. 1982. Cow's milk formula as a cause of infantile colic: A double-blind study. *Pediatrics* 70:7–10.

McGovern, J. P., and T. J. Haywood. 1970. Allergic headache. In *Allergy of the Nervous System,* edited by F. Speer. Springfield, Ill.: Charles C. Thomas.

McLaughlan, P., K. Anderson, and R. Cooms. 1981. An oral screening procedure to determine the sensitizing capacity of infant feeding formula. *Clinical Allergy* 11:311.

Matsumura, T., et al. 1966. Significance of food allergy in the etiology of orthostatic albuminuria. *J. Asthma Res.* 3:325.

May, C. 1981. Food sensitivity. *NESA Proceedings* 2:198–205.

May, C. 1982. Food allergy: Lessons from the past. *Journal of Allergy and Clinical Immunology* 69:255–259.

Null, G. 1992. *Clearer, Cleaner, Safer, Greener.* New York: Villard Books, Random House.

Oster, J. 1972. Recurrent abdominal pain, headache, and limb pain in children and adolescents. *Pediatrics* 50:429.

Pastorello, E., L. Stocchi, V. Prafettoni, A. Bigi, M. Schilke, C. Incorvaia, and C. Zanussi. 1989. Role of the elimination diet in adults with food allergy. *Journal of Allergy and Clinical Immunology* 84:475–483.

Pearson, D., K. Rix, and S. Benley. 1983. Food allergy: How much is in the mind? *Lancet* 1:1259–1261.

Pratt, E. L. 1958. Food allergy and food intolerance in relation to the development of good eating habits. *Pediatrics* 21:642.

Randolph, T. G., H. J. Rinkel, and M. Zeller. 1951. *Food Allergy.* Springfield, Ill., Charles C. Thomas.

Rapaport, H. G., and S. M. Linde. 1971. *The Complete Allergy Guide.* New York: Simon & Schuster.

Rapp, D. 1978. Hyperactivity and food allergy: Are they related? *Annals of Allergy* 40:297–298.

Rapp, D. 1980. Behavioral reactions following food challenges. *Annals of Allergy* 44:61.

Rapp, D. 1981. A prototype for food sensitivity studies in children. *Annals of Allergy* 47:123–124.

Rapp, D., J. McGovern, and F. Waikman. 1982. Video documentation of food and chemical sensitivities. *Annals of Allergy* 48:258.

Rapp, D. J. 1972. *Allergies and Your Child.* New York: Holt, Rinehart & Winston.

Rinkle, H. 1944. Food allergy: The role of food allergy in internal medicine. *Annals of Allergy* 2:115–124.

Rowe, A. H., Sr. 1930. Allergic toxemia and migraine due to food allergy. *Calif. West. Med.* 33:785.

Rowe, A. H., Sr. 1931. *Food Allergy: Its Manifestations, Diagnosis and Treatment.* Philadelphia: Lea & Febiger.

Sandberg, D. H. 1973. Recurrent abdominal pain: Recurrent controversy (letters). *Pediatrics* 51:307.

Scadding, G., R. Ayesh, J. Brostoff, S. Mitchell, R. Wring, and R. Smith. 1988. Poor sulphoxidation ability in patients with food sensitivity. *British Medical Journal* 297:105–107.

Schmitt, B. D. 1971. School phobia—the great imitator: The pediatrician's viewpoint. *Pediatrics* 48:433.

Shannon, W. R. 1922. Neuropathic manifestations in infants and children as a result of anaphylactic reactions to foods contained in their dietary. *Am. J. Dis. Child.* 24:89.

Speer, F. 1963. *The Allergic Child.* New York: Hoeber, Harper & Row.

Sternberg, L. 1942. Seasonal somnolence: A possible pollen allergy. *Journal of Allergy* 14:89.

Stone, R. T., and G. J. Barbero. 1970. Recurrent abdominal pain in childhood. *Pediatrics* 45:732.

Swanson, J. 1980. Behavioral responses to artificial color. *Science* 207: 28.

Taube, E. L. 1973. *Food Allergy and the Allergic Patient.* Springfield, Ill., Charles C. Thomas.

Taylor, E. 1984. Annotations: Diet and behavior. *Archives of Diseases in Childhood* 59:97–98.

Thorley, G. 1984. Pilot study to assess behavioral and cognitive effects of artificial food colors in a group of retarded children. *Developmental Medicine and Child Neurology* 26:56–61.

Tolber, S. G. 1981. Food Problems. *Cutis* 28:360.

Tsuei, J., et al. 1984. A food allergy study utilizing the EAV acupuncture technique. *American Journal of Acupuncture* 12(2):105–116.

Von Pirquet, C. 1906. Allergie. *Munch. Med. Wochenschr.* 53:1457.

Walker, W. A. 1987. Role of mucosal barrier in antigen handling by the gut. In *Food Allergy and Intolerance,* edited by J. Brostoff and S. J. Challacombe. London: Balliere-Tindall.

Weinberger, M. 1978. The diet wasn't controlled. *Pediatrics* 61:325–326.

GIARDIA

Bendig, B. 1989. Diagnosis of giardiasis in infants and children by endoscopic brush cytology. *Journal of Pediatric Gastroenterology and Nutrition* 8(2):204–206.

Edlind, T. 1989. Susceptibility of *Giardia lamblia* to aminoglycoside protein synthesis inhibitors: Correlation with RNA structure. *Antimicrobial Agents and Chemotherapy* 33(4):484–488.

Esrey, S., J. Collett, M. Miliotis, H. Koornhof, and P. Makhale. 1989. The risk of infection from *Giardia lamblia* due to drinking water supply, use of water, and latrines among preschool children in rural Lesotho. *International Journal of Epidemiology* 18(1):248–253.

Faulkner, C., S. Patton, and S. Johnson. 1989. Prehistoric parasitism in Tennessee: Evidence from the analysis of desiccated fecal material collected from Big Bone Cave, Van Buren County, Tennessee. *Journal of Parasitology* 75(3):461–463.

Holberton, D., D. Baker, and J. Marshall. 1989. Segmented alpha-helical coiled-coil structure of the protein giardin from the *Giardia* cytoskeleton. *Journal of Molecular Biology* 204(3):789–795.

Isaac-Renton, R., S. Byrne, and R. Pramey. 1989. Isoelectric focusing of ten strains of *Giardia duodenalis. Journal of Parasitology* 74(6):1054–1056.

Janoff, E., J. Craft, L. Pickering, T. Novotny, M. Blaser, C. Knisley, and L. Reller. 1989. Diagnosis of *Giardia lamblia* infections by detection of parasite-specific antigens. *Journal of Clinical Microbiology* 27(3):431–435.

Knisley, C., P. Englelkirk, L. Pickering, M. West, and E. Janoff. 1989. Rapid detection of giardia antigen in stool with the use of enzyme immunoassays. *American Journal of Clinical Pathology* 91:704–708.

Korman, S., E. Granot, and N. Ramu. 1989. Severe giardiasis in a child during cancer therapy (letter). *American Journal of Gastroenterology* 84(4):450–451.

Medical Letter. 1988. Drugs for parasitic infections. *Medical Letter* 30(759):15–24.

Rojas, L., D. Torres, B. Mediola, and C. Finlay. 1989. Detection of specific anti-giardia serum antibody by an immunofluorescence test in children with clinical giardiasis. *American Journal of Tropical Medicine and Hygiene* 40(5):477–479.

Senay, H., and D. MacPherson. 1989. Parasitology: Diagnostic yield of stool examination. *Canadian Medical Association* 140(11):1329–1331.

Sogin, M., J. Gunderson, H. Elwood, R. Alonso, and D. Peattie. 1989. Phylogenetic meaning of the kingdom concept: An unusual ribosomal RNA from *Giardia lamblia. Science* 243:75–77.

Spencer, M., L. Garcia, and M. Chapin. 1979. Dientamoeba fragilas. *American Journal of Disability in Children* 133:390–393.

Steketee, R., S. Reid, T. Cheng, J. Stoebig, R. Harrington, and J. Davis. 1989. Recurrent outbreaks of giardiasis in a child day-care center, Wisconsin. *American Journal of Public Health* 79(4):485–490.

HYPERACTIVITY

Abt, I. A. 1929. *System of Pediatrics.* Philadelphia: W. B. Saunders.

American Psychiatric Association. 1980. *Diagnostic and Statistical Manual of Mental Disorders,* 3d ed. Washington, D.C.: American Psychiatric Association.

Ayers, A. J. 1972. *Southern California Sensory Integration Tests.* Los Angeles: Western Psychological Services.

Baker, S. 1898. Fatigue in school children. *Educational Review* 15:34.

Bax, M., and R. MacKeith, eds. 1963. *Minimal Cerebral Dysfunction: Little Club Clinics in Developmental Medicine.* London: William Heinemann.

Beach, R. S., M. E. Gershwin, and L. S. Hurley. 1982. Gestational zinc deprivation in mice: Persistence of immunodeficiency for three generations. *Science* 218:469–471.

Beecher, H., and M. Boston. 1955. The powerful placebo. *JAMA* 159:-1602–1606.

Bell, I. 1976. A kinin model of mediation for food and chemical sensitivities: Biobehavioral implications. *Annals of Allergy* 35:206.

Benton, A. L. 1964–1965. Developmental aphasia and brain damage. *Cortex* 1:41–52.

Berry, C., S. Shaywitz, and B. Shaywitz. Girls with attention deficit disorder: A silent minority? *Pediatrics* 76:801–809.

Bock, S. 1980. Food sensitivity: A critical review and practical approach. *American Journal of Disabilities in Children* 134:973–982.

Bock, S. A. 1987. Prospective appraisal of complaints of adverse reactions to foods in children during the first three years of life. *Pediatrics* 79:683–688.

Bolton, R. 1973. Aggression and hypoglycaemia among the Qolla: A study in psychobiological anthropology. *Ethnology* 12:227–257.

Bowen, R., and R. M. Balyeat. 1934. Facial and dental deformities due to perennial nasal allergy in childhood. *Southern Medical Journal* 27:-933.

Brenner, A. 1977. A study of the efficacy of the Feingold diet on hyperkinetic children. *Clinical Pediatrics* 16:652–656.

Chandra, R. K. 1983. Nutrition, immunity, and infection: Present knowledge and future directions. *Lancet:* 668–691.

Charles, L., and R. Schain. 1981. A four-year follow-up study on the effects of methylphenidate on the behavior and academic achievement of hyperactive children. *Journal of Abnormal Child Psychology* 9:495–505.

Chobot, R., H. D. Dundy, and B. I. Pacella. 1950. The incidence of abnormal encephalographic patterns in allergic children. *Journal of Allergy* 21:334.

Clarke, T. W. 1944. Allergy of the central nervous system. *Annals of Allergy* 2:189.

Clements, S. D. 1966. *Minimal Brain Dysfunction in Children—Terminology and Identification.* Washington, D.C.: USPHS Publication 1415.

Cohen, L., and E. Kahn. 1934. Organic driveness: A brain stem syndrome and an experience. *New England Journal of Medicine* 210:748, 756.

Colquhoun, I., and S. Bunday. 1981. A lack of essential fatty acids as a possible cause of hyperactivity in children. *Medical Hypotheses* 7:673–679.

Conners, C. K. 1969. A teacher rating scale for use in drug studies with children. *American Journal of Psychiatry* 126:884.

Conners, C. K., C. M. Goyette, D. A. Southwick, J. M. Lees, and P. A. Andrulonis. 1976. Food additives and hyperkinesis: A controlled double-blind study. *Pediatrics* 58:154–166.

Cook, P. S., and J. M. Woodhill. 1976. The Feingold dietary treatment of the hyperkinetic syndrome. *Medical Journal of Australia* 2:85–90.

Crook, W. G. 1975. *Can Your Child Read? Is He Hyperactive?* Jackson, Tenn.: Pedicenter Press.

Crook, W. G. 1978. Adverse reactions to food can cause hyperkinesis (letters). *American Journal of the Disabled Child* 132:819.

Dees, S. C., and H. Lowenbach. 1951. Allergic epilepsy. *Annals of Allergy* 9:446.

DeToni, G. 1952. Unsere Erfahrung mit über 350 elektroencephalographischer Untersuchungen im Kindesalter. *Monatschrift Kinderheilkunde* 100:214.

Duke, W. W. 1930. Deformity of the face caused by nasal allergy in childhood. *Journal of Allergy* 1:466.

Egger, J., C. M. Carter, J. Wilson, M. W. Turner, and J. F. Soothill. 1983. *Is migraine food allergy? Lancet:* 865–869.

Egger, J., P. J. Graham, C. M. Carter, D. Gumley, and J. F. Soothill. 1985. Controlled trial of oligoantigenic treatment in the hyperkinetic syndrome. *Lancet* 1:540–545. Reprinted in *The Relationship of Food Sensitivities (and Other Dietary Factors) to Hyperactivity, Attention Deficits, and Other Nervous System Symptoms: A Compendium,* edited by W. G. Crook.

Feingold, B. F. 1975a. Hyperkinesis and learning disabilities linked to artificial food flavors and colors. *American Journal of Nursing* 75:797–803.

Feingold, B. F. 1975b. *Why Your Child Is Hyperactive.* New York: Random House.

Feingold, B. F., 1976. Hyperkinesis and learning disabilities linked to the ingestion of artificial food colors and flavors. *Journal of Learning Disabilities* 9:19–27. Reprinted in *The Relationship of Food Sensitivities (and Other Dietary Factors) to Hyperactivity, Attention Deficits, and Other Nervous System Symptoms: A Compendium,* edited by W. G. Crook.

Forman, J. 1939. Importance of mental hygiene in the management of the allergic child. *Ohio State Medical Journal* 35:747.

Freed, D. L. J., and R. Carter. 1982. Neuropathy due to monosodium glutamate intolerance. *Annals of Allergy* 48:96–97.

Gibson, S. 1937. Chorea. In Vol. 4 of *Practice of Pediatrics,* edited by J. Brenneman. Hagerstown, Md.: W. F. Prior.

Goyette, C. H., C. K. Conners, and R. H. Ulrich. 1978. Normative data on revised Conners parent and teacher rating scales. *Journal of Abnormal Child Psychology* 6:221–236.

Goyette, C. H., C. Connors, T. Petti, and L. Curtis. 1978. Effect of artificial colors on hyperkinetic children: A double-blind challenge study. *Psychopharmacology Bulletin* 14:139–140.

Green, M. 1974. Sublingual provocation testing for foods and FD&C dyes. *Annals of Allergy* 33:274.

Haavik, S., K. Altman, and C. Woelik. 1979. Effects of the Feingold diet on seizures and hyperactivity: A single-subject analysis. *Journal of Behavioral Medicine* 2:365–374.

Hagerman, D., and C. A. Villee. 1960. Transport functions of the placenta. *Physiological Reviews* 42:313.

Hagerman, R., and A. Falkenstein. 1987. An association between recurrent *otitis media* in infancy and later hyperactivity. *Clinical Pediatrics* 26:253–257.

Hall, K. 1976. Allergy of the nervous system: A review. *Annals of Allergy* 36:49.

Harley, J. P. 1976. Diet and hyperactivity: Any connection? *Nutrition Reviews* 34:49.

Harley J. P., R. S. Ray, L. Thomasi, et al. 1978. Hyperkinesis and food additives: Testing the Feingold hypothesis. *Pediatrics* 61:818–828.

Hawley, C., and R. E. Buckely. 1974. Food dyes and hyperkinetic children. *Academic Therapy* 10:27.

Helgason, T., and M. R. Jonasson. 1981. Evidence for a food additive as a cause of ketosis-prone diabetes. *Lancet:* 716–20.

Helgason, T., S. W. B. Ewen, I. S. Ross and J. M. Stowers. 1982. Diabetes produced in mice by smoked/cured mutton. *Lancet:* 1017.

Hertzog, C., and M. Rovine. 1985. Repeated-measures analysis of variance in developmental research: Selected issues. *Child Development* 56:787–809.

Hindle, R., and J. Priest. 1978. The management of hyperkinetic children: A trial of dietary therapy. *New Zealand Medical Journal* 88:43–45.

Hoffman, H. 1864. *The Story of Fidgety Philip*. From *Struwwelpeter*. New York: Frederick Warne.

Holmgren, B., and S. Kraepelien. 1953. Electroencephalographic studies of asthmatic children. *Acta Paediatrica* 43:432.

Jasper, H. H. 1949. Electroencephalography in child neurology and psychiatry. *Pediatrics* 3:783.

Kaplan, B. 1988. The relevance of food for children's cognitive and behavioral health. *Canadian Journal of Behavior and Science* 20(4):360–373.

Kaplan, B. J., et al. 1989. Dietary replacement in preschool-aged hyperactive boys. *Pediatrics* 83:7–17. Reprinted in *The Relationship of Food Sensitivities (and Other Dietary Factors) to Hyperactivity, Attention Deficits, and Other Nervous System Symptoms: A Compendium,* edited by W. G. Crook.

Kaplan, B. J., J. McNicol, R. A. Conte, et al. 1987a. Physical signs and symptoms in preschool-aged hyperactive and normal children. *J. Dev. Behav. Pediatr.* 8:305–310.

Kaplan, B. J., J. McNicol, R. A. Conte, et al. 1987b. Sleep disturbance in preschool-aged hyperactive and nonhyperactive children. *Pediatrics* 80:839–844.

King, D. S. 1981. Can allergic exposure provoke psychological symptoms? A double-blind test. *Biological Psychiatry* 16:3–19.

Kinsbourne, M. 1984. Hyperactivity management: The impact of special diets. In *Middle Childhood: Developmental Dysfunction,* edited by M. Levine and P. Saltz. Baltimore: University Park Press.

Kittler, F. G., and D. G. Baldwin. 1970. The role of allergic factors in the child with minimal brain dysfunction. *Annals of Allergy* 28:203–206.

Laroche, G., F. C. Richet, and F. Saint Girons. 1930. *Alimentary Anaphylaxis,* translated by A. H. Rowe. Berkeley: University of California Press.

Laufer, M. W., and E. Denhoff. 1957. Hyperkinetic behavior syndrome in children. *Journal of Pediatrics* 50:463–474.

McCarrison, R. 1982. *Nutrition and Health.* London: McCarrison Society.

Mandell, M., and G. Rose. 1968. May emotional reactions be precipitated by allergens? *Connecticut Medicine* 32:300–303.

Mattes, G., and R. Gittleman. 1981. The effects of artificial food coloring in children with hyperactive symptoms. *Archives of General Psychiatry* 38:714–718.

Mausner, J., and A. Bahn. 1974. *Epidemiology: An Introductory Test.* Philadelphia: W. B. Saunders.

Mayron, L. 1979. Allergy, learning, and behavioral problems. *Journal of Learning Disabilities* 12:32–42.

Mendelson, W., N. Johnson, and M. Stewart. 1971. Hyperactive children as teenagers: A follow-up study. *Journal of Nervous and Mental Disease* 153:237–239.

Menkes, M., J. Rowe, and J. Menkes. 1967. A twenty-five-year follow-up study on the hyperkinetic child with minimal brain dysfunction. *Pediatrics* 39:393–399.

Menzies, I. C. 1984a. Allergic and immunologic factors in child and family psychiatry. In *Recent Research in Developmental Psychopathology,* edited by J. E. Stevenson. No. 4 of *Journal of Child Psychology and Psychiatry Book Supplement* Oxford: Pergamon Press.

Menzies, I. C. 1984b. Disturbed children: the role of food and chemical sensitivities. *Nutrition and Health* 3(1–2):39–54. Reprinted in *The Relationship of Food Sensitivities (and Other Dietary Factors) to Hyperactivity, Attention Deficits, and Other Nervous System Symptoms: A Compendium,* edited by W. G. Crook.

Milich, R., M. Wolraich, and S. Lindgren. 1986. Sugar and hyperactivity: A critical review of empirical findings. *Clinical Psychology Review* 6:493–513.

Miller, J. B. 1977. A double-blind study of food extract injection therapy: A preliminary report. *Annals of Allergy* 38:185–191.

Millman, M. M., M. B. Campbell, K. Wright, and A. Johnston. 1976. Allergy and learning disability in children. *Annals of Allergy* 36:149.

Money, J., ed. 1962. *Reading Disability: Progress and Research Needs in Dyslexia.* Baltimore: Johns Hopkins University Press.

Morris, D. L. 1969. Use of sublingual antigen in diagnosis and treatment of food allergy. *Annals of Allergy* 27:289.

Moya, F., and B. E. Smith. 1965. Distribution and placental transport of drugs and anesthetics. *Anaesthesiology* 26:465.

Nair, V., and K. P. Dubois. 1968. Prenatal and early postnatal exposure to environmental contaminants. *Chicago Med. School Quart.* 27:75.

O'Shea, J. A., and S. F. Porter. 1981. Double-blind study of children with hyperkinetic syndrome treated with multi-allergen extract sublingually. *Journal of Learning Disabilities* 14:189–237.

Page, J. G., R. S. Janicki, J. I. Bernstein, C. F. Curran, and F. A. Michelli. 1974. Pemoline (Cylert) in the treatment of childhood hyperkinesis. *Journal of Learning Disabilities* 10:165–176.

Pellegrini, R., A. Schauss, and M. Miller. 1981. Room color and aggression in a criminal detention holding cell: A test of the "tranquilizing pink" hypothesis. *Orthomolecular Psychiatry* 10:174–181.

Prinz, R. J., W. A. Roberts, and E. Hantman. 1980. Dietary correlates of hyperactive behavior in children. *Journal of Consulting and Clinical Psychology* 48:760–769.

Randolph, T. G. 1945. Fatigue and weakness of allergic origin (allergic toxemia) to be differentiated from nervous fatigue and neurasthenia. *Annals of Allergy* 3:418.

Randolph, T. G. 1946. Fatigue of allergic origin. To be differentiated from "nervous fatigue" or neurasthenia. *Annals of Allergy* 3:418.

Randolph, T. G. 1947b. Blood studies in allergy IV: Variations in eosinophils following test feeding of foods. *Journal of Allergy* 18:199.

Randolph, T. G., and F. F. A. Rawling. 1946. Blood studies in allergy V: Variations in total leukocytes following test feeding of foods—An appraisal of the individual food test. *Annals of Allergy* 4:163.

Rapaport, J. I., and M. Benoit. 1975. The relation of direct home observations to the clinic evaluation of hyperactive school-age boys. *Journal of Childhood Psychology and Psychiatry and Allied Disciplines* 16:141–147.

Rapp, D. J. 1978. Does diet affect hyperactivity? *Journal of Learning Disabilities*: 56–62. Reprinted in *The Relationship of Food Sensitivities (and Other Dietary Factors) to Hyperactivity, Attention Deficits, and Other Nervous System Symptoms: A Compendium,* edited by W. G. Crook.

Rapp, D. J. 1979. *Allergy and the Hyperactive Child.* New York: Sovereign Books, Simon & Schuster.

Rapp, D. J. 1980. Hyperactivity and the tension-fatigue syndrome. In *Food Allergy: New Perspectives,* edited by J. W. Gerrard. Springfield, Ill.: Charles C. Thomas.

Rapp, D. J. 1981. Elimination diets and hyperactivity (letters). *Pediatrics* 67:937.

Ratner, B., and H. L. Gruehl. 1935. Anaphylactogenic properties of malted sugars and corn syrup. *Am. J. Disabled Child.* 49:307.

Ribon, A., and S. Joshi. 1982. Is there any relationship between food additives and hyperkinesis? *Annals of Allergy* 48:275–278.

Rinkel, H. J. 1944a. Food allergy I: The role of food allergy in internal medicine. *Annals of Allergy* 2:115.

Rinkel, H. J. 1944b. Food allergy II: The technique and clinical application of individual food tests. *Annals of Allergy* 2:504.

Rinkel, J. H. T. G. Randolph, and M. Zeller. 1951. *Food Allergy.* Springfield, Ill.: Charles C. Thomas.

Rogerson, C. A. 1937. The psychological factors in asthma-prurigo. *Quarterly Journal of Medicine* 6:367.

Rose T. 1978. The functional relationship between artificial food colors and hyperactivity. *Journal of Applied Behavior Analysis* 11:439–446.

Rowe, A. H. 1931. *Food Allergy, Its Manifestations, Diagnosis, and Treatment with a General Discussion of Bronchial Asthma.* Philadelphia: Lea & Febiger.

Rowe, A. H. 1937. *Clinical Allergy Due to Foods, Inhalants, Contactants, Bacteria, Fungi, and Other Causes: Management, Diagnosis and Treatment.* Philadelphia: Lea & Febiger.

Rowe, A. H. 1944. *Elimination Diets and the Patient's Allergies: A Handbook of Allergy,* 2d ed. Philadelphia: Lea & Febiger.

Rowe, K. 1988. Synthetic food colouring and "hyperactivity": A double-blind crossover study. *Australian Pediatrics* 24:143–147.

Rutter, M. L. 1970. Psycho-social disorders in childhood, and their outcome in adult life. *Journal of the Royal College of Physicians of London* 4:211–218.

Sabotka, T. J. 1978. Hyperkinesis and food additives. A review of experimental work. *FDA By-Laws* 4:493.

Safer, D., and J. Krager. 1988. A survey of medication treatment for hyperactive/inattentive students. *JAMA* 260:2256–2258.

Salzman, I. K. 1976. Allergy testing, psychological assessment, and dietary treatment of the hyperactive child syndrome. *Medical Journal of Australia* 2:248.

Scarnati, R. 1986. An outline of hazardous side effects of Ritalin (methylphenidate). *International Journal of the Addictions* 21(7):837–841.

Schauss, A. G. 1980. *Diet, Crime and Delinquency,* Calif.: Parker House.

Schauss, A. G. 1982. Nutrition and Behaviour: Implications for Criminology. Proceedings of the 112th Annual Conference of the American Correctional Association, Toronto, Canada.

Schauss, A. G. 1983. Nutrition and Behaviour. Paper presented at the McCarrison Society's Thirteenth Annual Conference, September 23–25, Oxford, England.

Schmidt, A. M. 1975. Statement of the Commissioner of the Food and Drug Administration before the U.S. Senate Committee on Labor and Public Welfare Subcommittee on Health, September 11.

Schneider, W. F. 1945. Psychiatric evaluation of the hyper-kinetic child. *Journal of Pediatrics* 26:559.

Sehan, M., and G. Sehan, 1926. *The Tired Child.* Philadelphia: J. B. Lippincott.

Shaywitz, B. 1978. Food coloring and animal studies. *Pediatric Notes* 2:1–4.

Smithells, R. W., M. J. Seller, R. Harris, D. W. Fielding, C. J. Schorah, N. C. Nevin, S. Sheppard, A. P. Read, S. Walker, and J. Wild. 1983. Further experience of vitamin supplementation for prevention of neural tube defect recurrences. *Lancet:* 1027–1031.

Speer, F. 1970. *Allergy of the Nervous System*. Springfield, Ill.: Charles C. Thomas.

Spyker, J. M. 1975. Behavioral toxicology and teratology. In *Behavioral Toxicology*, edited by B. Weiss and V. G. Luties. New York: Plenum.

Sternbergh, T. H., and G. D. Baldridge. 1948. Electroencephalographic abnormalities in patients with generalized neurodermatitis. *Journal of Investigative Dermatology* 11:401.

Stokes, J. H., and A. Beerman. 1940. Psychosomatic correlations in allergic conditions. *Psychosomatic Medicine* 2:438.

Strauss, A. A., and N. C. Kephart. 1955. *Psychopathology and Education of the Brain-Injured Child*, vol. 2. New York: Grune & Stratton.

Strauss, A. A., and L. E. Lehtinen. 1948. Psychopathology and Education of the Brain-Injured Child, vol. 1. New York: Grune & Stratton.

Swanson, J. M., and M. Kinsbourne. 1980. Food dyes impair performance of hyperactive children on a laboratory learning test. *Science* 207. Reprinted in *The Relationship of Food Sensitivities (and Other Dietary Factors) to Hyperactivity, Attention Deficits, and Other Nervous System Symptoms: A Compendium*, edited by W. G. Crook.

Thorley, G. 1983. Childhood hyperactivity and food additives. *Developmental Medicine and Child Neurology* 25:531–534.

Todd, T. W. 1938. The significance of developmental growth studies in evaluation of clinical allergy. *Journal of Allergy* 9:234.

United Kingdom. Ministry of Agriculture, Fisheries, and Food. Food Additives and Contaminants Committee. 1973. *Interim Report on the Review of the Colouring Matter in Food Regulations*. FAC/REP/29. H.M.S.O.

Wechsler, D. 1974. Wechsler Intelligence Scale for Children, rev. New York: Psychological Corporation.

Weiss, B. 1982. Food additives and environmental chemicals as sources of childhood behaviour disorders. *American Academy of Child Psychiatry. Journal* 21(2):144–152.

Weiss, B., et al. 1980. Behavioral responses to artificial food colors. *Science* 207. Reprinted in *The Relationship of Food Sensitivities (and Other Dietary Factors) to Hyperactivity, Attention Deficits, and Other Nervous System Symptoms: A Compendium*, edited by W. G. Crook.

Weiss, G., K. Minde, J. Werry, V. Douglas, and E. Nemeth. 1971. Studies on the hyperactive child: Five-year follow-up. *Archives of General Psychiatry* 24:409.

Wender, E. H. 1986. The food-additive-free diet in the treatment of behavior disorders: A review *J. Dev. Behav. Pediatr.* 6:493–513.

Werry, J. 1976. Food additives and hyperactivity. *Medical Journal of Australia* 2:281–282.

Woteki, C. E. 1986. Dietary survey data: Sources and limits to interpretation. *Nutrition Reviews* 44:204–213.

Wurtman, R. J. 1983. Behavioral effect of nutrients. *Lancet:* 1145–1147.

Yogman, M. W., and S. H. Zeisel. 1983. Diet and sleep patterns in newborn infants. *New England Journal of Medicine* 309:1147–1149.

Zametkin, A., and J. Rappaport. 1987. Neurobiology of attention deficit disorder with hyperactivity: Where have we come in fifty years? *American Academy of Child and Adolescent Psychiatry. Journal* 25(5):676–686.

Zentall, S.S., and T.R. Zentall. 1986. Hyperactivity ratings: Statistical regression provides an insufficient explanation of practice effects. J. Pediatr. Psychol. 11:393–396.

IMMUNOLOGY

Michael, F., J. Bousquet, Y. Coulomb, and M. Robinet-Levy. 1980. Comparison of clinical and immunologic parameters for the prediction of infant allergy. *Journal of Allergy and Clinical Immunology* 65:167.

Taudorf, E., L. Lauren, A. Lanner, B. Bjorksten, S. Dreborg, M. Soborg, and B. Weeke. 1987. Oral immunotherapy in birch pollen hayfever (Denmark and Sweden). *Journal of Allergy and Clinical Immunology* 80:153–161.

MIGRAINE

Brostoff, J. 1980. Food allergies in migraine. *Lancet:* 1–4.

Monro, J. C. Carini, and J. Brostoff. 1984. Migraine is a food allergic disease. *Lancet* 2:719–721.

O'Banion, D. 1981. Dietary control of headache pain: Five case studies. *Journal of Holistic Medicine* 3:14–20.

Rowe, A. H. 1930. Allergic toxemia and migraine due to food allergy: Report of cases. *Calif. and West. Med.* 33:785.

NERVOUS SYSTEM ALLERGIES

Bassoe, P. 1932. Auriculotemporal syndrome and other vasomotor disturbances about head: "Auriculotemporal syndrome" complicating disease of parotid gland; angioneurotic edema of brain. *Medical Clinics of North America* 16:409.

Cobb, S. 1936. Causes of epilepsy. *Medical Clinics of North America* 19:1583.

Criep, L. H. 1939. Allergic vertigo. Pennsylvania *Medical Journal* 43: 258.

Duke, W. R. 1927. Mental and neurologic reactions of asthma patient. *Journal of Laboratory and Clinical Medicine* 13:20.

Hinnant, I. M., and L. J. Halpin. 1936. Food allergy in mild and severe cyclic vomiting. *Medical Clinics of North America* 19:1931.

Kennedy, F. 1926. Cerebral symptoms induced by angioneurotic edema. *Arch. Neurol. & Psychiat.* 15:28.

Kennedy, F. 1936. Allergic manifestations in nervous system. New York State *Journal of Medicine* 36:469.

Kennedy, F. 1938. Allergy and its effect on the central nervous system. *Arch. Neurol. & Psychiat.* 15:1361.

Osler, W. 1914. The visceral lesions of purpura and allied conditions. *British Medical Journal* 517.

Pardee, I. 1938. Allergic reactions in the central nervous system. *Arch. Neurol. & Psychiat.*, 15:1360.

Quincke, H. 1921. Acute circumscribed edema and related conditions. *Med. Klin.* 17:675.

Ratner, B. 1943. Allergy, anaphylaxis, and immunotherapy: Basic principles and practice. Baltimore: Williams & Wilkins.

Rowe, A. H. 1927. Allergy in etiology of disease. *Journal of Laboratory and Clinical Medicine* 3:31.

Rowe, A. H. 1937. *Clinical Allergy.* Philadelphia: Lea & Febiger.

Shannon, W. R. 1922. Neuropathic manifestations as a result of anaphylactic reaction to foods contained in their dietary. *Am. J. Dis. Child.*, 24:89.

Speer, F. 1980. *Allergy of the Nervous System.* Springfield, Ill.: Charles C. Thomas.

Urbach, E. 1943. *Allergy.* New York: Grune & Stratton.

Vaughan, W. T., and E. K. Hawke. 1931. Angioneurotic edema with some unusual manifestations. *Journal of Allergy* 2:125.

Waldbott, G. L. 1934. "Allergic" shock from substances other than pollen and serum. *Annals of Internal Medicine* 7:1308.

Wilmer, H. B., and M. M. Miller. 1934. A case of epilepsy presenting unusual manifestations. *Journal of Allergy* 5:628.

NEUROLOGICAL ALLERGY IN CHILDREN

Andermann, F. 1987. Clinical features of migraine-epilepsy syndromes. In *Migraine and Epilepsy,* edited by F. Andermann and I. Lugaresi. London: Butterworth.

Anthony, M. 1982. Serotonin and cyclic nucleotides in migraine. *Neurology* 33:45–8.

Baier, W. K., and H. Doose. 1985. Petit mal—Absences of childhood onset: Familial prevalences of migraine and seizures. *Neuropediatrics* 16:80–3.

Baker, A. B., and H. H. Noran. 1945. Changes in the central nervous system associated with encephalitis complicating pneumonia. *Archives of Internal Medicine* 76:146.

Balyeat, R. M., and H. J. Rinkel. 1931. Allergic migraine in children. *Am. J. Dis. Child.* 42:1126.

Barnetson, R. S., R. A. Hardie, and T. G. Merrett. 1981. Late-onset atopic eczema and multiple food allergies after infectious mononucleosis. *British Medical Journal* 283:1086.

Barolin, G. 1966. Migraines and epilepsy: A relationship? *Epilepsia* 7:53–66.

Basser, L. S. 1969. The relation of migraine and epilepsy. *Brain* 92:-285–300.

Bladin, P. F. 1987. The association of benign Rolandic epilepsy with migraine. In *Migraine and Epilepsy,* edited by F. Andermann and E. Lugarsi. London: Butterworth.

Bladin, P. F., and G. Papworth. 1974. Chuckling and glugging seizures at night: Sylvian spike epilepsy. *Australian Association of Neurologists. Proceedings* 11:171–175.

Blatt, N. H., and M. H. Lepper. 1953. Reactions following antirabies prophylaxis. *Am. J. Dis. Child.* 86:395.

Brain, W. 1953. *Diseases of the Nervous System.* London: Oxford University Press.

Brantl, V., and H. A. Teschenmacher. 1979. A material with opioid activity in bovine milk and milk products. *Naunyn-Schmiedeberg's Archives of Pharmacology* 306:301–304.

Byers, R. K., and F. C. Mall. 1948. Encephalopathies following prophylactic pertussis vaccine. *Pediatrics* 1:437.

Camfield, P. R., K. Metrakos, and F. Anderman. 1978. Basilar migraine, seizures, and severe epileptiform EEG abnormalities: A relatively benign syndrome in adolescents. *Neurology* 28:584–588.

Carter, C. M., J. Egger, and J. F. Soothill. 1985. A dietary management of severe childhood migraine. *Human Nutrition. Applied Nutrition* 39A:294–303.

Casale, T. B., S. Bowman, and M. Kaliner. 1984. Induction of human cutaneous mast cell degranulation by opiates and endogenous opioid peptides: Evidence for opiate and non-opiate receptor participation. *Journal of Allergy and Clinical Immunology* 73:775.

Chobot, R., H. D. Dundy, and B. L. Pacella. 1950. The incidence of abnormal electroencephalographic patterns in allergic children. *Journal of Allergy* 21:334.

Churchill, J. A., and G. D. Gammon. 1949. The effect of antihistamine drugs in convulsive seizures. JAMA 141:18.

Clarke, T. W. 1948. Neuro-allergy in childhood. *New York State Journal of Medicine* 48:393.

Clein, N. W. 1937. Epilepsy of allergic origin. *Northwest Medicine* 36:378.

David, T. J. 1984. Anaphylactic shock during elimination diets for severe atopic eczema. *Arch. Dis. Child.* 59:983–986.

Davison, H. M. 1952. Allergy of the nervous system. *Quarterly Review of Allergy* 6:157.

Dees, S. C. 1945. Inter-relationships of allergic and psychosomatic factors in allergic children. Woods School *Bulletin* 12:59.

Dees, S. C. 1951. Neurological allergy. In *Allergy in Relation to Pediatrics,* edited by B. Ratner. St. Paul, Minn.: Bruce.

Dees, S. C. 1953. Electroencephalography in allergic epilepsy. *Southern Medical Journal* 46:618.

Dees, S. C. 1954. Neurologic allergy in childhood. *Pediatric Clinics of North America* 1:1017–1027. Reprinted in *The Relationship of Food Sensitivities (and Other Dietary Factors) to Hyperactivity, Attention Deficits, and Other Nervous System Symptoms: A Compendium,* edited by W. G. Crook.

Dees, S. C., and H. Lowenbach. 1948. The electroencephalograms of allergic children. *Annals of Allergy* 6:99.

Duke, W. W. 1893. Ueber Meningitis Scrosa. *Samml. klin. Vortrage innere Medicin* 5:655.

Egger, J., C. M. Carter, P. J. Graham, D. Gumley, and J. F. Soothill. 1985. A controlled trial of oligoantigenic diet treatment in the hyperkinetic syndrome. *Lancet* 1:940–945.

Egger, J., C. M. Carter, J. Wilson, M. W. Turner, and J. F. Soothill. 1983. Is migraine a food allergy? A double-blind controlled trial of oligoantigenic diet treatment. *Lancet* 2:865–869.

Egger, J., et al. 1989. Oligoantigenic diet treatment of children with epilepsy and migraine. *Journal of Pediatrics:* 51–58. Reprinted in *The Relationship of Food Sensitivities (and Other Dietary Factors) to Hyperactivity, Attention Deficits, and Other Nervous System Symptoms. A Compendium,* edited by W. G. Crook.

Ely, F. A. 1930. The migraine-epilepsy syndrome: A statistical study of heredity. *Arch. Neurol. Psychiatry* 24:943–949.

Erickson, T. C., W. J. Bleckwenn, and C. N. Woolsey. 1952. Observations on the post central gyrus in relation to pain. *Trans. Am. Neurol. Assoc.* 77:57–59.

Eyerman, C. H. 1931. Allergic headache. *Journal of Allergy* 2:106.

Fanchamps, A. 1982. The evolution of thinking about the role of site of action of serotonin in migraine. *Advances in Neurology* 33:31–33.

Finley, K. H. 1938. Pathogenesis of encephalitis occurring with vaccination, variola, and measles. *Arch. Neurol. & Psychiat.* 39:1047.

Ferraro, A. 1944. Pathology of demyelinating diseases as an allergic reaction of the brain. *Arch. Neurol. & Psychiat.* 52:443.

Frenk, H., J. Engel, Jr., R. F. Ackerman, Y. Shavit, and J. C. Liebeskind. 1979. Endogenous opiods may mediate post-ictal behavioral depression in amygdaloid kindled rats. *Brain Research* 167:435–440.

Frick, O. L., D. F. German, and J. Mills. 1979. Development of allergy in children: Association with virus infections. *Journal of Allergy and Clinical Immunology* 68:228–41.

Gardere, M., and M. Gaugolphe. 1908. Nervite au cours d'un cas de tetanos traite par la serum therapie. *Lyon Med.* 110:497.

Gayle, R. F., Jr., and R. L. Bowen. 1933. Acute ascending myelitis following the administration of typhoid vaccine: Report of a case with necropsy findings. *Journal of Nervous and Mental Disease* 78:221.

Goltman, A. M. 1936. Mechanism of migraine. *Journal of Allergy* 7:351.

Goodridge, M. G., and S. D. Shovron. 1983. Epileptic seizures in a population of six thousand. *British Medical Journal* 287:641–647.

Gowers, W. R. 1901. *Epilepsy and Other Convulsive Disorders: Their Causes, Symptoms, and Treatment.* London: Churchill.

Gowers, W. R. 1907. *The Borderland of Epilepsy: Faints, Vagal Attacks, Vertigo, Migraine, Sleep Symptoms, and Their Treatment.* London: Churchill.

Hamby, W. B. 1961. Reversible central pain. *Archives of Neurology* 5:82–86.

Hansel, F. K. 1949. The treatment of headache. *Annals of Allergy* 7:155.

Hills, M., and P. Armitage. The two period cross-over trial. *British Journal of Clinical Pharmacology* 8:7–20.

Hoeffel, G., and M. Moriarty. 1924. The effect of fasting on the metabolism of epileptic children. *Am. J. Dis. Child.* 28:16–24.

Hurst, E. W. 1942. Experimental demyelination of the central nervous system III: Poisoning with potassium cyanide, sodium azide, hydroxylamine, narcotics, carbon monoxide, etc., with some consideration of bilateral necrosis occurring in the basal nuclei. *Australian Journal of Experimental Biology and Medical Sciences* 20:297.

Huttenlocher, P. R., A. J. Wilbourn, and J. M. Signore. 1971. Medium-chain triglycerides as therapy for intractable childhood epilepsy. *Neurology* 21:1097–1103.

Jackson, J. H. 1875. Hospital for the epileptic and paralyzed: Case illustrating the relation between certain cases of migraine and epilepsy. *Lancet* 2:244–245.

Jenkins, C. M. 1949. Cerebral oedema due to phenobarbital sensitivity. *Annals of Allergy* 7:346.

Klee, W. A., et al. 1979. Exorphins: Peptides with opioid activity isolated from wheat gluten, and their possible role in the etiology of schizophrenia. In *Endorphins in Mental Health Research,* edited by E. Usdin, W. E. Bunney, and N. S. Kline. New York: Oxford University Press.

Lane, S. L., A. H. Kutscher, and R. Segall. 1953. Unusual toxic reactions to sulfonamides and antibiotic therapy: A review of the literature from 1936 to 1953. *Annals of Allergy* 11:615.

Lapin, J. H., and I. Mond. 1951. Serum sickness-like syndrome from penicillin. *Am. J. Dis. Child.* 82:335.

Laplante, P., J. M. Saint-Hilaire, and G. Bouvier. 1983. Headache as an epileptic manifestation. *Neurology* 33:1493–1495.

Lauritzen, M., T. S. Olsen, N. Lassen, and O. B. Paulson. 1983. Regulation of regional cerebral blood flow during and between migraine attacks. *Annals of Neurology* 14:569–572.

Lende, R. A., W. M. Kirsch, and R. Druckman. 1971. Relief of facial pain after combined removal of precentral and postcentral cortex. *Journal of Neurosurgery* 34:537–543.

Lennox, W. G., and M. A. Lennox. 1960. *Epilepsy and Related Disorders.* Boston: Little, Brown.

Lewin, W., and C. G. Phillips. 1952. Observations on partial removal of the post central gyrus for pain. *Journal of Neurology, Neurosurgery, and Psychiatry* 15:143–147.

Lewis, H. M., J. V. Parry, R. P. Parry, et al., 1979. Role of viruses in febrile convulsions. *Archives of Diseases in Childhood.* 54:869–876.

Lou, H. C., L. Henriksen, P. Bruhn. 1984. Focal cerebral hypoperfusion in children with dysphasia and/or attention deficit disorder. *Archives of Neurology* 41:825–828.

McGovern, J. P. 1948. An unusual case of hypersensitivity to cold complicated by paroxysmal diarrhea. *Journal of Allergy* 19:408.

Mason, V. R. 1922. Optic neuritis in serum sickness. *JAMA* 78:88.

Newton, R., and J. Aicardi. 1983. Clinical findings in children with occipital spike-wave complexes suppressed by eye opening. *Neurology* 33:1526–1529.

Ninck, B. 1970. Migraine and epilepsy. *European Neurology* 3:168–178.

Olesen, J., B. Larsen, and M. Lauritzen. 1981. Focal hyperemia followed by spreading oligemia and impaired activation of rCBF in classic migraine. *Annals of Neurology* 9:344–352.

Ounsted, C. 1955. The hyperkinetic syndrome in epileptic children. *Lancet* 2:303–311.

Panayitopoulos, C. P. 1980. Basilar migraine? Seizures and severe EEG abnormalities. *Neurology* 30:1122–1125.

Paskind, H. A. 1934. The relationship of migraine and epilepsy and some other neuropsychiatric disorders. *Arch. Neurol. Psychiatry* 32:45–50.

Ratner, B. 1948. Allergic manifestations in the central nervous system. *Am. J. Dis. Child.* 75:747.

Saint-Hilaire, J. M., P. Laplante, and G. Bouvier. 1984. Epileptic headache (letter). *Neurology* 34:988.

Scott, T. F., L. Coriell, H. Blank, and C. F. Burgoon. 1952. Some comments on herpetic infection in children with special emphasis on unusual clinical manifestations. *Journal of Pediatrics* 41:835.

Selby, G., and J. W. Lance. 1960. Observations on five hundred cases of migraine and allied vascular headaches. *Journal of Neurology, Neurosurgery, and Psychiatry* 23:23–32.

Seshia, S. S., J. D. Reggin, and R. S. Stanvick, 1985. Migraine and complex seizures in children. *Epilepsia* 26:232–236.

Shannon, W. R. 1922. Neuropathic manifestations in infants and children as a result of anaphylactic reactions to foods contained in the dietary. *Am. J. Dis. Child.* 24:89.

Sheldon, J. M., R. G. Lovell, and K. P. Matthews. 1953. *A Manual of Clinical Allergy*. Philadelphia: W. B. Saunders.

Sheppe, W. M. 1931. Reaction of the meninges to therapeutic serum. *American Journal of Clinical Pathology* 1:77.

Shovron, S. D. 1984. The temporal aspects of prognosis in epilepsy. *Journal of Neurology, Neurosurgery, and Psychiatry* 47:1157–1165.

Sicuteri, F. 1982. Natural opioids in migraine. In *Advances in Neurology*, vol. 33, edited by M. Critchley, A. P. Friedman, S. Gorini, and F. Sicuteri New York: Raven Press.

Slatter, K. H. 1968. Some clinical and EEG findings in patients with migraines. *Brain* 91:85–98.

Spangler, R. H. 1931. Some allergic factors in essential epilepsy. *Journal of Allergy* 1:39.

Sprick, U., M. S. Oitzl, K. Ornstein, and J. P. Huston, 1981. Spreading depression induced by microinjection of encephalins into the hippocampus and neocortex. *Brain Research* 210:243–252.

Staffieri, D., L. Bentoliala, and L. Levit. 1952. Hemiplegia and allergic symptoms following ingestion of certain foods: A case report. *Annals of Allergy* 10:38.

Sternberg, T. H., and G. D. Baldridge. 1948. Electroencephalographic abnormalities in patients with generalized neurodermatitis. *Journal of Investigative Dermatology* 11:401.

Stoesser, A. V., and L. S. Nelson. 1954. Incidence and treatment of headaches due to allergy in children. Paper presented before a Meeting of the American College of Allergists, April 9, Miami, Fla.

Thompson, J. 1921. Clinical types of convulsive seizures in very young babies. *British Medical Journal* 2:679.

Tripp, J. H., D. E. Francis, J. A. Knight, and J. T. Harries. 1979. Infant feeding practices: A cause for concern. *British Medical Journal* 2:707–709.

Turner, M. W., J. F. Mowbray, B. A. M. Harvey, J. Brostoff, R. S. Wells, and J. F. Soothill. 1978. Defective yeast opsonization and C2 deficiency in atopic patients. *Clinical and Experimental Immunology* 34:253–259.

Turner, M. W., J. Yalcin, J. F. Soothill, et al. In vitro investigations in asthmatic children undergoing hyposensitization with tyrosine-absorbed D. pteronyssinus antigen. *Clinical Allergy* 14:221–231.

Valquist, B., and G. Hackzell. 1948. Migraine of early onset. *Acta Paediatricia* 38:622.

Vaughan, W. T. 1927. Allergic migraine. *JAMA* 88:1383.

Walker, D. C. 1952. Serum neuritis secondary to tetanus antitoxin. *Bulletin of the Springer Clinic* (Tulsa, Okla.) 3:3.

Ward, J. F. 1922. Protein sensitization as a possible cause for epilepsy and cancer. New York, *Med. J. Rec.* 115:592.

Wieser, H. G., and H. Isler. 1983. Headache as epileptic manifestation. *Schweizerische Rundschau fuer Medezin Praxis* 24:844–848.

Wilder, R. M. 1921. Effect of ketonuria on course of epilepsy. *Mayo Clin. Bull.* 2:307.

Winkleman, N. W., and N. Gotten. 1935. Encephalomyelitis following the use of serum and vaccine: Report of two cases, one with autopsy. *Am. J. Syph. & Neurol.* 19:414.

Wurtman, R. J. 1983. Behavioural effects of nutrients. *Lancet* 1:1145–1147.

Young, F. 1932. Peripheral nerve paralysis following the use of various serums. *JAMA* 98:1139.

Young, G. B., and W. T. Blume. Painful epileptic seizures. *Brain* 106:-537–554.

Ziegler, D. K., and G. Wong. 1967. Migraine in children: Clinical and electroencephalographic study of families—the possible relation to epilepsy. *Epilepsia* 8:171–187.

NUTRITION

Benton, D. 1990. Vitamin/mineral supplementation and intelligence. *Lancet* 335:1158–1160.

Benton, D., and G. Roberts. 1988. The effect of vitamin and mineral supplementation on intelligence of a sample of school children. *Lancet:* 140–143.

Cheek, D., G. McIntosh, V. O'Brien, D. Ness, and R. Green. 1989. Malnutrition in aboriginal children at Yalata, South Australia. *European Journal of Clinical Nutrition* 43(3):161–168.

Newbold, H. 1988. Reducing the serum cholesterol level with a diet high in animal fat. *Southern Medical Journal* 81:61–63.

Newbold, H. 1988. Vitamin B_{12}, megaloblastic madness, and the founding of Duke University. *Medical Hypotheses* 27:231–240.

Poilos, C. 1981. What effects do corrective nutritional practices have on alcoholics? *Orthomolecular Psychiatry* 10:61–64.

Schauss, A. 1985. Research links nutrition to behavior disorders. *School Safety* 3:20–28.

Schauss, A. 1986. Nutrition, student achievement, and behavior: Insights from new research. *Intermediate Teacher* (Canada) 20:5–14.

Schoenthaler, S., W. Doraz, and J. Wakefield. 1986. The testing of various hypotheses as explanations for the gains in national standardized academic test scores in the 1978–1983 New York City Nutrition Policy Modification Project. *International Journal for Biosocial Research* 8(2):196–203.

PROVOCATION/NEUTRALIZATION TESTING

Bock, S., J. Buckley, A. Holst, and C. May 1977. Proper use of skin tests with food extracts in diagnosis of hypersensitivity to foods in children. *Clinical Allergy* 7:375–383.

Brown, S. 1922. Studies in specific hypersensitiveness I: The diagnostic cutaneous reaction in allergy; comparison of the intradermal method (Cooke) and the scratch method (Schloss). *Journal of Immunology* 7:97–111.

Caplin, I. 1973. Report of the committee on provocative food testing. *Annals of Allergy* 31:375–381.

Fineman, A. 1926. Studies in hypersensitiveness XXIII: A comparative study of intradermal, scratch, and conjuctival tests in determining the degree of pollen sensitivity. *Journal of Immunology* 11:465–476.

Hardman, P., J. Clay, and A. Liberman. 1989. The effects of diet and sublingual provocative testing on eye movements with dyslexic individuals. *American Optometric Association. Journal* 60(1):10–13.

Jewett, D., et al. 1990. A double-blind study of symptom provocation to determine food sensitivity. *JAMA* 323:429–433.

King, D. 1988. The reliability and validity of provocative food testing: A critical review. *Medical Hypotheses* 25:7–16.

Radcliffe, M., et al. 1974. Sublingual provocation testing for foods and F, D, and C dyes. *Annals of Allergy* 33:274.

Rapp, D. 1978. Herpes progenitalis responding to influenza vaccine. *Annals of Allergy* 40:302.

Rapp, D. 1981. Sublingual provocative food testing. *Annals of Allergy* 46:44.

Rea, W., R. Podell, M. Williams, E. Fenvyes, D. Sprague, and A. Johnson. 1984. Intracutaneous neutralization of food sensitivity: A double-blind evaluation. *Archives of Otolaryngology* 110:248–252.

PSYCHOLOGICAL DISORDERS

Campbell, M. B. 1973. Neurological manifestations of allergic disease. *Annals of Allergy* 31:485–498.

Coleman, M. 1979. Physiology and the neurosciences (editorial). *Biological Psychiatry* 14:1–2.

Rogers, M., K. Bloomingdale, B. Murawski, N. Soter, P. Reich, and F. Austen. 1986. Mixed organic brain syndrome as a manifestation of systemis mastocytosis. *Psychosomatic Medicine* 6:437–447.

Shaw, H. B. 1912. Hypersensitiveness: The parallelism in the phenomena of hypersensitiveness and certain clinical manifestations of obscure nature. *Lancet* 1:713–719.

SEROUS OTITIS

Berstein, J. M. 1981. Recognizing and managing otitis media with effusion. *Journal of Respiratory Diseases* 2:15.

Bernstein, J. M. 1984. The role of IgE-mediated hypersensitivity in otitis media with effusion. *Otolaryngology—Head Neck Surgery* 89:874.

Bluestone, C. D. 1982. Current concepts in otolaryngology—Otitis media in children: To treat or not to treat? *New England Journal of Medicine* 306:1399.

Coca, A. F. 1942. *Familial Non-reaginic Food Allergy*. Springfield, Ill.: Charles C. Thomas.

Harrell, M., and J. Shea. 1978. Hazards of ventilation tubes. *Advances in Otolaryngology* 23:22.

Hagerman, R. J., and A. R. Falkenstein. 1987. An association between recurrent otitis media in infancy and later hyperactivity. *Clinical Pediatrics* 26:253–257.

Naunton, R. F. 1981. Panel on experiences with middle ear ventilating tubes: The conservative approach. *Annals of Otology, Rhinology, and Laryngology* 90:529.

TENSION FATIGUE SYNDROME

Alvarez, W. C. 1946. Puzzling "nervous storms" due to food allergy. *Gastroenterology* 7:241.

Bowen, R. 1945. Some practical suggestions in the management of asthmatic children. *Med. Rec. & Ann.* 39:1189.

Clarke, T. W. 1948. The relation of allergy to childhood neuroses. *Journal of Child Psychiatry* 1:177.

Clein, N. W. 1952. Influence of tonsillectomy and adenoidectomy on children, with special reference to the allergic implications on respiratory symptoms. *Annals of Allergy* 10:568.

Clein, N. W. 1954. Cow's milk allergy in infants. *Pediatric Clinics of North America* 1:949.

Conners, C. K., C. H. Goyette, P. A. Southwick, J. M. Lees, and P. A. Andrulonis. 1976. Food additives and hyperkinesis: A controlled double-blind experiment. *Pediatrics* 58:165–166.

Cook, P. S., and J. M. Woodhill. 1976. The Feingold dietary treatment of the hyperkinetic syndrome. *Medical Journal of Australia.* 2:85.

Crook, W. G. 1977. *Can Your Child Read? Is He Hyperactive?* Jackson, Tenn.: Professional Books.

Crook, W. G. 1980. Can what a child eats make him dull, stupid, or hyperactive? *Journal of Learning Disabilities* 13:53–58. Reprinted in *The Relationship of Food Sensitivities (and Other Dietary Factors) to Hyperactivity, Attention Deficits, and Other Nervous System Symptoms: A Compendium,* edited by W. G. Crook.

Crook, W. G., et al. 1961. Systemic manifestations due to allergy: Report of fifty patients and a review of the literature on the subject (sometimes referred to as allergic toxemia and the allergic tension-fatigue syndrome). *Pediatrics* 27:790–799.

Davison, H. M. 1947. Cerebral allergy. *Southern Medical Journal* 42:-712.

Davison, H. M. 1950. In discussion of T. W. Clarke, The relation of allergy to character problems in children: A survey. *Annals of Allergy* 8:175.

Duke, W. W. 1923. Food allergy as a cause of illness. *JAMA* 81:886.

Duke, W. W. 1925. *Allergy, Asthma, Hayfever, Urticaria, and Other Allied Manifestations of Reaction.* St. Louis: Mosby.

Greenbaum, J. V., and L. A. Lurie. 1948. Encephalitis and behavior disorders. *JAMA* 136:923.

Harley, J. P., C. G. Matthews, and P. Eichman. 1978. Synthetic food colors and hyperactivity in children: A double-blind challenge experiment. *Pediatrics* 62:975–983.

Hoobler, B. R. 1916. Some early symptoms suggesting protein sensitization in infancy. *Amer. J. Dis. Child.* 12:129.

Horesh, A. J. 1946. Allergy in children. *Clinics* 5:678.

Karnosh, L. J. 1944. Psychosomatic aspects of allergy. *Psychiatric Quarterly* 18:618.

Kaufman, W. 1952. *Primary Food-Induced Allergic Syndromes and Their Secondary Psychopathological Accompaniments.* Basel: S. Karger.

Lynch, J. D., and W. D. Snively, Jr. 1951. Hypoproteinosis of childhood. *JAMA* 147:115.

May, E. 1923. Attacks of unnatural somnolence of anaphylactic origin. *Société Médicale des Hospitaux de Paris. Bulletins et Mémoires* 47:704.

May, E. 1923. Unnatural somnolence. *Société Medicale des Hospitaux de Paris. Bulletins et Mémoires* 47:704.

Mayron, L. A. 1979. Allergy, learning, and behavior problems. *Journal of Learning Disabilities* 12:32–42.

Miller, J. B. 1972. *Food Allergy.* Springfield, Ill.: Charles C. Thomas.

Miller, J. B. 1977. A double-blind study of food extract injection therapy: A preliminary report. *Annals of Allergy* 38:185–191.

Moore, M. W. 1958. Extra-respiratory tract symptoms of pollinosis. *Annals of Allergy* 16:152.

O'Banion, D., B. Armstrong, R. A. Cummings, and J. Stang. 1978. Disruptive behavior: The dietary approach. *Journal of Autism and Childhood Schizophrenia* 8:325.

O'Shea, J. A. 1978. Sublingual immunotherapy of hyperkinetic children with food, chemical, and inhalant allergies: A double-blind study. Paper presented at the Thirteenth Annual Meeting of the Society for Clinical Ecology, November 19, Key Biscayne, Fla.

Piness, G., and H. Miller. 1925. Allergic manifestations in infancy and childhood. *Arch. Pediat.* 42:557.

Pounders, C. M. 1952. The life cycle of the allergic individual. *Southern Medical Journal* 45:875.

Randolph, T. G. 1945. Fatigue and weakness of allergic origin (allergic toxemia) to be differentiated from nervous fatigue and neurasthenia. *Annals of Allergy* 3:418.

Randolph, T. G. 1947. Allergy as a causative factor of fatigue, irritability, and behavior problems of children. *Journal of Pediatrics* 31:560.

Randolph, T. G. 1948. The fatigue syndrome of allergic origin. *Mississippi V. Med. J.* 70:105.

Randolph, T. G. 1950. Allergy as a cause of acute torticollis. *Amer. Practit.* 1:1062.

Randolph, T. G. 1959. Musculoskeletal allergy in children. *Int. Arch. Allergy* 14:84.

Rapp, D. 1978. Double-blind study and treatment of milk sensitivity. *Medical Journal of Australia* 1:571–572.

Rapp, D. 1979. *Allergies and the Hyperactive Child.* New York: Sovereign Books, Simon & Schuster.

Ratner, B. 1953. Bone maturation and capillary microscopy as indications for the use of thyroid in childhood allergy. *Annals of Allergy* 11:419.

Rinkel, H. J., T. G. Randolph, and M. Zeller. 1951. *Food Allergy*. Springfield, Ill.: Charles C. Thomas.

Rowe, A. H. 1930. Allergic toxemia and migraine due to food allergy. *Calif. West. Med.* 33:785.

Rowe, A. H. 1944. Clinical allergy in the nervous system. *Journal of Nervous and Mental Disease* 99:834.

Rowe, A. H. 1944. *Elimination Diets and the Patient's Allergies.* Philadelphia: Lea & Febiger.

Rowe, A. H. 1950. Allergic toxemia and fatigue. *Annals of Allergy* 8:72.

Rowe, A. H. 1959. Allergic toxemia and fatigue. *Annals of Allergy* 17:9.

Schorer, E. H. 1912. Idiosyncrasy to common foods. *Journal of the Missouri Medical Society* (December).

Shannon, W. R. 1922. Neuropathic manifestations in infants and children as a result of anaphylactic reactions to foods contained in their dietary. *Amer. J. Dis. Child.* 24:89.

Sheldon, J. M. 1953. *A Manual of Clinical Allergy.* Philadelphia: W. B. Saunders.

Speer, F. 1954. Allergic tension-fatigue in children. *Annals of Allergy* 12:168.

Speer, F. 1954a. The allergic tension-fatigue syndrome. *Pediatric Clinics of North America* 1:1029–1037.

Speer, F. 1954b. Allergic tension-fatigue in children. *Annals of Allergy* 12:168–171. Reprinted in *The Relationship of Food Sensitivities (and Other Dietary Factors) to Hyperactivity, Attention Deficits, and Other Nervous System Symptoms: A compendium,* edited by W. G. Crook.

Speer, F. 1958. The allergic tension-fatigue syndrome in children. *Int. Arch. Allergy* 12:207.

Sternberg, L. 1942. Seasonal somnolence: A possible pollen allergy. *Journal of Allergy* 14:89.

Stewart, M. A. 1970. Hyperactive children. *Scientific American* 4:1222.

Swanton, J., and M. Kinsbourne. 1978. Artificial food colors impair the learning performance of hyperactive children: Laboratory evaluations of in-patients. Paper presented at the American College of Allergists, Second International Food Allergy Symposium, Mexico City.

Weinberg, W., and R. Brumback. 1990. Primary disorder of vigilance: A novel explanation of inattentiveness, daydreaming, boredom, restlessness, and sleepiness. *Journal of Pediatrics* 116:720–725.

Wender, E. 1977. Food additives and hyperkinesis. *American Journal of Diseases of Children* 131:1204.

Winkelman, N. W., and M. T. Moore. 1941. Allergy and nervous diseases. *Journal of Nervous and Mental Disease* 93:736.

TOURETTE'S SYNDROME

Comings, D., and B. Comings. 1985. Tourette syndrome: Clinical and psychological aspects of 250 cases. *American Journal of Human Genetics* 37:435–450.

Mandell, M. 1984. Unsuspected allergies play a major role in Tourette's syndrome. Presented at the Society for Clinical Ecology, November.

Nee, L., E. Caine, R. Polinsky, R. Eldridge, and M. Ebert. 1980. Gilles de la Tourette syndrome: Clinical and family study of fifty cases. *Annals of Neurology* 7:41–49.

O'Quinn, A., and R. Thompson. 1980. Tourette's syndrome: An expanded view. *Pediatrics* 66:420–424.

Singer, H. 1982. Tics and Tourette syndrome. *Johns Hopkins Medical Journal* 151:30–35.

Singer, H., I. Butler, L. Tune, W. Seifert, and J. Coyle. 1982. Dopaminergic dysfunction in Tourette syndrome. *Annals of Neurology* 12:361–336.

Singer, H., L. Tune, I. Butler, R. Zaczek, and J. Coyle. 1982. Clinical symptomatology, CSF neurotransmitter metabolites, and serum haloperidol levels in Tourette's syndrome. *Advances in Neurology* 35:-177–183.

TRIMETHYLAMINURIA (FISH-ODOR SYNDROME)

Arbuthnot J. 1735. *An Essay Concerning the Nature of Ailments.* London: J. Tonson.

Blumenthal, I., G. T. Lealman, and P. P. Franklyn. 1980. Fracture of the femur, fish odour, and copper deficiency in a preterm infant. *Archives of Diseases in Childhood.* 55:229–231.

Brewster, M. A., and H. Schedewie. 1983. Trimethylaminuria. *Annals of Clinical and Laboratory Science* 13:20–24.

Calvert, G. D. 1973. Trimethylaminuria and inherited Noonan's syndrome. *Lancet* 1:320–321.

Danks, D. M., J. Hammond, P. Schlesinger, K. Fach, D. Burke, and B. Halpern. 1976. Trimethylaminuria: Diet does not always control the fishy odor. *New England Journal of Medicine* 295:962.

Higgins, T., S. Chagkin, K. B. Hammond, and J. R. Humbert. 1972. Trimethylamine N-oxide synthesis: Human variant. *Biochemical Medicine* 6:392–396.

Humbert, J. R., K. B. Hammond, W. E. Hathaway, J. G. Marcoux, and D. O'Brien. 1970. Trimethylaminuria: The fish odour syndrome. *Lancet* 2:770–771.

Lee, C. W. G., J. S. Yu, B. B. Turner, and K. E. Murray. 1976. Trimethylaminuria: Fishy odours in children. *New England Journal of Medicine* 295:937–938.

Lintzel, W. 1934. Trimethylaminoxyd Im Menschlichen Harn. *Klinische Wochenschrift* 13:304–305.

Mahgoub, A., J. R. Idle, L. G. Dring, R. Lancaster, and R. L. Smith. 1977. The polymorphic hydroxylation of debrisoquine in man. *Lancet* 2:584–586.

Marks, R., M. W. Greaves, C. Prottey, and P. J. Hartop. 1977. Trimethylaminuria: The use of choline as an aid to diagnosis. *British Journal of Dermatology* 96:399–402.

Mitchell, S. C., R. H. Waring, C. S. Haley, J. R. Idle, and R. L. Smith. 1984. Genetic aspects of the polymorphically distributed sulphoxidation of S-carboxymethyl-L-cysteine in man. *British Journal of Clinical Pharmacology.* 18:507–521.

Muller, M., and I. Immendorfer. 1942. Ein Beitrag zum Verhalten des Trimethylamins und des Trimethylaminoxyds im Stotfwechsel. *Hoppe-Seyler's Zeitschrift für Physiologische Chemie* 275:267–276.

Shelley, E. D., and W. B. Shelley. 1984. The fish-odour syndrome, *JAMA* trimethylaminuria. 251:253–255.

Simenhoff, M. L., S. R. Dunn, A. Asatoor, and M. D. Milne. 1977. Determination of trimethylamine and trimethylamine N-oxide in urine. Proceedings of the 173rd Meeting of the American Chemical Society.

Spector, W. S. 1950. Acute toxicities. In Vol. 1 of *Handbook of Toxicology,* edited by W. S. Spector. Philadelphia: W. B. Saunders.

Spellacy, E., R. W. E. Watts, and S. K. Goolamali. 1979. Trimethylaminuria. *Journal of Inherited Metabolic Disease* 2:85–88.

Todd, W. A. 1979. Psychosocial problems as the major complication of an adolescent with trimethylaminuria. *Journal of Pediatrics* 94:936–937.

Al-Waiz, M., S. C. Mitchell, J. R. Idle, and R. L. Smith. 1986. Variation of trimethylamine N-oxidation in man. *Acta Pharmacologica et Toxicologica* 59:218.

Al-Waiz, M., et al. 1988. Trimethylaminuria ("fish-odour syndrome"): A study of an affected family. *Clinical Science* 74:231–236.

Ziegler M.D., and H.C. Mitchell. 1972. Microsomal oxidase IV: properties of a mixed function amine oxidase isolated from pig liver microsomes. *Archives of Biochemistry and Biophysics* 150:116–125.

URTICARIA

August, P., and J. O'Driscoll. 1989. Urticaria successfully treated by desensitization with grass-pollen extract. *British Journal of Dermatology* 120:409–410.

Baumgardner, D. 1989. Persistent urticaria caused by a common coloring agent. *Postgraduate Medicine* 85:265–266.

Berger, T., and J. Tappero. 1989. Traumatic plantar urticaria or plantar erythema nodosum (letter). *American Academy of Dermatology. Journal* 20(4):701–702.

Bressler, R., K. Sowell, and D. Huston. 1989. Therapy of chronic idiopathic urticaria with nifedipine: Demonstration of beneficial effect in a double-blinded placebo-controlled, crossover trial. *Journal of Allergy and Clinical Immunology* 83:756–763.

Clyne, C., and G. Eliopoulos. 1989. Fever and urticaria in acute giardiasis. *Archives of Internal Medicine* 149:939–940.

Collins, D. 1989. Pancytopenia, rash, and fever caused by diethylstilbestrol used for prostate cancer. *Journal of Rheumatology* 16:408–409.

Janier, M., D. Bonvalet, M. Blanc, F. Lemarchand, B. Cavelier, A. Ribrioux, B. Aguenier, and J. Civette. 1989. Chronic urticaria and macroglobulinemia (Schnitzler's syndrome): Report of two cases. *American Academy of Dermatology. Journal* 20:206–211.

Kamide, R., M. Nimiira, H. Ueda, S. Yamamoto, H. Yoshida, and K. Kukita. 1989. Clinical evaluation of ketotifen for chronic urticaria: Multicenter double-blind comparative study of clemastine. *Annals of Allergy* 62:322–325.

Lanf, D., S. Sugimoto, J. Curd, S. Christiansen, and B. Zuraw. 1989. High molecular weight kininogen is cleaved in active erythema multiforme. *Journal of Allergy and Clinical Immunology* 83:802–810.

Lawlor, F., A. Black, A. Ward, R. Morris, and M. Greaves. 1989. Delayed pressure urticaria: Objective evaluation of a variable disease using a dermographometer and assessment of treatment using colchicine. *British Journal of Dermatology* 120:403–408.

McLean, S., E. Arreaza, M. Lett-Brown, and J. Grant. 1989. Refractory cholinergic urticaria successfully treated with ketotifen. *Journal of Allergy and Clinical Immunology* 83:738–741.

Paul, E., and R. Bodeker, 1989. Comparative study of astemizole and terfenadine in the treatment of chronic idiopathic urticaria: A randomized double-blind study of forty patients. *Annals of Allergy* 62:318–320.

Pujol, R., M. Barnadas, S. Brunet, and J. DeMoragas. 1989. Urticarial dermatosis associated with Waldenstrom's macroglobulinemia (letter). *American Academy of Dermatology. Journal* 20:855–857.

Quaranta, J., A. Rohr, G. Rachelefsky, S. Siegel, R. Katz, L. Spector, and M. Mickey. 1989. The natural history and response to therapy of chronic urticaria and angioedema. *Annals of Allergy* 62:421–424.

Saurat, J. 1989. Immunofluorescence biopsy for pruritic urticarial papules and plaques of pregnancy (letter). *American Academy of Dermatology. Journal* 20:711.

Weiner, M. 1989. Methotrexate in cortocisteroid-resistant urticari (letter). *Annals of Internal Medicine* 110:848.

MISCELLANEOUS

Anderson, S., H. Chinn, and K. Fisher. 1982. History and current status of infant formulas. *American Journal of Clinical Nutrition* 35:381.

Bagnato, A., P. Brovedani, P. Comina, P. Milinaro, C. Scalzo, V. Triolo, and G. Milani. 1989. Long-term treatment with thymomodulin reduces airway hyperresponsiveness to methacholine. *Annals of Allergy* 62:-425–428.

Barish, C., W. Wu, and D. Castell. 1985. Respiratory complications of gastroesophageal reflux. *Archives of Internal Medicine* 145:1882–1888.

Baxter, P., J. Dickson, S. Variend, and C. Taylor. 1989. Intestinal disease in cystic fibrosis. *Archives of Disability in Children* 63:1496–1497.

Jones, B., F. Hoffner, R. Teele, and R. Lebowitz. 1990. Pitfalls in pediatric urinary sonography. *Urology* 35(1):38–44.

Laseter, J. 1990. Monitoring of aromatic and chlorinated solvents in blood following inhalant abuse in juveniles. Paper presented at the National Inhalant Abuse Prevention Conference, March 13–16, San Antonio, Tex.

Leonard, J., G. Haffenden, W. Tucker, J. Unsworth, F. Swain, R. McMinn, J. Holobrow, and L. Fry. 1983. Gluten challenge in *dermatitis hepetiformis. New England Journal of Medicine* 308:816–819.

Norgaard, J., S. Rittig, and J. Djurhuus. 1989. Nocturnal enuresis: An approach to treatment based on pathogenesis. *Journal of Pediatrics* 114:705–709.

Pearson, D. 1988. Psychologic and somnatic interrelationships in allergy and pseudoallergy. *Journal of Allergy and Clinical Immunology* 81:351–360.

Pounders, C. 1952. The life cycle of the allergic individual. *Southern Medical Journal* 45:857–861.

Rea, W., et al. 1986. The environmental aspects of the Post-Polio Syndrome. World Conference on Post-Polio.

Roper, W., W. Winkerwerder, J. Hackbarth, and H. Krakauer. 1988. Effectiveness in health care: An initiative to evaluate and improve medical practice. *New England Journal of Medicine* 319:1197–1202.

Russell, M., K. Dark, R. Cummins, G. Ellman, E. Callaway, and H. Peeke. 1984. Learned histamine release. *Science* 23:733–734.

Schumacher, M. 1988. Fiberoptic nasopharyngolaryngoscopy: A procedure for allergists? *Journal of Allergy and Clinical Immunology* 81:-960–962.

Shaw, H., M. Lond, and F. Lond. 1912. Hypersensitiveness: The parallelism in the phenomena of hypersensitiveness and certain clinical manifestations of obscure nature. *Lancet* 1:713–719.

Sjovall, P., O. Christensen, H. Moller, and M. Malmo 1987. Oral hyposensitization in nickel allergy. *American Academy of Dermatology. Journal* 17:774–778.

Slutsker, L., et al. 1990. Eosinophilia-Myalgia syndrome associated with exposure to tryptophan from a single manufacturer. *JAMA* 264:-213–217.

Spencer, M., L. Garcia, and M. Chapin. 1979. Dietamoeba fragilis. *American Journal of Disability in Children* 133:390–393.

Wortham, D., R. Lufkin, W. Hanafee, and P. Ward. 1987. Magnetic resonance imaging of the head and neck. *American Academy of Otolaryngology—Head and Neck Surgery* 2:255–265.

Glossary of Medical Terminology

acetaldehyde — A by-product of yeast as it ferments carbohydrates. This can be harmful when it occurs in the human digestive tract as a result of candida.

adrenergic — Releasing or activated by epinephrine (adrenaline) when stimulated, as in adrenergic nerve fibers.

albicans — Type of candida organism that causes thrush when allowed to multiply unchecked.

allergen — A substance that induces an allergic reaction.

allergenic — Allergy causing.

alpha-adrenergic receptor — Site in autonomic nervous system where nerve impulses are aroused when allergy-causing agents such as norepinephrine and epinephrine are released.

amenorrhea — The abnormal cessation of menstruation.

antigen — A substance that stimulates an immune response.

antioxidants — Substances such as vitamins A, C, E, and beta carotene that decrease oxidation or free-radical damage to tissues.

arteriosclerosis (atherosclerosis)	Chronic diseases characterized by thickening and hardening of the arteries due to a buildup of fatty substances and plaque.
autoantibodies	Immune cells that attack the body.
autoimmune condition	The condition in which cells of the immune system attack normal tissue.
basophile	Type of white blood cell.
beta-adrenergic receptor	A site in the nervous system where inhibitory responses occur when allergy-causing agents such as epinephrine and norepinephrine are released.
blood-brain barrier	A concept involving the relative inability of many substances to pass from the brain capillaries into the brain tissues.
bradykinin	A kinin that is formed locally in injured tissue. (See kinin.)
candida	A yeastlike flora normally present in the mouth, skin, intestinal tract, and vagina. The word has also come to mean the condition in which candida flora have abnormally multiplied, causing various health problems such as thrush.
dysmenorrhea	Painful menstruation.
effusion process	Intravenous administration of a substance.
epidemiologist	A person who specializes in the relationships between disease frequency and the distribution of disease.
Epstein-Barr virus	A herpes virus, discovered in 1964, that causes infectious mononucleosis.
eosinophile	Type of white blood cell.
Environmental Medicine	Branch of medicine involved in the treatment and study of the effects of the environment on health.

free radical	An atom or groups of atoms having one or more unpaired electrons that reacts to and can damage bodily tissue.
hydrocephalus	A condition in which cerebrospinal fluid accumulates within the brain.
hyperthyroidism	The increased release, production, or function of the thyroid gland or hormone.
hypothyroidism	The decreased release, production, or function of the thyroid gland or hormone.
IgE	An antibody (immune cell) that binds to an irritant (pollen, food, etc.). High IgE levels are confirmations of allergy.
immune dysfunction	Decreased ability for the immune system to operate normally or effectively. A deficiency in nutrients, such as vitamin B_6, zinc, or protein, can decrease immune function.
kinin	Molecular chains of amino acids having considerable biological activity. They are capable of influencing smooth muscle contractions, inducing hypotension, increasing blood flow and permeability of small blood capillaries, and inciting pain.
Metabolite	An organic compound essential to the chemical changes in living cells by which energy is provided for vital processes and activities and new material is assimilated.
Nightshade	A family of plants known as Solanaceae that includes such crops as tomatoes, potatoes, and eggplants.
pathogen	A disease-causing substance.
pathological immune response	Immune reaction causing illness or disease.
pollutant injury	Refers to the free-radical damage incurred upon normal, healthy cells from such pollutants as chemicals and smoke.

RAST	Radio Allergo Sorbency Test, a blood test that is done to determine antibody IgE response to a substance.
smooth muscle	Muscle tissue capable of involuntary movement.
status asthmaticus	A life-threatening asthmatic attack.
stress	Forces that disrupt balance. It is generally believed that some stress is beneficial in helping an organism produce change while too much stress is harmful.
stressors	Stress-causing stimuli that can adversely or beneficially affect body function such as worry, alcohol, or exercise.
sublingual drops	Drops given under the tongue that can enter the bloodstream quickly, bypassing the digestive tract.

Notes

CHAPTER 1. ALLERGIES AND THE OVERAGRESSIVE IMMUNE SYSTEM

1. Gary Null interview with Dr. Warren Levin.
2. Gary Null interview with Dr. John Trowbridge.
3. Gary Null interview with Dr. William Rea.
4. Gary Null interview with Dr. William Philpott.
5. Gary Null interview with Dr. Albert Robbins.

CHAPTER 2. ALLERGIES VS. CHEMICAL POISONING

1. Gary Null interview with Dr. A. Lockyer.
2. Gary Null interview with Dr. John Boyles.
3. Gary Null interview with Dr. Marjorie Siebert.
4. Gary Null interview with Dr. William Rea.
5. Gary Null interview with Dr. I-Tsu Chao.
6. Gary Null interview with Dr. I-Tsu Chao.
7. Gary Null interview with Dr. Albert Robbins.

CHAPTER 3. HOW ALLERGIES CAN MANIFEST

1. Gary Null interview with Dr. James Miller.
2. Robert Atkins interview with Dr. Magid Ali.
3. Gary Null interview with Dr. Albert Robbins.
4. Gary Null interview with Dr. John Boyles.
5. Gary Null interview with Dr. John Trowbridge.
6. Gary Null interview with Dr. William Rea.
7. Gary Null interview with Dr. Michael Schachter.
8. Gary Null interview with Dr. A. Lockyer.
9. Gary Null interview with Dr. Alfred Zamm.
10. Gary Null interview with Dr. James Miller.
11. Gary Null interview with Dr. Marjorie Siebert.
12. Gary Null interview with Dr. Dr. Marjorie Siebert.

CHAPTER 4. CHILDHOOD ALLERGIES

1. Gary Null interview with Dr. Doris Rapp.
2. Gary Null interview with Dr. Doris Rapp.
3. Gary Null interview with Dr. William Rea.
4. Gary Null interview with Dr. Albert Robbins.

CHAPTER 5. ALLERGY-PROVOKING SUBSTANCES

1. Gary Null interview with Dr. Albert Robbins.
2. Gary Null interview with Dr. William Rea.
3. Gary Null interview with Dr. I-Tsu Chao.
4. Gary Null interview with Dr. Alfred Zamm.

5. Gary Null interview with Dr. Doris Rapp.
6. Gary Null interview with Dr. A. Lockyer.
7. Gary Null interview with Dr. Alan Levin.
8. Gary Null interview with Dr. Alan Levin.
9. Gary Null interview with Dr. Alan Levin.

CHAPTER 6. TESTING FOR AND TREATING FOOD ALLERGIES AND CHEMICAL SENSITIVITIES

1. Gary Null interview with Dr. Doris Rapp.
2. Gary Null interview with Dr. Albert Robbins.
3. Gary Null interview with Dr. Joseph Wojcik.
4. Gary Null interview with Dr. Michael Galante.
5. Gary Null interview with Dr. Michael Galante.
6. Gary Null interview with Dr. Michael Galante.
7. Gary Null interview with Dr. Michael Galante.
8. Gary Null interview with Dr. Michael Schachter.
9. Gary Null interview with caller.
10. Gary Null interview with Dr. Richard Podell.
11. Gary Null interview with Mary LaMiele.

CHAPTER 7. THE TRADITIONAL VS. THE ENVIRONMENTAL APPROACHES TO ALLERGY MEDICINE

1. Gary Null interview with Dr. John Boyles.
2. Gary Null interview with Rob McCaleb.
3. Gary Null interview with Dr. John Trowbridge.
4. Gary Null interview with Dr. John Trowbridge.
5. Gary Null interview with Dr. Joseph Wojcik.

6. Gary Null interview with Dr. Joseph Wojcik.
7. Gary Null interview with Dr. John Trowbridge.
8. Gary Null interview with Dr. Richard Podell.
9. Gary Null interview with Dr. Marshall Mandell.
10. Gary Null interview with Dr. Christopher Calapai.
11. Gary Null interview with Dr. Christopher Calapai.
12. Gary Null interview with Dr. Christopher Calapai.
13. Gary Null interview with Dr. Alfred Zamm.
14. Gary Null interview with Dr. John Boyles.
15. Gary Null interview with Dr. Michael Schachter.
16. Gary Null interview with Dr. Alan Levin.
17. Gary Null interview with Dr. Doris Rapp.
18. Gary Null interview with Dr. Doris Rapp.
19. Gary Null interview with Dr. Gary Oberg.
20. Gary Null interview with Dr. Doris Rapp.
21. Gary Null interview with Dr. Doris Rapp.
22. Gary Null interview with Dr. Dorothy Calabrese.
23. Gary Null interview with Dr. Alan Levin.
24. Gary Null interview with Dr. Marshall Mandell.
25. Gary Null interview with Dr. John Boyles.
26. Gary Null interview with Dr. Christopher Calapai.
27. Gary Null interview with Dr. William Rea.
28. Gary Null interview with Dr. John Boyles.
29. Gary Null interview with Dr. Gary Oberg.
30. Gary Null interview with Dr. Michael Galante.
31. Gary Null interview with Dr. Gary Oberg.
32. Gary Null interview with Dr. James Miller.

33. Gary Null interview with Dr. Richard Podell.

34. Gary Null interview with Dr. Dorothy Calabrese.

35. Gary Null interview with Dr. John Trowbridge.

36. Gary Null interview with Dr. Warren Levin.

CHAPTER 8. PERSONAL TESTIMONIALS

1. Gary Null interview with caller.

2. Gary Null interview with caller.

3. Gary Null interview with caller.

4. Gary Null interview with Kevin.

5. Gary Null interview with caller.

6. Gary Null interview with James Howard.

7. Gary Null interview with Jim.

8. Gary Null interview with Barbara.

9. Gary Null interview with Linda.

10. Gary Null interview with Irene.

11. Gary Null interview with Glen.

12. Gary Null interview with Lillian.

13. Gary Null interview with Katie.

14. Gary Null interview with Melody.

15. Gary Null interview with John.

16. Gary Null interview with Mrs. Minor.

17. Gary Null interview with Sarah.

18. Gary Null interview with Maria.

19. Gary Null interview with Charlotte.

20. Gary Null interview with Lisa.

21. Gary Null interview with Jennifer's father.

22. Gary Null interview with Patty Brandt.

23. Gary Null interview with Pat Byrnes.

24. Gary Null interview with Cheryl.

25. Gary Null interview with Cathy.

26. Gary Null interview with Allison.

Index

ABOUT THE AUTHOR

GARY NULL hosts a series of nationally syndicated one-minute health-and-nutrition radio spots, "Total Health," as well as a television show carried in 97 cities across the country. His radio talk show, *The Gary Null Show,* is carried nationwide by the American Radio Network.

He holds a Ph.D. in human nutrition and public health science, is a nutritionist, consumer advocate, and environmental activist who has written over twenty books as well as numerous articles for national magazines on health, diet, and nutrition, and lectures on these topics around the country. In addition, he has been involved with the environmental movement for over twenty years. His most recent books include *Gary Null's Complete Guide to Healing Your Body Naturally* and *The Complete Guide to Health and Nutrition.* He is a national champion racewalker who lives in New York City.